Thanks Again!

I've often said that writing books is a little like making babies. You conceive. You do some seriously heavy lifting. Expend a lot of energy. Lose a lot of sleep. And finally . . . you deliver (hopefully, on time).

And you can't do either one on your own. Fortunately, I've never had to try. From day (and book) one, I've had support I could count on from more amazing people than I can count. But as always, I'll try. Thanks a million to:

Erik, literally What to Expect's baby daddy – the man who made me a mum to Emma and Wyatt, and with that, a mum to What to Expect, and a mum on a mission (a mission we've shared since the very beginning). You're my partner in life, love, work, advocacy and everything What to Expect. Not to mention the best partner in parenting (and grandparenting) a mum could ever have.

Maisie Tivnan, who has fearlessly stepped into some pretty big shoes, picking up the mantle for my editor-forever, Suzanne Rafer, without missing a beat. Nobody said it was going to be easy to go with my frenetic flow of edits or take my pickiness (okay, nitpickiness) in stride, but you kind of make it look that way. And to Suzanne, whose contribution to What to Expect – and friendship – will always be treasured.

Everyone else at Workman who has helped birth this baby: to Vaughn Andrews and Lisa Hollander for designing a book that's easy to read and good enough to eat, and for sifting through all those melons, muffins, shades of blue and Emmas to create a cover that will make readers hungry for more. To Barbara Peragine, as always, for magically making text fit and getting us out of some serious deadline tight spots. Beth Levy and Doug Wolf for your production values under endless pressure. My forever Workman family, Jenny Mandel and Emily Krasner. Peter Workman for creating the house my books have been born in, and Suzie Bolotin for growing and nurturing it.

Eating Well's first recipe consultant, Rena Coyle, for her dedication to all things delicious and nutritious. And to our latest one, Brierley Horton, for developing yummy recipes to fit a time-challenged mum's reality, and bringing a fresh perspective to cooking well (with a minimum of cooking). Who ever said that too many cooks spoiled the broth (or in this case, the carrot-ginger soup)?

Alan Nevins, of Renaissance Literary & Talent, for always going that extra mile (say, to Romania with us), for your friendship and support, and for always being so much fun to drink wine (or pretty much anything) with. To Marc Chamlin for taking such good care of me, and more importantly, for caring so much about me – you're my friend and my lawyer, and that's an unlikely combination!

Our WhatToExpect.com dream team, led by Heidi Cho, Christine Mattheis, Michele Calhoun and, hopefully always, Kyle Humphries and Sara Stefanik for endless energy, enthusiasm, innovation, integrity, creativity, conviction, patience, passion and shared purpose (and for believing in the power of purple). And for never forgetting the most important part of the Quarterly Business Review: big hugs and big reds.

American College of Obstetricians and Gynecologists (ACOG) for being tireless advocates for mums and babies everywhere, and all the obstetritians, midwives, nurses, doulas and lactation consultants around the world helping to deliver a healthy beginning and a healthy future for our mums and babies. To the experts and advocates at the US Centers for Disease Control and Prevention (CDC) – an organisation devoted to the health and well-being of our global family, especially when it comes to our most vulnerable – for your shared mission and commitment to improving maternal and infant health.

Dr Erika Werner for your thoughtful, thorough review of *Eating Well,* for making sure the facts about the impact of maternal nutrition on the health of mums and babies are stated, not overstated.

Howie Mandel for always being the voice of reason and delivering compassionate care (and Lennox). Lauren Crosby for being an invaluable source of information and common sense for so many parents (including Emma and Simon) and the What to Expect family, as well your friendship.

The What to Expect Project, our incredibly passionate leader, Annie Toro, and our director of policy, strategy, research and everything else, Wyatt Murkoff. Together, and in partnership with organisations who care just as much about maternal health (and nutrition) as WTEP does, we will make the world a healthier, happier, more nurtured place for mums and the babies they love to live in.

For inspiration and love, Wyatt, Emma, Simon, Lennox and Sebastien (who would happily eat this book if he could). Victor Shargai (I'll never stop missing you) and Craig Pascal (we'll never stop inviting you for Christmas).

Arlene Eisenberg, for everything you've given me and continue to give to me every day. Your legacy lives on; you'll always be loved and never forgotten.

And most of all, to every mum and every baby, everywhere. You inspire me to do what I do and to never stop doing it, and I love you all (and only wish I could hug you all).

Thanks again, everybody, and big hugs,

heidi

Contents

INTRODUCTION: The Dish on Eating Well...viii

PART 1
EATING WELL

Chapter 1: Why Eat Well?..2

Eating Well: What's in It for Baby 3

Eating Well: What's in It for You 7

Chapter 2: The Nutrients That Make a Baby 10

From A to Zinc: An Encyclopedia of Vitamins and Minerals 10

Beyond Vitamins and Minerals 24

Chapter 3: The Pregnancy Diet...26

Nine Ways to Eat Well When You're Expecting – and Beyond 26

The Pregnancy Daily Dozen 32

Chapter 4: Selecting Well to Eat Well.....................................57

Shopping for Two 57

Selecting for Two 60

Chapter 5: Shelved for Two 69

What to Limit When You're Expecting 69

What to Omit When You're Expecting 78

Chapter 6: Gaining for Two: Baby and You............................... 85

How Much to Gain? 85

Gaining Weight at the Right Rate 88

The Downside of Too Little Weight Gain 90

The Downside of Too Much Weight Gain 91

Weighing In 93

If You're Gaining Too Fast 96

If You're Gaining Too Slowly 99

If You're Gaining for Multiples 101

Chapter 7: Eating Well When You're Feeling Unwell 105

Morning Sickness 106

Food Cravings 113

Food Aversions 117

Constipation 119

Wind and Bloating 122

Heartburn 123

Fatigue 125

Other Pregnancy Symptoms 127

Chapter 8: Eating Well Whenever, Wherever, Whatever 130

On the Job 131

On a Budget 132

When Time Is Tight 135

When Eating Out 140

While Travelling 143

At Parties 146

Chapter 9: Eating Well When Eating Is Complicated 148

If You Can't Handle Dairy 148

If You Have Coeliac Disease (or Gluten Sensitivity) 150

If You Have Irritable Bowel Syndrome 152

If You Have Food Allergies 153

If You Have Gestational Diabetes 154

If You're Carrying Multiples 156

When You're Sick 158

When You're on Activity Restriction 160

Chapter 10: Eating Well Postnatal 162

The Postnatal Diet 163

Eating Well When You're Breastfeeding 168

Chapter 11: Safe Cooking and Prepping When You're Expecting ... 177

Keeping Your Kitchen Safe 178

Keeping Your Foods Safe 179

Safe Produce 181

Safe Meat, Poultry and Fish 183

Safe Dairy 186

Safe Eggs 186

PART 2
COOKING WELL

Breakfast 191

Muffins 204

Sandwiches 210

Soups 222

Pasta 235

Salads 247

Meat 269

Poultry 280

Fish and Seafood 294

Veggies, Beans and Grains 314

'Mocktails' and Smoothies 342

Desserts 352

Conversion Table 361

Index 362

Recipe Index 378

The Dish on Eating Well

Ever notice that when it comes to nutrition, the more things change, the more they stay the same? Sure, you can yo-yo with fad diets (low-carb? That's so last week . . . low-fat? Week before last . . . raw foods? . . . raw deal), but if you step off the diet treadmill and think about it, you'll notice that the basics of healthy eating haven't changed all that much over time. A balanced diet of lean protein, calcium-rich foods, wholegrains, fruits and vegetables, and healthy fats is what nutritionists, doctors and Mum herself have been quietly touting for years while the conflicting nutrition books fight it out on the bestseller lists, only to be forgotten the moment the newest diet craze makes headlines.

And what about for pregnant mums? Have the fundamentals of eating well when you're expecting changed much over the years? They haven't really – and mostly because eating well for two isn't all that much different from eating well for one. The proportions may shift a bit (to accommodate a growing baby's proportions), but the basics are still very much basic.

So if eating well when you're expecting is really just a matter of sticking to a balanced diet, why would you need a book to show you how?

To answer that question, let me go back a few years. Make that 30-plus years. Six weeks into my first pregnancy (due to some cycle wrinkles, it was a little late in the game when I first got the news), I was determined to make up for lost time – and make the most of the rest of my seven-and-a-half months of baby growing. I was a healthy 23-year-old who lived a healthy lifestyle and ate a healthy diet – and I was pretty sure I knew what it took to feed myself and my baby healthfully. So I stocked our fridge and prepared our meals with nature's best baby-building materials: fresh chicken breasts, fish, dairy, wholegrains and a plethora of produce.

And then I ran to the toilet and vomited.

The chicken breasts, my usual protein of choice, were the first to go – victim of a sudden aversion to flesh foods (funny, I'd never thought of chicken as flesh before). The salmon didn't stand a chance, of course – the smell (that's before I even took the fillets out of the wrapper) sent me reeling (and back to the toilet). Got milk? I did, but definitely couldn't bear the thought of drinking it. The wholegrains were welcome to stay (in bread form, toasted within an inch of their life, thank you very much), as was the fruit (with the possible exception of the honeydew, which had somehow become a honey-don't). But the broccoli I used to gobble with a rabbit's abandon turned my stomach.

I knew that I was supposed to eat a certain number of green vegetables a day, but nobody (not even my doctor) could tell me how to eat them without turning greener than they were. I knew protein was the building block of human cells (which meant that building a baby would take protein aplenty), but I had no idea that cottage cheese could stand in for those dreaded flesh foods until the first-trimester aversions had worn off. Or that microwaving the salmon zapped its offensive odour. Or that calcium did not have to come with a white moustache (and a side of bloat). Or that dried apricots quelled the queasies while simultaneously satisfying my baby's requirement for vitamin A (turns out babies don't need broccoli after all) or that I could drink my vitamin C in a smoothie instead of a glass of tummy-churning orange juice. Or that I could take my baby out to eat almost anywhere (except maybe that Italian place, where just a whiff of the scampi could inflict third-degree heartburn).

So I spent the rest of my pregnancy eating the best I could – gagging down the milk, choking down the chicken and, most of the time, worrying that my best wasn't nearly good enough. If only I knew then what I know now. That eating well when you're expecting doesn't have to be torture – and that it doesn't even have to be challenging. It can be fun, easy and, most of all, delicious – no matter what pregnancy symptom has got you down (or is keeping food from staying down). You can coddle your cravings, pander to your aversions, mollify your morning sickness, indulge your indigestion – and still feed yourself and your growing baby exceptionally well.

Enter (way too late for me, but hopefully right on time for you) *Eating Well When You're Expecting*, everything you need to know to feed yourself and your baby well in the real world – the world where nausea dictates what's on the menu (even if that's two crackers and an extra-cold glass of ginger ale); where heartburn can burn a hole in your resolve to eat your vegetables; where temptations (glazed, iced, fried, chocolate-covered, creamed, or supersized) lurk around every corner; where 'lunch' meetings in the conference room are catered by Doughnuts-by-the-Dozen; where airline flights aren't catered at all. Everything you need to make eating for two half the effort and twice the pleasure – from savvy shopping to smart snacking, dining out strategies to pregnant party protocol, packed lunches to breakfasts on the fly. Everything you need to put it all together, including 175 recipes that neatly package all your nutritional requirements into gourmet – yet quick and easy – dishes, while taking into account the special needs of your often tender tummy. In short, everything you need to eat well when you're expecting.

Wishing you a delicious and nutritious nine months of eating well!

heidi

PART 1

Eating Well

Why Eat Well?

Congratulations! The pregnancy test (and the three you took afterwards, just to be sure) is positive – and the big (but still very little) news has started to sink in. You're pregnant. As you sit back and take it all in, you're probably equal parts overjoyed and overwhelmed by the enormity of what has just happened . . . and what is about to happen. That and, more than likely, a little queasy.

Ready or not, you're about to grow a baby – from a shapeless blob of cells not yet visible to the human eye to a dimpled, suitable-for-snuggling newborn.

Much of that work will take place without you lifting a finger – or a fork. In many ways, your pregnant body (especially if it's a healthy one) will rely on biological-business-as-usual to transform the rapidly dividing bundle of cells that's just burrowed into your uterus into a warm bundle of baby you'll hold in your arms in about eight months' time, give or take. Nature is good at what it does, no matter what a mum does or doesn't do – which means your baby already has an excellent chance of arriving in those welcoming arms of yours fully developed and completely healthy.

Still, there's no reason to take a back seat to your body's pregnancy autopilot. In fact, there are many convincing reasons to jump up front (while you can still jump), take the wheel and help guide your baby to a healthy start in life and a healthy future.

How? Chances are you probably know many of the basics of healthy baby making – and if you were planning this pregnancy, you may have implemented many (or all) of them before sperm even met egg: see your GP or a midwife for a preconception check-up, adjust your lifestyle as needed (cut back on caffeine, cut out alcohol, smoking, marijuana and any other recreational drug use), finesse your fitness routine, and take a close look at the supplements and medications you take, adjusting as recommended by your antenatal healthcare professional. And, of course, eat well.

Seeing as you've picked up this book, you're probably already committed to eating well when you're expecting – or at least, you're curious why you should think about committing. Maybe you don't need any facts or figures to convince you that feeding yourself and

My Baby, the Parasite?

Myth: A baby takes all the nutrients needed for growth and development from mum, no matter what she eats or doesn't eat.

Fact: It's true that most babies develop and grow well even when their mums don't eat particularly well. But they aren't parasites. When there aren't enough nutrients to go around – because mum's stores are low and she's not eating well enough to replenish them – mum gets first dibs. To ensure the survival of the species, Mother Nature swings in favour of the mother (who can live to reproduce again if she's well nourished and healthy) – not in favour of her baby. In fact, babies can be born with vitamin deficiencies to mums who show no signs of deficiency. The exception: when it comes to calcium, a developing baby's needs will be met first when mum doesn't tuck away enough – even if it means draining her bones of this vital mineral to build her baby's bones.

your baby right during pregnancy is a priority.

But the connection between pregnancy eating and pregnancy health may be even more compelling and far-reaching than you'd imagine. And it's growing, too. Almost daily, scientists make a stronger case, discovering just how many aspects of a baby's development and future well-being can be influenced by a mum-to-be's diet. What's more, what's good for a baby is also good for mum. Research continues to show that healthy eating can make pregnancy safer, less likely to become complicated and (importantly from where you're sitting, queasy, tired, windy, constipated and bloated) more comfortable. Talk about win-win . . . and more win!

Eating Well: What's in It for Baby

No news flash here: your body will be changing plenty during the 40 weeks of pregnancy. And growing, too – in places you'd expect (your breasts, your tummy) and in places you probably wouldn't (like your feet). But consider how much your baby will be changing and growing over those same 40 weeks (really, 38 weeks counting from conception). Cells dividing at an unbelievable rate, organs (that heart, that brain, those lungs, that stomach) and systems (circulatory, urinary, digestive) rapidly developing, the senses (hearing, sight, taste and smell) taking shape, along with those perfect ten little fingers, ten little toes, and those little girl and boy parts. Bones, muscle, skin and eventually fat forming, hair sprouting. All in life's first and most fantastic journey, taking fertilised egg to blastocyst to embryo to foetus and finally, to ready-to-deliver baby.

CHEW ON THIS. If there's one thing that every culture and every generation shares – from the East to the West, from the ancient to the contemporary – it's the tradition of telling pregnant women what they should and shouldn't eat. Pregnancy is fertile ground for superstitions, folklore and tales from old wives from around the world and through the ages . . . not to mention sketchy internet rumours, social media shaming and public pregnancy policing ('you're going to eat *that?*').

The truth is you can pass up most of that passed-along pregnancy advice, as well meaning or time honoured (by old-timers) as it might be. Among the pregnancy food myths you can definitely discount:

- Eat salty or sour foods and your baby will be born with a sour personality.

- Spicy foods will make your baby hot tempered.

- Chow down on chillies and other spicy foods and your baby will be born bald.

- A teaspoon each of honey and vinegar, taken every morning during pregnancy, will help your baby grow more hair.

- Dark-coloured foods will make a baby's skin darker, while light-coloured foods (some say milk) will turn a baby's skin lighter.

- Eat fish and your baby could end up stupid as a salmon. (Ironically, of course, eating salmon and many other types of fish is linked to optimal baby brain development.)

- Eat rabbit and your baby might sleep with his or her eyes open.

Hungry for more pregnancy food fiction? You'll find 'Chew on This' boxes throughout this book.

What fuels that journey? Actually, the fuel source is you. Your baby – and the complex, ingeniously designed baby-making factory your body runs – is fuelled primarily by what you eat and what you drink. Vitamins, minerals, calories, protein, fluids and other nutrients necessary for healthy baby production – and a healthy pregnancy – come mostly from your diet. Though your body can use backup reserves of some resources, such as calcium from your bones and calories from stored fat, it'll spoon up (or suck up) most from what you're eating and drinking – and the more nutrients you take in, the more you'll dish out to your baby. Though most babies grow and develop normally even when their mums don't eat all that well, study after study shows that, on average, healthier eaters have healthier pregnancies and healthier babies.

Think of healthy eating as one of the first and best gifts you can give your baby-to-be. And it's a gift that keeps on giving. Your diet can impact many components of your little one's health in many ways – in both the short and the long term – including:

Your baby's organ development. With all those body parts developing from tiny cells (the heart, liver, lungs, kidneys and nervous system, just to name a few), and only nine months in which to accomplish this phenomenal growth, your baby-making factory is working full steam, day and night. Most of the raw materials needed to turn a fertilised egg into a fully equipped bouncing baby are supplied through your diet.

Fortunately, those raw materials aren't hard to come by. The average British diet provides enough of most nutrients to ensure a healthy, bouncing baby – but, not surprisingly, extra-good nutrition can offer extra insurance that all will develop according to plan. At the other extreme, a diet that is severely deficient in certain types of nutrients (which is uncommon in the UK) increases the risk that a baby may not develop normally. For instance, a deficiency in folic acid can result in neural tube defects (defects in the brain or spinal cord), such as spina bifida. Happily, the number of babies born with these defects has decreased since folic acid supplementation has become routinely recommended for women of childbearing age – a great case for taking an antenatal vitamin before and during pregnancy.

Your baby's brain development. While the development of most organs is relatively complete midway through pregnancy, your baby's brain will have its greatest growth spurt during the last trimester and beyond (brain development continues at a mind-boggling pace for the first three years of a baby's life). Since protein, calories and omega-3 fatty acids are particularly crucial to optimal brain development, taking in enough of these nutrients – especially during those final three months of baby growing – may boost your baby's brainpower. So it's smart to reach for that bowl of walnuts or that dish of fish.

Your baby's birthweight. How much and how well you eat can impact how your baby measures up – and weighs in – at delivery. While genetics definitely plays a role in baby's birthweight and beyond, a mum's diet during pregnancy does, too. Eating too little can keep a baby from growing to potential in the uterus, sometimes resulting in a low birthweight (also known as small for gestational age, or SGA). Eating too

much can lead to a baby growing too much too fast, and being born too large for gestational age. Very small babies have an increased risk of complications and health problems at birth and sometimes later on. Extra-large babies are more likely to arrive early and/or via caesarean section (because they're too big to fit through mum's pelvis) and are more likely to have complications and health problems, including low scores on the Apgar test (which measures a baby's well-being at birth), an increased risk of breathing problems and hypoglycaemia, and a greater chance of needing a stay in the neonatal intensive care unit, or NICU. Very large babies are also predisposed to obesity and type 2 diabetes later in life. Not surprisingly, following a just-right formula – eating a healthy number of calories and gaining about the right amount of weight – can help fuel just the right amount of growth for your baby. See Chapter 6 for more on weight gain.

But it's not only the quantity of food (or calories) you eat that matters to your baby's nutritional intake. The quality matters, too. Too little iron can slow a baby's growth. So can too little zinc. Falling short on folate (folic acid) or being generally malnourished can lead to restricted foetal growth (aka intrauterine growth restriction, or IUGR) and a baby being born small or even with signs of malnutrition. Eating the right amounts of the right foods will help give your baby what he or she needs to grow on – and contribute to a bouncing baby birthweight.

Your baby's arrival time. There are many reasons why a mum might deliver prematurely that have nothing to do with diet. Still, on average, mums who lack enough key nutrients like iron, zinc, vitamin C, vitamin D and magnesium may be more likely to have a preterm birth than well-nourished mums. Ditto for mums who don't get enough folate in their diets. On the other hand, mums who eat well and gain the right amount of weight can boost their chances of carrying to term. Not surprisingly, full-term babies are more likely to be healthy babies.

Your baby's sleep habits. There's some evidence that newborns whose mums get their fill of omega-3 fatty acids during the last trimester are better overall sleepers than other babies. So does feasting on fish late in pregnancy guarantee you a full night's sleep in your baby's first months? No – and in fact, spoiler alert: newborns aren't supposed to sleep through the night. But it may promote healthier sleep patterns. So may having a daily serving of dark chocolate during your last trimester, which some research links to babies who sleep better and cry less (and, obviously, to happier mums).

Your baby's eating habits. Fast-forward to future family dinners, and you can definitely see how your tastes might affect your baby's. After all, little monkeys tend to mimic their mums and dads in many ways, including whether they savour salad or favour chips. But did you know that how you eat during pregnancy can also help shape your baby's future eating habits? Because your baby's taste buds develop at about 16 weeks of pregnancy, he or she can become accustomed to flavours that make their way from your meals into the amniotic fluid he or she swallows. Which means that baby's food favourites can form before he or she even takes a first bite of solids. This concept, sometimes referred to as flavour learning, has been boosted not only by word of mum ('I ate nothing but watermelon, and my baby loves watermelon!'

or 'I craved hot sauce and so does my child!'), but also by studies. For instance, one study found that babies of mums who drank a lot of carrot juice during pregnancy were more likely to lap up cereal mixed with carrot juice than those whose mums didn't touch the orange stuff. Other studies have shown that babies of mums who couldn't get enough garlic and other strong flavours while they were expecting were more likely to scarf down scampi or curry, and those of mums who brought on the broccoli and other 'bitter' vegetables were more likely to be sweet on those bitter tastes. The moral of these studies: if you'd like your baby to eat his or her leafy green vegetables later, consider going green now. And keep going green later, too, since flavour learning continues as baby becomes acclimated to the changing taste of breast milk, which is also flavoured by a mum's diet.

Your baby's long-term health. So you know your baby has a lot of growing and developing to do during those nine months in your womb. And you know that your little one is a miraculous work in progress – and that you can help that progress along by eating well and eating enough. But did you know that this early progress – and your efforts to fuel it – may go a long way beyond birth, laying the foundation not only for a healthy start in life, but also a healthy lifetime?

Researchers have provided plenty of food for thought on how a mum's diet during pregnancy (and even, to a certain extent, before conception) can affect her baby's long-term health. A person's predisposition to certain diseases (cancer, for instance, or schizophrenia) or to chronic conditions such as diabetes, hypertension and heart disease may be related to his or her mum's nutritional intake during pregnancy. A striking example: studies show that babies who are undernourished in the first trimester or who are overfed in the third trimester may be at greater risk for obesity later in life. Other research has suggested a link between a mum's low intake of calcium and other bone-building nutrients and her child's risk for osteoporosis later in life. Nutrition during pregnancy, say researchers, may influence a baby's health not only at birth, but years later, even into adulthood.

Eating Well: What's in It for You

Baby's not the only one benefiting every time you brake for breakfast, crunch on carrots or choose the grilled chicken salad over the finger-licking nuggets and chips. There's plenty in eating well for you, too. Among the many possible perks of healthy pregnancy eating for mums-to-be:

More comfort. Let's face it: the average pregnant woman doesn't really walk around for nine months with a rosy glow. In fact, in the first few months, she's more likely to walk around with a greenish tint. And morning sickness is just one of the many miseries pregnancy can serve up. Other uncomfortable symptoms your body may have in store for you: fatigue, constipation, haemorrhoids, heartburn, headaches, backaches, varicose veins, pregnancy spots (even the dreaded bacne), bleeding gums, swollen ankles – and that's just naming a few. Will you have every symptom in the book or just a handful? Will they be majorly miserable or just moderately? Your individual pregnancy comfort (or discomfort) quotient will largely be decided by factors you can't control, like your genes (thanks, Mum!), the work you do (say, standing all day on the job) or the weather you're weathering (like sweltering heat and humidity). But at least some of it will be up to you – and influenced, to some extent, by how you eat. Grazing on the energy-boosting combo of protein and complex carbs can ease fatigue, minimise headaches and mood swings, even keep some of the queasies at bay. Filling up on fibre and fluids can clear up constipation, and curbing sugar while focusing on healthy fats may help clear up your complexion. Cutting the grease can cut back on heartburn. For more on eating well to feel well during pregnancy, see Chapter 7.

Fewer complications. It's as simple as this: pregnancy complications are less common among mums who eat well. For instance, good dietary habits – eating plenty of fruits and vegetables, lean protein, beans and wholegrains, and limiting sugar and refined grains may lower the risk of gestational diabetes. Top-notch nutrition – including enough magnesium – may reduce the chances of developing pre-eclampsia.

Staying well hydrated can help prevent excessive swelling and preterm contractions. Getting enough iron can help reduce the risk of anaemia and postnatal complications. And because eating well is likely to lead to healthy weight gain, the risks of all kinds of pregnancy complications, from developing gestational diabetes to having a caesarean section, are lowered. The main point: a healthy pregnancy diet gives you the right balance of vitamins, minerals and other vital nutrients, paving the way for a healthier pregnancy.

Birthing benefits. Can eating well help you order up an easier labour and delivery? Not exactly (though wouldn't that be a nice app to have?). But an overall healthy diet – one that provides a balance of baby-friendly nutrients and about the right number of calories (leading to the right amount of weight gain) – may help prevent a too-early birth. Especially beneficial when it comes to keeping a baby bun baking until term: iron, zinc, vitamin C, vitamin D and magnesium. Deficiencies in those nutrients have been linked to premature labour. And though there are definitely no sure things when it comes to labour and delivery, here's another possible birthing room benefit: in general, mums who are well nourished handle whatever childbirth happens to hand them better than those who are low on nutrient stores – just as a well-nourished athlete is able to perform better and endure better than one who's nutrient-deprived. (And when it comes to athletic events, there's none more challenging than childbirth. Just ask any Iron Woman who's also a mum.)

A faster route to recovery. A baby's not the only thing you can expect after delivery, though it's definitely the best thing. No, you'll also take home a host of postnatal symptoms as your body attempts to recover from nine long months of pregnancy, the gruelling marathon of labour and the pounding it might have taken while delivering 7, 8 or even more pounds of baby (or having major surgery, if you end up with a caesarean section). Add to your body's challenges overall exhaustion and the cumulative toll of

new-parent sleep deprivation – plus the energy needed to care for and feed your baby (particularly if you're breastfeeding) – and you'll understand why it'll need all the help it can get. Eating well during pregnancy allows your body to store resources that will help you meet the physical and emotional challenges of new-mum life, speed your postnatal recovery and provide the get-up-and-go you'll need to keep on getting-up-and-going. That, and help supply your little one's fast-growing demand for breast milk. (See Chapter 10 for more on eating well postnatal.)

Better bone health. All ready to put your baby's needs ahead of your own? The truth is that your pregnant body has other plans when it comes to divvying up the nutrients from incoming food – giving you first dibs on most of them, then serving leftovers to your baby. One nutrient this mum-first policy doesn't cover: that essential bone-builder, calcium. If you don't take in enough calcium when you're pregnant, your body will drain this vital mineral from your own bones to help build baby's. This potential shortfall could set you up for bone loss later in life, and even for osteoporosis.

Better overall health. It's probably not a shocker, but healthy eating habits can improve overall health. Embracing healthy eating habits for baby's sake now can – if you stick with them later – gift you with a lowered risk of all kinds of diseases, from chronic hypertension to heart disease, type 2 diabetes to cancer. Share those healthy eating habits at home, and you'll be sharing those possible long-term health benefits with your whole family – including your baby-to-be.

Ready to Get Started?

So now you know the 'why' of eating well – it's best for you, your baby and your pregnancy. But what about the 'how' – and the know-how – you'll need to make it happen? It's all here in the pages that follow: the nutrition facts, and the facts about nutrition. The tips, advice and recipes you'll need to eat your way through a healthy and comfortable pregnancy. How to prepare (or order up) meals and snacks that satisfy your cravings, tempt your taste buds and fill your pregnant body's requirements while nurturing your baby's growth and development. Plus, how to keep your weight gain on the track that's right for you and your pregnancy.

Ready to get started? Sit back, sip a fruit smoothie and read on to learn how to eat well when you're expecting.

CHAPTER 2

The Nutrients That Make a Baby

....

Y ou can't see them. You can't smell them. You can't even taste them. But they're in just about every bite you take. They're nutrients, substances your body needs to survive and thrive – the vitamins, minerals, protein, carbohydrates and fats in the salmon and strawberries and broccoli and cereal (and yes, even in the ice cream, crisps and chocolate bars) you eat. Whether these nutrients find their way into foods naturally (like the vitamin C and lycopene in that juicy vine-ripened tomato) or thanks to fortification (for instance, the vitamin D in that dairy-free milk alternative, the B vitamins added to that slice of bread), whether they're found in the healthiest sources (that kale salad) or the least healthy ones (those gummy bear sweets), they all play an important role in the making of your little baby bun. Wondering how? Read on to learn what's behind all the nutrients in the foods you eat every day and what makes them so vital to the growth and development of a foetus. Don't want to get into the details about your nutrients and just want to get busy eating well? Jump ahead to Chapter 3, 'The Pregnancy Diet'.

From A to Zinc: An Encyclopedia of Vitamins and Minerals

F ew people digging into their morning porridge or tucking into their lunchtime sandwich give a first – never mind second – thought to the vitamins and minerals they're about to consume and absorb. But every food you eat

What's an RNI, Anyway?

The British Nutrition Foundation is the organisation that establishes principles and guidelines for approximately how much of each nutrient an average person requires – and approximately how many mouthfuls of a certain food you'll need to eat to meet that requirement. These guidelines are called the Dietary Reference Values, or DRVs. For the most part, they're also TMI (too much information). That's because they're just a little too specific for most consumers, even especially health-conscious ones, and definitely too specific for those who'd rather just consume food, not analyse the nutrients in it.

Still, there are two DRVs that apply in this chapter at least, if you choose to apply them (you can also just look for foods that are high in a certain essential nutrient, and leave the analysis to the pros):

Reference Nutrient Intakes (RNI). An RNI is the amount of a nutrient needed per day to meet the nutrient requirements of nearly all healthy people (divided by sex) in a particular life stage (infant or child, for instance, or during pregnancy or lactation). (If you are reading up on nutrients in US sources, they're called Recommended Daily Allowances, or RDAs.)

Safe Intake (SI). An SI is the amount of a nutrient recommended per day when there is insufficient scientific evidence to develop an RNI. The SI is set at a level assumed to ensure nutritional adequacy, so it's not as reliable as an RNI, which is based on solid evidence, but it still gives good guidance.

For the latest nutrient information, visit the British Nutrition Foundation's website at www.nutrition.org.uk.

---

contains at least some of these essential nutrients, each of them vital to your health (clearly some foods deliver more nutrients and come in more nutritious packages than others). During pregnancy, the mission of the nutrients you consume becomes even more important, since they must fuel the needs of two bodies, including a rapidly growing one. Which means you'll need to take in more vitamins and minerals than ever before. You'll get a good supply from your antenatal vitamin-mineral supplement, but you'll benefit even more from getting nutrients from their natural sources. Knowing how each vitamin and mineral contributes to making a healthy baby – and where you can find them – can help inform (and, hey, inspire!) the food choices you make. Here's a guide to the most important nutrients your body needs.

Vitamins

Vitamins play leading roles when it comes to metabolism, cell production, tissue repair and a variety of other vital processes. And while vitamins themselves are not sources of energy, they also help convert the carbs, fats and proteins that you eat into energy. Quite simply, you can't live without them, and neither can your baby.

Not surprisingly, mums-to-be – who are nourishing not only themselves but also a rapidly growing baby – require more vitamins than the average adult

Can Your Body Store Vitamins?

Here's a fast fact about vitamins: they can be either fat-soluble or water-soluble.

Fat-soluble vitamins – vitamins A, D, E and K, for instance – can be stored in the body, which means that you don't necessarily need a daily dose of them, assuming your body has backup to draw from. That's the good news. The bad news is that because the body can store these vitamins, taking too much of them (for instance, taking mega-doses of A or D supplements) can lead to toxic levels in your system, which can be particularly danger-ous if you're pregnant or planning to become pregnant. But (back to the good news) you can't overdose on these vitamins by eating foods that are naturally rich in them, even if you're also taking an antenatal.

Water-soluble vitamins – such as vitamins B and C – dissolve in water and therefore can't be stored in the body. Your body uses what it needs for the day and then gets rid of the rest via urine. So you'll have to make sure you restock those water-soluble vitamins daily by eating a healthy, vitamin-rich diet and taking that vital antenatal supplement.

female. Popping an antenatal vitamin supplement is always a good place to start, but eating well will also help you get your pregnancy share of vitamins.

Vitamin A. Vitamin A is a nutritional powerhouse – essential to many aspects of baby making, including the growth and development of cells, bones, skin, eyes (especially important for night vision), teeth and immunity. Too little vitamin A in a mum-to-be's diet (plus the absence of an antenatal vitamin) has been linked to premature delivery and to slow growth in her baby, as well as to skin disorders and eye damage. But as with other fat-soluble vitamins, when taken in supplement form in very high doses for long periods of time, vitamin A can be toxic. Pregnant women who take very high doses of vitamin A (beyond what is included in an antenatal supple-ment) may increase the risk of birth defects in their unborn babies. But don't let that stand between you and the salad bar. You can't get too much vitamin A from your diet – not even if you pile your plate high with broccoli, carrots and other vitamin A–rich foods.

The reference nutrient intake (RNI) for vitamin A during pregnancy is 700 mcg, but there's no need to calcu-late. It's easy to get what you need from a well-balanced diet, though your ante-natal supplement will offer insurance in the form of beta-carotene. You'll find the best sources in the produce department (or in the frozen fruit and vegetable section), and hue will clue you in: look for vitamin A in yellow and orange vegetables and fruits (carrots, squash and pumpkin, sweet potatoes, cantaloupe, papaya, apricots) and dark green vegetables (spinach, kale, broc-coli, spring greens). You'll also score smaller amounts of A in oatmeal and other wholegrains, as well as in some animal sources, including eggs.

Vitamin B$_1$ (thiamin or thiamine). Nothing B-list about this B vitamin, which helps convert carbohydrates into energy, regulate the supply of carbo-hydrates to your baby, aid in the produc-tion of red blood cells (which you and your baby need plenty of), and assist in the functioning of the nervous system. Thiamin also promotes a healthy appe-tite – something that can definitely come

Ugh … What's an Ug?

Maybe you're wondering how many bananas you'll need to eat to reach your goal of 1.2 mg of vitamin B_6 or how many carrots equal 770 mcg of vitamin A. And wait – why do you sometimes see vitamin measurements in 'ug's? What on earth is an 'ug'?

Reading food labels (see the box on page 58) – provide some nutritional information such as energy, fat, fibre, protein and salt – but don't normally provide mg, mcg and ug recommendations for vitamins and minerals. However, the Daily Dozen (page 32) lets you dispense with all the ug, mg and mcg measurements, making meeting your nutritional needs much easier.

But if you're still curious, this chart should help you make sense of what all these measurements mean:

g	gram	A unit of weight equal to about 0.03 of an ounce
mg	milligram	One-thousandth of a gram
mcg	microgram	One-millionth of a gram
ug	same as mcg	One-millionth of a gram

Now for some perspective: A paper clip weighs 1 g. A single grain of salt is equal to approximately 120 mcg or 120 ug. (So 770 mcg isn't looking so daunting after all, is it?) In terms you can appreciate, and eat: a bowl of cereal and a banana has your B_6 bases covered for the day. Ugs . . . without the ugh.

---

in handy when you're nourishing for two. Deficiencies (something that won't happen if you're taking your antenatal vitamin) can cause fatigue and weakness in a mum and slowed growth and heart irregularities in her baby.

The RNI for thiamin during pregnancy is 0.9 mg in the last trimester; your antenatal will offer cover, but you can easily get it by eating wholegrains, brown rice, oats, pork, fish, beans, peas, peanuts, raisins, cauliflower, sweetcorn, acorn squash, nuts and sunflower seeds, among other healthy foods in your diet.

Vitamin B_2 (riboflavin). Riboflavin helps release energy (something every mum-to-be can always use more of) from fats, proteins and carbohydrates. It also helps in cell division (remember, baby's cells are dividing at a remarkable rate), and in the growth and repair of tissues (those tiny baby tissues!). Finally, riboflavin stabilises appetite, promotes healthy skin and eyes for you, and the development of healthy skin and eyes for baby, and boosts baby's brain growth (making a steady supply of this vital vitamin especially important in the third trimester). Deficiencies of riboflavin (something that won't happen if you're taking an antenatal vitamin) can cause problems with the formation of foetal bones, poor digestive function in the foetus and a suppressed foetal immune system. For mum, a deficiency can lead to poor appetite and mouth sores. There's also some evidence that a deficiency may increase the risk of pre-eclampsia, but again, if you're taking an antenatal vitamin and eating healthy foods, you don't have to worry about a riboflavin deficiency.

The RNI for riboflavin during pregnancy is 1.4 mg. You'll find it in eggs (it's in both the yolk and the white),

A Baby in the Making

In approximately 266 days, your baby is transformed from a single cell to a complete human being. During that time, miraculous changes are occurring, sometimes on an hourly basis – from the formation of crucial organs (heart, lungs, stomach) to the formation of vital systems (digestive system, urinary system, circulatory system), from the development of arms and legs (including those tiny fingers and toes!) to the development of the central nervous system and brain. Here are some highlights of that transformation:

The First Trimester. Soon after sperm meets egg, the fertilised ovum begins dividing rapidly as it moves down your fallopian tube. Approximately five days post-conception, the bundle of cells (already more than 100 cells) implants in your uterus. The outer cells will form the placenta, while the inner cells (made up of three layers) will form your baby.

The cells of that newly implanted embryo are already starting to specialise, getting organised into distinct tissues and organs. The outer layer of cells (the ectoderm) will develop into the brain, nervous system, hair, eyes and skin. The middle layer of cells (the mesoderm) will develop into the muscle, bones and cardiovascular and excretory systems. The inner layer of cells (endoderm) will develop into the digestive tract, lungs and glands.

As your pregnancy progresses, your baby will develop a rudimentary brain and the beginnings of a spinal column. The heart starts to beat somewhere around the middle of week 5. Arm buds and leg buds begin to form. As the embryo grows to the size of a grain of rice, the liver, kidneys and thyroid gland become visible. The eyelids begin to appear, as do the nose, ears, lips, gums and jaws. Towards the middle of the first trimester, the kidneys begin to function, blood forms in the liver and the stomach begins to produce some digestive juices. By the time the foetus has reached the size of a coffee bean,

milk, yogurt, meat, chicken, mushrooms, peas, beans, asparagus, broccoli, spinach and quinoa.

Vitamin B$_3$ (niacin). Not only is niacin involved in releasing much-needed energy from the foods you eat, but it also boosts blood flow – and the circulation of nutrients to your baby – by widening blood vessels. The right amount of niacin helps build a healthy nervous system and digestive tract for your baby while promoting healthier skin for you. But watch out for overdoses – which, once again, you can't get from eating healthy foods, only from taking too much in supplement form. Too much niacin can trigger itchy skin (something pregnant women definitely don't need more of) and tummy troubles (something else pregnant women don't need more of).

The RNI for niacin during pregnancy is 13 mg. Good sources include meat, chicken, fish, milk, eggs (there's more in the whites than the yolks), legumes (aka pulses) and mushrooms.

Vitamin B$_6$ (pyridoxine). Vitamin B$_6$ helps the body use protein to build tissue – a very good thing when there's so much tissue to build. Because it plays a major role in baby's brain and nervous system, adequate intake of B$_6$ reduces the risk of neural tube defects. It also helps form red and white blood cells and is involved in immune function.

your baby bean's skeleton has already formed, and fingers and toes have begun to form. Fingerprints appear, and internal organs continue to mature. By the end of the first trimester, your baby, looking more like a human being now, can make facial expressions. Vocal cords are developing, bones are beginning to calcify, nails are forming and tiny tooth buds are present. Sex organs are also developing.

The Second Trimester. Bones continue to develop and harden, causing the foetus to straighten from its curled position. Hair is beginning to grow, and muscles are more developed. (You'll probably begin feeling those first kicks sometime around weeks 16 to 20.) Your baby can hear by the sixth month, and will react to loud noises with a startle. Lanugo (a downy coat of hair) appears on the skin, as does vernix caseosa, a waxy covering that protects the baby's skin during its long soak in an amniotic bath. By the end of the second trimester, your still very little one has regular periods of wakefulness and sleep and is making more coordinated movements. Baby's eyes open and close, reacting to light. A baby boy's testicles begin their descent from the abdominal cavity into the scrotum.

The Third Trimester. Your baby will gain an average of 225–350 g (8–12 oz) each week during this trimester (almost as much as you're gaining). As the weight accumulates, baby fat develops under the skin, filling out that cute little form and ironing out that wrinkled look. Hair on that sweet head is starting to fill in (more in some babies than in others), eyebrows and eyelashes are present, and nails are already set for a manicure, having grown beyond the tips of the fingers and toes. The lungs and the digestive tract are reaching the final stages of maturity, but the most remarkable growth is in the brain, which is working overtime on its development. Your baby's immune system is also getting stronger. And 38 weeks or so after the amazing transformation began, it's showtime: baby is ready to be born.

And an added bonus: B_6 has been shown to reduce morning sickness symptoms, as well as help clear up skin unsettled by pregnancy hormones.

The RNI for pyridoxine during pregnancy is 1.2 mg. Feasting on many of your favourites will ensure that intake: bananas, avocados, tomatoes, spinach, watermelon, potatoes, brown rice, bulgar wheat, soya beans, chickpeas, oatmeal, chicken, meat and fish.

Vitamin B_7 (biotin). Biotin is involved in the production of amino acids and helps digest fats, carbohydrates and proteins. Even more importantly when growing a baby: the rapidly dividing cells of the developing foetus require biotin for DNA replication. Deficiencies (if you're not taking an antenatal or eating well) can exacerbate several pregnancy symptoms, including fatigue, nausea, skin problems and muscle pain. It can also trigger something that isn't common during pregnancy: hair loss.

In the UK there is no RNI for biotin, but you'll find biotin aplenty in many favourites, including egg yolks, fish, soya beans, seeds, nuts, sweet potatoes, spinach and broccoli.

Vitamin B_{12}. Vitamin B_{12} is fundamental in the formation of red blood cells, for building genetic material, and for the proper development and functioning of the nervous system – in other words,

The Placenta at Work

The placenta is what makes the making-of-a-baby possible – sort of the mission control of the baby factory. A complex network of blood vessels and tissues attached to the uterine lining and to the baby via his or her umbilical cord, the placenta contains two blood supplies: yours and baby's. These blood supplies communicate but never touch.

The placenta takes on many important roles, including producing several of the hormones that regulate growth and development. But its most significant function is as a vital pipeline, shipping nutrients from you to your baby and waste products from your baby back to you for disposal. Here's how that pipeline works.

When you eat something, your body digests it, taking available nutrients and transferring them into your bloodstream. Once your body takes what it needs (mum gets first dibs on most nutrients), it sends the rest to the placenta, where the foetus's blood vessels distribute them, along with fluids, oxygen and other important substances. After baby's been fed, the placenta deposits waste products that are eventually shipped back for excretion via your kidneys (so, you really are urinating for two).

As baby grows, the placenta grows – but not without your help. The growth of your baby's placenta is directly related to the quality and quantity of what you eat. A better-nourished mum, on average, produces a bigger, more productive placenta (and when it comes to placentas, size does matter).

for the making of a healthy baby. It also partners with folate (keep reading) – another essential baby building block. Deficiencies can cause neural tube defects (such as spina bifida), digestive tract disorders or neurological disorders in the foetus, as well as severe fatigue and anaemia in the mother.

The pregnancy RNI for vitamin B_{12} is 1.5 mcg. The only natural dietary sources are animal products such as meat, chicken, dairy products and fish. If you're a vegan, you'll need to get your vitamin B_{12} from a supplement taken in addition to your antenatal supplement (ask your healthcare professional for guidelines) and/or from nutritional yeast or B_{12}-fortified soya milk.

Choline. It starts with a C, but choline is a valued (if not well-known) member of the vitamin B family, essential for a baby's neural tube and brain development. It will also help give your brain a boost (you'll say 'thanks for the memory' when pregnancy forgetfulness kicks in). Low levels of choline during pregnancy increase the risk of birth defects in the newborn, which is why most antenatal vitamins contain this essential nutrient in their portfolio.

There is no RNI for choline in the UK, but the European Food Safety Authority (EFSA) says the safe intake (SI) during pregnancy is 480 mg a day. Sources include egg yolks, meat, poultry, fish, dairy, nuts, seeds, legumes, wholegrains, quinoa, mushrooms, potatoes, beans, cauliflower and Brussels sprouts.

Folate (folic acid). Another member of the B team (and probably one of the most valuable players on Team Baby), folate is crucial in the proper

Folate versus Folic Acid

Wondering why folate and folic acid are often used interchangeably? Confused about the difference between the two? So are many people, especially after a Google search. Here's the short explanation of how these two terms for the same nutrient (actually B₉) differ:

Folate. Folate is the name of the naturally occurring vitamin. It comes from the Latin word *folium*, which means 'leaf' – something that makes a lot of sense, since some of the best dietary sources of folate are leafy vegetables.

Folic acid. Folic acid is the synthetic form of vitamin B₉ and is what's used in supplements and added to processed- and fortified-food products, such as cereals.

Glad that's cleared up? Great. Now comes the potential for more confusion. Many experts now believe that lumping folate and folic acid together is a false equivalency, at least for part of the population. And it all comes down to genes. Mums-to-be with a mutation in their MTHFR gene (and no, that's not shorthand for an expletive, it's just the name of a gene) have a difficult time properly metabolising folic acid into usable folate. People with a mutation are better served getting most of their folate/folic acid from foods (in the form of folate) than relying only on an antenatal supplement to provide folic acid. And that's why (whether you have the gene mutation or not, or if you're not sure whether you have the mutation or not) it's so important not only to take an antenatal supplement that contains folic acid, but also to eat a diet rich in folate foods. There are also some antenatal supplements that provide folate in the form of 'folinic acid' (you may also see it listed as 'folate' on the label). This form (the 'active' form of folic acid) may provide better absorption of this vital vitamin.

---

development of the neural tube (the embryonic structure that develops into the brain and spinal cord). In fact, studies show that low levels of folate in the first months of pregnancy are responsible for about 70 per cent of all neural tube defects – which is why it's so important that you get the right amount of folic acid before and during pregnancy. But folate does more than prevent birth defects, and its starring role doesn't end in the first trimester either. Folate also aids in cell division and in the formation of red blood cells (yours and baby's), which is why getting too little can lead to anaemia. Getting plenty of folate later in pregnancy is associated with a lower risk of slow foetal growth and an increased birthweight for baby, and has been linked in some situations to lower rates of premature birth, congenital heart defects and possibly pre-eclampsia. Some research has suggested that adequate folate intake might help prevent Down's syndrome. Other research suggests that too little folate during pregnancy may be linked to attention deficit hyperactivity disorder or future obesity in a child.

Aim to get 400 mcg of folic acid daily both before and during the first 12 weeks of pregnancy. Good sources are most leafy green vegetables, romaine lettuce, Brussels sprouts, asparagus, avocados, bananas, oranges and grapefruit (a glass of orange or grapefruit juice

Don't Do the Maths

Just skimming through this chapter, you can clearly see how vitamins, minerals and other nutrients help build a healthier baby. But remember that good nutrition is not just about numbers – it's about food. So instead of whipping out your calculator to see if your RNIs for this mineral or that vitamin add up, just follow the Pregnancy Diet in Chapter 3. It does all the calculating for you. Follow the guidelines there (no need to do the maths), and you and your baby will get your share of every nutrient from A to zinc. Try the recipes in Part 2, and you'll get more delight in every nutritious bite.

will score more), tomatoes (and tomato juice), black-eyed beans, green peas, beans and peanuts. Most grain products are also fortified with folic acid.

Vitamin C. Probably the best known of all vitamins, vitamin C has a remarkable CV. For one thing, it's essential to the production of collagen. This protein is what gives structure and strength to a developing baby's cartilage, muscles, blood vessels and bones, and it's also found in skin and eyes. For another, it's needed (by both you and baby) for tissue repair, wound healing and various other metabolic processes. And there's more to C: it helps in the absorption of iron and may help you resist infection. Getting enough vitamin C during pregnancy has been linked to a healthy birthweight and a decreased risk of preterm premature rupture of the membranes (when a mum's water breaks too early, leading to preterm birth). Deficiencies of vitamin C (not usually an issue if you're popping an antenatal daily) can

cause periodontal disease, aka gum disease (which pregnant women are more susceptible to anyway).

The safe intake for vitamin C during pregnancy is 50 mg – and you'll need a fresh supply daily. Besides the obvious orange, sources include other citrus fruits, broccoli, Brussels sprouts, raw cabbage, cauliflower, kale, red and green peppers, sweet potatoes, tomatoes, cantaloupe, cranberries, honeydew, kiwi fruit, mangoes, papayas, peaches, strawberries and watermelon.

Vitamin D. Essential for maintaining healthy teeth and bone structure, vitamin D helps in the absorption of calcium and is very important during pregnancy. A severe vitamin D deficiency (something that is rare these days) can lead to rickets (a softening of bones), muscle disease and seizures in a newborn. Some research suggests a link between a deficiency of D and an increased risk for pre-eclampsia and a caesarean delivery. Women who get enough D may be less likely to go into preterm labour, deliver prematurely or develop infections – though the evidence for these isn't so strong and more research is ongoing.

The pregnancy RNI for vitamin D is 10 mcg. While the body produces vitamin D when exposed to sunlight, making enough can be challenging – especially for those with darker skin and those who live in less-sunny climates, don't get outdoors enough, wear sunscreen or cover their skin. Can you eat your D? Not easily, since it isn't found naturally in large amounts in any food. Fortified dairy-free milk alternatives and mushrooms contain some, as do salmon, sardines and egg yolks (plus some eggs are fortified too), but not enough to prevent a D deficit. Your best bet is to fill in any D gaps with your antenatal vitamin, plus possibly an additional D supplement recommended by your healthcare provider.

Vitamin E. Vitamin E helps ward off cell-membrane damage. There is also some preliminary evidence that an adequate intake of vitamin E for a mum during pregnancy may help prevent allergies in her child later on. However, too much of this fat-soluble vitamin can be toxic, so be sure to get your E from food sources and from your antenatal supplement only – don't take any extra supplements.

There is no RDI for vitamin E in the UK. The Department of Health advises you get your fill from your diet. Good sources are rapeseed and olive oils, nuts, seeds, green leafies (like kale, rocket, spinach, lettuce), broccoli, kiwi fruit, mangoes and tomatoes.

Vitamin K. Vitamin K is essential for blood clotting and prevents excess blood loss after injuries (and after childbirth). It also maintains healthy bones and helps heal bone fractures. Not getting enough vitamin K (something that's unlikely if you're taking an antenatal) can cause easy bleeding and bruising in both you and the baby. Too much vitamin K (which you could get only from over-supplementation, not from foods you eat) can be toxic. Because little vitamin K gets transferred from mum to foetus during pregnancy, newborn babies receive a vitamin K injection soon after birth.

The Department of Health says you should get enough vitamin K from your diet. Good sources are rapeseed oil, olive oil, beef, broccoli, kale, spinach, turnip tops and spring greens, rocket, lettuce, edamame, green beans, asparagus, avocados, kiwi fruit, blueberries, pomegranates and bananas.

Pantothenic acid. Pantothenic acid, yet another member of the vitamin B family (B5, if you're keeping score), is important for the metabolism of fats, carbohydrates and proteins and the production of steroid hormones. It also regulates the body's adrenal activity, helps make antibodies and stimulates wound healing.

There is no RDI for pantothenic acid in the UK. Sources include beef, chicken, dairy products, eggs, wholegrains, potatoes, broccoli and mushrooms.

Minerals

Vitamins may get all the buzz, but you wouldn't get very far without minerals – elements that are necessary for the health and proper functioning of many systems in your body. Though they tend to get lumped together with vitamins (did your parents ever tell you to 'take your minerals'?), minerals are different, and they're important in different ways. The body (including your baby's body) contains about 25 essential minerals. Not surprisingly, the need for certain minerals increases when you're pregnant.

Calcium. Calcium is well known for its contribution to strong bones and teeth (including tiny baby bones and teeth) – but this vital mineral is also necessary for muscle contraction, blood clotting and normal heart rhythm, as well as nerve development and enzyme activity. While mum gets first dibs on most vitamins and minerals (if there's not enough to go around, mum's needs will be met before baby's), that's not so with calcium. If your calcium intake is low, your body will drain your bones in order to supply calcium to your growing baby – and that can set you up for bone loss later on in life. Still, deficiencies can cause bone problems for both mother and baby. Another reason to bone up on calcium during pregnancy: optimal intake has been associated with a decreased risk of pre-eclampsia.

The RNI for calcium during pregnancy is 700 mg. Milk may be the

CHEW ON THIS. Here's a tart tall tale from the old wives' club: drinking lime water frequently while you're pregnant will build strong teeth in the unborn baby. There's only one problem with that one. Even if it did strengthen baby's teeth (and it does not), it might weaken yours – that is, if you're sucking on limes often or drinking lime water 24/7. That's because the acid from the limes can wear away enamel over time – unless, of course, you brush after drinking lime water or sucking on limes.

obvious source (cow's or goat's milk or fortified soya, almond and other nut milks all contain approximately the same amount, glass for glass), but you can also claim calcium from yogurt, cheese and other dairy products, sardines, tinned salmon with bones, sesame seeds, tofu, almonds, dark green leafy vegetables, pak choi, broccoli, fortified fruit juice and dried figs.

Chromium. Chromium works with other substances to control insulin and maintain the normal regulation of blood sugar – a process that's particularly important during pregnancy, when baby needs a steady supply of fuel for growth and development. This versatile mineral also stimulates the synthesis of protein in tissues and is necessary for baby's muscle strength, brain function and immunity. Deficiencies (which are rare) can lead to weight loss and poor blood glucose control in the mum (which can then lead to gestational diabetes and its associated risks) and glucose intolerance in the baby.

The Department of Health advises getting chromium from your diet, and most antenatal supplements don't contain it. You can get your share of chromium

from food sources such as cheese, wholegrains, meat, poultry, spinach, mushrooms, peas, broccoli and beans.

Copper. Copper allies with iron to form red blood cells (though iron usually gets all the credit). It also aids tissue growth, glucose metabolism and growth of healthy hair, and is essential for the development of the foetus's heart, arteries, blood vessels, skeletal system, brain and nervous system. Deficiencies, which are rare, can cause seizures and neurological abnormalities in the baby and anaemia in the mum. Excess amounts of copper can be toxic.

The RNI for copper during pregnancy is 1.5 mg. You can cash in on copper with your antenatal supplement (but check to make sure yours contains it, since not all do) and by eating lobster, crab, cooked oysters, potatoes, dark green leafy vegetables, mushrooms, prunes, barley, beans, wholegrains, brown rice, nuts and seeds.

Fluoride. Everyone knows that fluoride is a tooth's best friend, helping to strengthen enamel and prevent cavities. But bones depend on fluoride, too, since it acts as a bonding agent for calcium and phosphorus. With baby building up a storm in the tooth and bone departments, getting enough fluoride in your diet helps get those important jobs done. It'll also help protect your bones and teeth (bear in mind that teeth during pregnancy are more susceptible to decay). However, too much fluoride can cause fluorosis (mottling of teeth), especially in young children.

There is no RNI for fluoride in the UK. You will find it in your toothpaste, but you won't be swallowing it anyway. However, it also shows up in kale, spinach, milk, seafood and tinned fish with bones, as well as in green and black tea. The easiest way to access fluoride: drink tap water, which contains fluoride.

Iodine. A component of the thyroid hormone thyroxine, iodine is needed for the proper functioning of the thyroid gland (responsible for regulating metabolism), as well as for a baby's nervous system development. Deficiencies (an intake of less than 10 to 20 mcg of iodine a day) can cause thyroxine levels to drop, resulting in a condition called goitre in the mum and possibly in her baby, too. Low iodine intake is associated with restricted growth and neuro-developmental problems in the uterus, as well as with a lowered IQ or learning problems later on for a child. Severe iodine deficiency (rare in the UK) is also linked with miscarriage and stillbirth.

The RNI for iodine during pregnancy is 140 mcg. Many people get what they need from a varied and balanced diet. The mineral is available in seafood, seaweed and dairy products as well as cereals and grains, depending on the iodine level in the soil in which they were grown. Bear in mind that some antenatal supplements may not contain iodine (see the box on this page).

Iron. Getting enough iron, the must-have mineral used to produce red blood cells and distribute oxygen throughout the body, is the greatest nutritional challenge a woman faces during her reproductive life, full stop – and not only because of those monthly periods. In fact, the challenges multiply when you're pregnant and not getting those periods. That's because of the dramatic increase in blood production during pregnancy, which requires more iron than ever. Low iron levels can result in iron-deficiency anaemia, with symptoms that include feeling extremely weak, fatigued and/or breathless (beyond what's normal in pregnancy).

Get Your Iodine – But Not Too Much

According to the Association of UK Dietitians, young women are not getting enough iodine, and the organisation recommends women ensure they have enough iodine in their diet several months before trying to conceive, during pregnancy and when breastfeeding.

It's difficult to estimate the amount of iodine in food because it varies depending on the soil, seasons and farming practices. In general, seafood, milk and dairy products are the best sources, but bear in mind dairy-free substitutes are not fortified. White fish, such as haddock and cod, is a better source for iodine than oily fish, and scampi is also a good source.

Seaweed is a concentrated source, especially kelp and other brown seaweeds. However, too much iodine can cause thyroid problems, so seaweed should be consumed no more than once a week, especially during pregnancy.

For some mums-to-be it may be difficult to fill the pregnancy requirement for this must-have mineral through diet alone, or even from the iron that's added to a standard antenatal supplement. If a blood test shows you have a low iron level during pregancy, your GP or midwife will recommend an iron supplement. Taking a slow-release supplement can be easier on your stomach.

The RNI for iron during pregnancy is 14.8 mg. You can get additional iron (beyond what's in your antenatal and/ or the supplement prescribed by your healthcare provider) by eating beef, seafood, beans, lentils, chickpeas, tofu, peas, spinach, potatoes, dried apricots, prunes, dark chocolate and oatmeal.

Magnesium. Another mineral that gives calcium an assist in the bone-building department, magnesium is also needed for nerve and muscle function, as well as for helping the body process carbohydrates. What's more, it's essential in the regulation of insulin and blood-sugar levels (so important during pregnancy) and needed for the removal of toxins from the body (ditto). Because magnesium relaxes muscles (as opposed to calcium, which stimulates muscles to contract), adequate levels of magnesium during pregnancy may help prevent premature contractions of the uterus (aka premature labour). Getting enough magnesium may help ward off leg cramps, constipation and even morning sickness. Severe deficiencies are rare but can increase the risk of pre-eclampsia in a mum and stunted growth, muscle spasms and congenital malformations in her baby.

The pregnancy RNI for magnesium is 270 mg. Most antenatals contain magnesium only in small amounts, so be sure to fill your requirement the natural way as well. Tasty sources include legumes, beans, nuts, seeds, tofu, yogurt, milk, wholegrains, dried apricots, prunes, bananas and dark green leafy vegetables.

Manganese. Not on many people's mineral radar (and often confused with magnesium), manganese is vital for the development of baby's bones, cartilage and hearing. It's also necessary for good reproductive function. Deficiencies (very rare) can cause growth restriction in the foetus. Not all antenatal supplements contain manganese, so check the label to see if yours does.

There is no RNI for manganese during pregnancy. Sources include strawberries, bananas, raisins, spinach, carrots, broccoli, wholegrains, brown rice, legumes, nuts and seeds.

Molybdenum. You probably haven't heard of this mineral before (and you almost certainly can't pronounce it), but humble molybdenum is thought to help in a monumentally important task: the transfer of oxygen from one molecule to another. It is also required for protein and fat metabolism, and it helps the baby use iron.

The is no RNI for molybdenum during pregnancy. You can find it in legumes, beans, wholegrains and nuts. It can also be found in some antenatal supplements – check the labels.

Phosphorus. Another comrade of calcium, phosphorus is a component of healthy teeth and bones. It's also needed to maintain the right balance of body fluids and is essential for muscle contractions, normal heart rhythm and blood clotting. Deficiencies, which are uncommon, can cause a loss of appetite (no good when you're pregnant), weakness (you're tired enough) and a loss of calcium from bones (your bones). Too

---

Another Strike Against Fizzy Drinks

Need one more reason to limit fizzy drinks (besides all that sugar or all those artificial sweeteners)? Most fizzy drinks are loaded with phosphorus (listed as phosphoric acid), which lowers the level of calcium in the blood – with some offering up to 500 mg of phosphorus per serving. So not only can a serious soda habit keep you from drinking your calcium-loaded milk, but it also prevents the absorption of whatever calcium you do get from other sources.

The Food Fortification Frenzy

Food enrichment (adding vitamins and minerals lost in processing back into a product) and fortification (adding extra vitamins and minerals that weren't naturally occurring in the first place) was introduced in the UK during the Second World War when calcium was added to flour due to a possible dairy shortage. Worldwide fortification has prevented thousands of deaths in the 20th century that would have resulted from severe vitamin and mineral deficiencies. It worked, big-time – such deficiencies have been virtually eradicated.

Fast-forward to the 21st century and while enrichment is still humming away (replacing vital nutrients in white rice, white bread and other refined bakes), fortification is really on a roll. With manufacturers keen to cash in on the fortification frenzy, you'll find fortified foods and beverages in just about every aisle of your supermarket: calcium, vitamins A through to E, zinc, even plant stanols (for a 'heart healthy' bonus) in your yogurt drink, added omega-3s in your dairy-free spread, phytochemicals in those gummies, amino acids in that chocolate, and electrolytes plus protein (yes, protein) in that bottle of water.

Do the benefits of added nutrients add up? Sometimes – as when adding iron, thiamin and niacin to white and brown flour or calcium to milk substitutes. But often those added nutrients add only to the product's cost – not its health benefits. They won't make an already nutritious food significantly more nutritious. And they definitely won't make an otherwise unwholesome food a health food.

The key point: eating a diet of naturally healthy foods is the best way to fill your nutritional requirements and, now that you're expecting, your baby's. There's no harm in chowing down on enriched and fortified foods (and in some cases, there are significant protective perks, especially for the pregnant). But there's no reason to go out of your way – or out of your budget – to load up on them either.

much phosphorus (which you might get from drinking too many fizzy drinks; see the box on the opposite page) can interfere with your body's ability to properly use both calcium and iron.

The RNI for phosphorus during pregnancy is 550 mg. Look for it in yogurt and cheese (where you'll also find your calcium), fish, meat, poultry, eggs, oatmeal and butter beans.

Potassium. Potassium works with sodium to maintain fluid balance in cells (which is so vital during pregnancy, when fluid levels must increase significantly) and regulate blood pressure. It also maintains muscle tone, key in minimising pregnancy aches and pains, aiding in delivery and speeding up postnatal recovery.

The RNI for pregnant women is 3,500 mg of potassium a day. There are many delicious sources of potassium, including avocados, bananas, dried apricots, oranges, peaches, pears, raisins, prunes, tomatoes, carrots, peas, pumpkin, spinach, squash, potatoes, lentils, kidney beans, peanuts, meat, fish, poultry and dairy products.

Selenium. Selenium is important for your body's defence against disease – preventing cell damage, working with vitamin E as an antioxidant and binding with toxins in the body, thereby rendering them harmless (and protecting baby from them).

The pregnancy RNI for selenium is 60 mcg. Sources include Brazil nuts (half a nut supplies all the selenium you need for the day), fish, meat, poultry, eggs, dairy products and wholegrains.

Sodium. Sodium generally gets a bad rap – and not without good reason. But while too much sodium is a diet-don't for any body, so is too little sodium, especially when it comes to pregnant bodies. The right amount of sodium is needed to maintain the right amount of water in the body (essential when blood and fluid volumes are expanding rapidly), as well as the perfect balance of acids and bases in body fluids. It also helps nutrients cross cell membranes, a very valuable skill when there's a baby to be nourished.

Though your need for sodium increases slightly during pregnancy, it's unlikely you'll need to shake up your salt intake (though many mums-to-be find themselves craving salty foods such as pickles). After all, the average British diet includes more than enough (way more than enough) sodium to keep you covered. That said, unless your healthcare provider suggests otherwise, there's no need to restrict your sodium intake.

The RNI for sodium during pregnancy is 1,600 mg per day. You'll find sodium – a main component of salt – in almost every food in some amount (even unlikely sources such as celery), and in generous amounts in processed foods, pickles, sauces and, of course, your salt shaker.

Zinc. Zinc is one of a developing baby's best mineral buddies, essential for cell division and tissue growth, as well as for hair, skin and proper bone growth. It also helps in the perception of taste and works with insulin to regulate blood sugar. Touted for its reproductive benefits (boosting fertility in both women and men), some research has suggested pregnancy benefits, too. Deficiencies in this vital mineral can increase the risk of miscarriage, preterm delivery, low birthweight and possibly birth defects such as spina bifida, cleft lip or palate (or both), and visual impairment. Luckily, a daily antenatal supplement will have you covered in the zinc department.

The RNI for zinc during pregnancy is 7 mg. Good sources include turkey, beef, cooked oysters and other shellfish, eggs (mostly in the yolk), yogurt, sweetcorn, wheatgerm, oatmeal and cashews.

> **CHEW ON THIS.** Old wives in Indonesia have spooned this theory up: a superstition there advises expectant mothers to avoid putting a spoon in the salt container. According to the tale, failure to keep their salt shaken, not stirred, may cause them to have problems in labour. Clearly, another one to be taken with a grain (or a shake, or a spoonful) of salt.

Beyond Vitamins and Minerals

Now that you know everything you could possibly ever know about vitamins and minerals and how they nourish bodies, both big (yours) and tiny (baby's), is your nutrition education complete? Not quite yet. There are many other nutrients that benefit your body and your baby's, including:

Fibre. Fibre is a nutrient that your body doesn't actually digest – but it's key to digestion. The most famous part of fibre's job description, and one a constipation-prone pregnant mum can really appreciate: it helps move waste through the intestines. But fibre has other talents, too, including the ability to help regulate blood sugar, possibly reducing the risk of gestational diabetes and pre-eclampsia. Sources of fibre include fruit, vegetables, beans, legumes and wholegrains.

Omega-3 fatty acids. These good fats are essential in the production of cell membranes, hormones and prostaglandins. But they've received the most kudos for their important work in baby brain and eye development. Enough DHA (a type of omega-3) during pregnancy may reduce the chances of baby being born too early or being born at a low birthweight. Research also shows that eating foods rich in omega-3 may help boost your mood. There is no recommended daily intake of omega-3s in the UK, but you can get them in your diet by chowing down on fish, nuts and nut oil, and omega-3 eggs. Your antenatal supplement may also contain some. Read more on page 51.

Phytonutrients. They've been around since the first little sprout – but they're big news, for good reason. Phytonutrients is a broad name for compounds (beyond vitamins and minerals) that are found in plants – fruits, vegetables, grains. Each type of phytonutrient – and there are thousands – is believed to have different benefits for the body. You may have heard of phytonutrients by some of their names: antioxidants, phytochemicals, flavonoids, isoflavones and carotenoids, for instance. Research has shown that phytonutrients help reduce disease risk and stimulate immunities. Every day, researchers are uncovering more and more benefits of these and other natural components of plants, which you can't find in supplements. Fruits and vegetables are super sources of phytochemicals.

Probiotics. It's all in the name: probiotics are beneficial (or 'pro') bacteria that bulk up the numbers of helpful bacteria and crowd out illness-causing bacteria. Beyond helping to counterbalance the negative effects of antibiotics (such as diarrhoea), probiotics may stimulate the intestinal bacteria to break down food better, aiding the digestive tract in its efforts to keep things moving. They also help strengthen the intestinal lining so that bad bugs can't cross into the bloodstream, and even change the intestinal environment, making it more acidic and therefore less hospitable to bad bacteria. Research suggests that probiotics may possibly combat sinus, respiratory and urinary infections (all more common in pregnant women), as well as boost the immune system in general. Studies have also shown that probiotics during pregnancy (and breastfeeding) may reduce the risk of food allergies and eczema in early childhood. You'll find plenty of probiotics in yogurt and yogurt drinks that contain active cultures. You can also ask your healthcare provider to recommend a good probiotic supplement – in capsules, chewables or a powder form.

CHAPTER 3

The Pregnancy Diet

What does it take to make a healthy baby? Nutrients, and lots of them. From the vitamin A that'll help those little eyes see you for the first time . . . to the manganese that'll help those little ears hear you. From the calcium that will build strong bones and teeth (and make those tiny finger- and toenails grow!) . . . to the omega-3 fatty acids that will boost the development of a brain that has so many things to learn in a lifetime.

But just how do you take all the nutrients you and your baby need during the next nine months and put them together in an eating plan that's easy to follow, practical to live and work with, as nutritious as can be – and as delicious as possible, so you can have fun feeding yourself and your baby well? Welcome to the Pregnancy Diet.

Nine Ways to Eat Well When You're Expecting - and Beyond

Eating well may not be rocket science – but there are times when it can seem just as complicated. Pregnancy is one of those times – what with all those recommendations that need following (Don't eat sushi! Drink your milk! Limit your caffeine!), those requirements that need filling, and those symptoms getting in the way of eating altogether. But eating well doesn't have to be so complicated, even when you're trying to eat well for two. In fact, it can be easily broken down into nine basic principles. Follow these steps even loosely, and you can't help but feed your pregnant body and your growing baby well during the nine months ahead. Stick with them after delivery, and you and your family will continue to collect benefits that can last a lifetime.

Choose calories you can count on. While it's true that a calorie is a calorie, it's also true that not all calories are created equal. Some calories are packed with nutrients (the calories in an avocado, for instance), but others are essentially empty of nutrients (the calories in a glazed doughnut). With pregnancy awarding you only about 200 extra calories a day (over your regular daily intake), and with requirements for protein, calcium, vitamins and minerals increased, it's smart to spend most of your calories on foods with nutritional cachet. To snack on a 100-calorie bag of almonds instead of a 100-calorie bag of jelly beans. To invest 200 calories in a cheese toastie with wholemeal bread instead of a sausage roll in puff pastry. And to choose the 35 calories in a tablespoon of hummus and a handful of baby carrots over the same number of calories from munching on a handful or so of potato crisps (who can stop at a handful anyway?).

Be an efficient eater. Packing all those recommended nutrients into a day's worth of eating can seem overwhelming – a stretch for even the hungriest (let alone the queasiest) and definitely a stretch for your time, your tummy, your budget and possibly your weight-gain goals.

How to meet this challenge? By becoming an efficient eater: focus on foods that over-achieve in overall nutrients and multitask in nutritional categories (filling two or more food groups in the same serving), and don't waste too many calories or too much space in your stomach.

For instance, looking for a calorie-efficient way to score a serving of protein? Choose 225 g of low-fat cottage cheese (weighing in at 180 calories) over 225 g of the full-fat variety (240 calories). Seeking a zesty topping for your chilli that will also add calcium to your diet? Reach for low-fat yogurt instead of soured cream – you'll get about twice the calcium for a quarter of the calories.

Another way to eat efficiently: choose foods that do double (or even triple) nutritional duty, filling two or more buckets in a single serving. Like a serving of mango or cantaloupe, which serves up both vitamin C and vitamin A. Broccoli or kale, which do the same (with a calcium bonus), or dried apricots, which deliver iron, too. Greek yogurt, which ticks off calcium and protein. Salmon, which satisfies protein and omega-3s (plus calcium, if you eat the tinned variety mashed with the bones). High-protein wholegrain pasta, which provides protein plus complex carbs. Chickpea or lentil pasta, which adds even more protein.

If you're having trouble gaining weight, being an efficiency expert will come in handy as well, with a switch in strategy: choose foods that are dense both nutritionally and in calories (see page 99).

Feed yourself, feed your baby. Maybe you've been skipping meals since secondary school. Or maybe it's a habit you've picked up on the job. Or maybe you're too nauseous or too tired these pregnant days to even think about preparing or eating those three squares a day. Still, while you may not miss the breakfasts (or lunches, or dinners) you're skipping, your baby will – especially as those growth-intensive second and third trimesters roll around. Once growing really gets going, your little one counts on you for a steady supply of energy and nutrients around the clock – he or she can't order in when you don't eat lunch. In fact, 'more often' may actually be 'more' when it comes to eating regularly.

Putting the Natural in Sugar Substitutes

Trying to put less sugar and fewer calories into your diet naturally? There are many low-cal natural sugar substitutes to choose from, derived from fruits and vegetables instead of chemicals. Options that are probably safe for pregnancy (check with your healthcare provider before reaching for these and others) include monk fruit sweetener (derived from, you guessed it, monk fruit), BochaSweet (derived from kabocha, a pumpkin native to Japan) and allulose (a rare sugar found in fruits like raisins and figs), all available online. Calories aren't your concern? Then you'll have even more natural, pregnancy-safe sugar substitutes to choose from, including honey (ask your healthcare provider before using raw, unpasteurised honey), agave, fruit juice concentrate, coconut sugar, molasses, barley malt syrup, maple syrup or rice syrup. Run these options by your doctor or dietitian if you have gestational diabetes, since all can impact blood-glucose levels, some more than others. For information about the safety of artificial sweeteners, see page 74.

Research suggests that eating frequently as pregnancy progresses (three meals plus snacks or six small meals a day) may boost the odds of a mum-to-be carrying to term. Plus, eating early and often every day will help keep your blood sugar level (minimising headaches, fatigue, mood slumps and more), and ease queasiness and other digestive troubles.

Know the benefits of eating regularly, but have a hard time fitting frequent meals into your schedule and your tummy? Or can't stomach the idea of eating at all, never mind eating often? See Chapter 7 for strategies to help you get around obstacles to regular eating.

Be complex with carbs. Complex carbohydrates (such as wholegrain breads and cereals, brown rice, fruits and vegetables, beans and legumes/aka pulses) contain energy-yielding and energy-sustaining nutrients that every pregnant body needs – especially those B (for baby-building!) vitamins. Complex carbs also pack a natural punch of fibre, which can not only kick constipation in the buttocks but may reduce the risk of gestational diabetes. On the other, less healthy hand, simple carbs (like white rice, white bread and other bakes made with refined flour, and sugary foods) have lost their natural nutritional edge in processing or (in the case of sugar) never had any. So when going for carbs (as you should every day; see the box on page 30), go complex whenever you can.

Spare the sugar. Easily sweet-talked by sugary treats? Listen to this: calories that come from refined sugar actually come without benefits. Yes, they're often found in foods that provide pleasure (in some cases, lots and lots of pleasure), but too often those foods don't contain much in the way of nutritional value. Which means too much sugar can add up quickly in calories without adding to your nutritional intake, or your baby's. Fine as a treat, not so fine as a staple of a healthy diet, especially a healthy pregnancy diet. Plus, another minus: research shows that mums-to-be who consume too many sugary foods and drinks during pregnancy increase the risk of their babies developing allergies and asthma.

Does this mean you have to cut your sweet tooth off entirely? Absolutely not. Cutting back on sugar is certainly a smart move to make, but cutting it out entirely isn't necessary unless you want to (or you know you're the kind of sweets addict who can't stop popping the sweeties once you start). Plus, sweet foods don't always come in empty packages, or even in sugary ones, especially if they've come by their sweetness naturally (think a juicy summer peach, a slice of ripe melon, a perfect banana – hey, spread with peanut butter and dipped in dark chocolate if that helps make the case). Or if their package is wholegrain (like the Triple Blueberry Muffins on page 205 or a batch of the oat biscuits on page 352). So that you can have your cake . . . and nutrients, too.

Feature fruits and vegetables. Everyone knows that fruits and vegetables are the mainstay of a healthy diet – and that everyone can benefit from eating more of them, especially a mum-to-be who needs all the vitamins (vitamins A, B and C, folate . . .), minerals (including the ever-important potassium), fibre and phytochemicals those yummy fruits and vegetables provide. Need another reason to up your veggie intake? Researchers have found that children born to women who eat plenty of vegetables during pregnancy have a lower risk of developing type 1 diabetes. An added bonus: most vegetables and many fruits are naturally low in fat and calories. Another bonus: they fight constipation.

The best way to make sure you're getting the most out of your diet is to follow the rainbow – at least the one in your produce aisle. If your food palate is mostly brown and beige (as in burgers and chips, not as in brown bread or walnuts), it's time to add some colour to your life – and to your dinner plate – by loading up on fruits and vegetables. The more vibrantly coloured the fruits and vegetables are on the inside, the better – those are the ones packed with the nutrients most valued in baby making.

Produce-Phobic?

I s a fear of pesticide residue keeping you and produce apart? Don't let it. As long as you follow the basic principles of fruit and vegetable safety (always wash fruits and vegetables, choose organic when you can, vary the produce you eat and, when in doubt, peel), you won't have to pay the price in pesticides. In fact, many types of fruits and vegetables actually contain natural substances that protect you and your baby against the effects of chemical contamination (not only from the produce you eat, but also from other sources in your environment). So fear not your produce. For more information on chemical residue and pesticides on produce, visit the Food Standards Agency website on 'Pesticides in food' at www.food.gov. uk/business-guidance/pesticides -in-food. For more on choosing organic produce, see page 66.

Start early in the day by blending a fruit (or veggie) smoothie. Toss some spinach and peppers into your eggs. Top your yogurt or porridge with a bounty of berries. Explore recipes that include more vegetables – say, soups, salads and stir-fries. Think green (or red, yellow, orange, purple) by prepping some of your produce ahead (or buying it prepped) and storing cut-up fruits and veggies in sealed containers in the fridge, alongside a container of dip for extra incentive. Freeze bananas so they're smoothie ready, and grapes for easy popping.

Choose foods that remember their roots. What separates the peach you're about to eat from the day it was picked? A week at the farmers market, ripening

The Lowdown on Low-carb, Raw and Paleo

Are you paleo-friendly? Keto curious? Raring to go raw? There's a reason why low is not the way to go when it comes to carbs, why you should aim for better balance in your diet (not higher protein) and why you shouldn't revisit the raw roots of your prehistoric ancestors now that you're expecting.

Low-carb. A diet short on carbs (especially the complex kind) may be short on vital baby-making ingredients such as the folate and other vitamins and minerals found in grains, fruits and vegetables. It can also pack far more protein than your body needs, even when you're pregnant. Other downsides to downsizing your carbs: you'll be skimping on constipation-fighting fibre and on the B vitamins believed to battle morning sickness and pregnancy-unsettled skin. A balanced diet may not be buzz-worthy, but it's definitely baby-worthy.

Keto. Taking low-carb to a new low is the keto diet, which eliminates nearly all carbs, including fruits, wholegrains and some vegetables. The thinking behind the keto craze? Carbs are the body's preferred energy source, and when the body runs out of carbs to burn, it burns fat instead, a state called ketosis. This can lead to rapid weight loss – something that's never recommended during pregnancy. Another downside to ketosis: ketones (the by-products of that fat breakdown) can cross the placenta, and it's unclear how a build-up of ketones can affect a developing baby. Adding to the case against keto for you: while the general science about this eating plan is very limited, the research is even scarcer when it comes to pregnancy. There haven't been any controlled studies done in pregnant humans, but babies of pregnant mice fed a ketogenic diet had complications, including slower growth and behavioural changes after birth. Need more convincing? It's a given that the lack of fibre in a keto diet will compound pregnancy constipation. By all means, choose your carbs carefully when you're making a baby, but for healthiest results, don't choose to cut out all carbs.

Paleo. What's old (really, really old) is new again, thanks to the much-hyped

in the sun? Or months in transport from overseas, cold storage in a warehouse, then more travel to the supermarket? Was it cut and flash-frozen or freeze-dried fresh days after picking, or cut, cooked with water, glucose-fructose syrup and sugars, and canned? No shocker here: nature's finest doesn't fall far from the tree – and is at its finest when served up with its just-harvested goodness still intact (even if it was frozen or freeze-dried or minimally processed and canned just after harvest and served much later). Picking up that produce at a farm stall? Chances are the vegetable or fruit you're choosing remembers its roots. Shopping at a supermarket produce section? Gauge the freshness factor by checking not only a product's source (is it local . . . or did it come from cross-country . . . or around the world?), but also its colour, texture and condition. Is the broccoli soft, pale and anaemic from its journey, or vibrant green and firm (almost certainly packing more nutrients, stalk for stalk)? Are the carrots soft, split and faded, or brilliantly hued and begging to be crunched? Tomatoes or strawberries washed out from premature picking and subsequent storage

paleo diet, which takes eaters back (way, way back) to the days when meat ruled and foraging was limited to whatever grew on bushes and trees. While some of the principles of the paleo diet, like cutting out refined sugar and processed foods, are good diet values in general (and in pregnancy), going all hunter-gatherer when you're growing a baby may not be so smart. Studies show that eating high amounts of red meat while going low on carbs during pregnancy can lead to low birthweight. Other risks for women who eat paleo while pregnant: low blood sugar and constipation (because of the lack of grains and the excess of protein). A modified paleo diet – lower on the proteins and higher on the carbs, particularly wholegrains, beans and legumes (aka pulses) – can fit the bill during pregnancy (and will look similar to the Pregnancy Diet). Another positive takeaway from the paleo diet you can feel free to take with you into pregnancy: eat more nuts and seeds.

Raw. Another blast from our primitive past, eating a completely raw diet was a pregnant woman's only choice BC (before cooking). Today, of course, with dozens of cooking techniques at your fingertips (along with apps to deliver your food fully cooked), you've got options. Which is a good thing, because eating a raw-only diet may be a raw deal for you and your baby. First reason: because some vitamins and minerals are absorbed only when they're cooked, it's hard to get all the nutrients you need during pregnancy when you're eating only raw. Second reason – and perhaps most important: there's always the possibility that raw foods may be contaminated with bacteria that cooking or pasteurising (both taboo among raw eaters) would otherwise kill. That holds true not only for the obvious suspects – the ones you're not supposed to eat anyway during pregnancy (raw dairy products, raw juice, raw meat and fish) – but also for 'raw' prepared foods sold in health-food markets that aren't prepared or stored safely. So dig into those raw veggies (also have cooked vegetables to optimise absorption), savour those salads and by all means eat that apple (and fresh peach, and fresh mango) a day – but also remember that some foods were made to be cooked (or heat-pasteurised), at least when you're baking a baby bun.

and transport – or blushing a deep, vine-ripened red? When you can't find produce that's as fresh as nature intended, don't change your menu, just head to the frozen-food aisle. Quick-freezing is done almost immediately after harvesting, when produce is at the height of its nutritive value, so most frozen fruits and vegetables have as much to offer as their 'fresh' counterparts – or even more. Just read labels to be sure nothing has been added to your frozen produce picks, such as sauces, sugar, salt or other unwanted ingredients. Canned fruits and vegetables (without added salt or sugar) can be nutrition-packed and handy in a pinch, too. Also explore the growing assortment of crunchy freeze-dried fruits and vegetables, which offer the same nutritional benefits as fresh, with a far longer shelf life – not to mention a long life in your car, your handbag, the deepest recesses of your office drawer and, ultimately, your nappy bag.

Carry the freshness principle over to the other aisles of the supermarket, too. When possible, select porridge oats over packets of instant, fresh potatoes for mashing over flakes, natural cheese over those plastic-wrapped slices.

Cave to the crave. Maybe you've always thought about food in two categories: food you want to eat (I shouldn't . . . but yum), and food you're supposed to eat (I should . . . but yuck). And now, with the responsibility of growing a healthy baby weighing heavily on your growing tummy, maybe you're assuming your focus needs to be only on the foods you're supposed to eat. Not so. Always denying yourself the foods you want to eat will just leave you feeling grumpy – and hungry. So don't deprive yourself. Find ways to substitute like for like (see page 114 for some suggestions). Or, if you're craving ice cream, have a scoop or two (and choose your ice cream with an eye on calcium content – some varieties contain more than others, often for fewer calories). Longing for a chocolate bar? Munch on a mini instead of a jumbo-sized (or try switching to dark chocolate, which comes with health benefits). Just keep the amount of healthy foods higher than the less healthy ones, and add nutrition where you can (choose the brownie with walnuts instead of the one with chocolate chips, switch from a caramel topping to fresh berries on your ice cream). Of course, if you find you can't stop once the lid's off the ice cream – or you can't stop at one brownie if there's a tray in front of you – it's smart to curb your enthusiasm . . . and your cravings.

Eat well family-style. How well you and your baby eat isn't directly impacted by how well the rest of your family is eating – but there's definitely a connection that goes both ways. First, it's always easier to eat well when those around you (at least those who live with you) eat well, too – chowing down on a packet of crunchy kale crisps instead of sour-cream-and-chives potato crisps, or savouring the salmon and brown rice bowl instead of the bowl of chicken wings and chips. Secondly, it's win-win-win if eating well during pregnancy becomes a lasting family tradition: a win for baby (nurtured on a healthy pregnancy diet, then weaned on healthy foods and raised in a home where healthy eating habits are second nature). A win for you (no surprise, you'll be left with a healthier postnatal body if you eat well during pregnancy, and if those habits you develop now stick, you'll have a healthier body for life). And a win for your partner (who will be healthier, too – now and in the future). If your new and improved eating style becomes the new and improved family norm, everyone stands to gain long-term health benefits – including not gaining too many pounds over the years to come. Encouraging healthy eating habits can also lower your family's future risk of diet-influenced (and weight-influenced) diseases such as diabetes and high blood pressure.

The Pregnancy Daily Dozen

No need to keep track of your K, add up your A, chart your chromium, monitor your magnesium or follow your fibre. The Pregnancy Daily Dozen serves up all the vitamins, minerals and nutrients you and baby need in 12 easy food groups. Just eat about the number of recommended servings from each of the 12 categories (bearing in mind that many foods overlap in two or more categories, cutting down on the number of portions you'll have to eat from each), and you're done for the day.

Calories: Approximately 200 extra daily. Never thought of calories as your friend? It's time to rethink that relationship. Calories represent the amount of energy supplied by the carbohydrates, protein and fats in foods. They're essential to life, but especially essential in the life of a pregnant woman, who needs energy for so many things – from just staying on her feet (no easy feat when pregnancy has you beat) to fuelling that baby-making factory.

Does your need for extra energy require you to eat extra calories? Yes – just maybe not as many as you might expect (or as the phrase 'eating for two' suggests). Believe it or not, the making of a baby requires only about 200 extra calories a day (added to the number of daily calories required to maintain pre-pregnancy weight; see the box on page 34), and fewer than that during early pregnancy. A bonus, true, but not exactly the all-access ice-cream pass you might have been hoping for.

Now that you know how many calories you'll need every day for the rest of your pregnancy, forget it. Instead of keeping track of calories, just keep track of your weight gain. If you're gaining about the right amount of weight, you're eating about the right number of

---

The Pregnancy Daily Dozen in a Nutshell

Here are the 12 food groups that make up the Pregnancy Diet – the Pregnancy Daily Dozen:

Calories: Approximately 200 extra daily

Protein: 3 servings daily

Calcium: 4 servings daily

Vitamin C: 3 servings daily

Vitamin A: 3 to 4 servings daily

Other fruits and vegetables: 1 to 2 servings daily

Wholegrains and legumes: 6 or more servings daily

Iron-rich foods: Some daily

Fat and high-fat foods: Some daily

Omega-3 fatty acids: Some daily

Fluids: At least 10 x 240-ml glasses daily

Antenatal vitamin supplement: A pregnancy formula taken daily

---

Pregnancy Calorie Count

Over the course of 40 weeks, it takes an estimated 75,000 calories to make a baby. Just don't try to eat them all in one sitting.

---

calories. If you're not gaining enough weight, you're eating too few calories. If you're gaining too much weight (or gaining it too quickly), you're getting too many. Adjust as needed – and you're done and done.

Mums carrying more than one baby need more calories. See page 156 for details.

Protein: three servings daily. There's no material more essential to the making of a baby than protein's amino acids, the

The Truth About Eating for Two

Myth: You're eating for two during pregnancy. So that means you should take everything you usually eat and then double it.

Fact: While it's true you're eating for two people – you and your baby – remember that one of those two is very, very small. Feeding your baby and fuelling your baby-making factory won't require extra calories during the first two trimesters, when your little one is extra little. As baby grows and your body works harder in the third trimester, you'll need to add about 200 calories – more, but definitely not double your usual.

building blocks of human tissue (your little human's tissues included). But does that mean you'll have to pack in extra protein when you're building a baby?

That depends on how much protein you're already getting. The pregnancy requirement for protein is about 75 g, or three servings, a day – but many women eat at least that much protein without even trying, and those on high-protein diets consume much more. Chances are you too fit that protein-plentiful profile (unless you're a vegetarian, or especially if you're a vegan; see the box on page 42).

Here's how easy it is to get your fill of protein. Have just one serving at each meal (for example, a cheese omelette for breakfast, a salad topped with grilled chicken for lunch and a fish fillet for dinner), and you're done. Prefer to graze your day away? Six half servings of protein will fill the bill. Can't contemplate so much protein first thing in the morning? Fill in the protein gaps later on in the day – say, with 225 g of chicken for lunch or dinner. And if 225 g sounds like a lot, consider that it's just an average serving in most restaurants.

Not in a meat-eating mood? Look for protein in the dairy case – you'll find a third of a serving in every glass of milk, every 28 g of cheese or a 110-g serving (about 6 tablespoons) of Greek yogurt. Score additional protein from wholegrain bread, cereal and pasta (especially high-protein pastas, like those made from beans).

If You're Counting

You know you're supposed to add 200 calories to your daily intake at six months, but what number are you supposed to add them to? Start with your pre-pregnancy weight and change it to pounds (1 stone = 14 lb; 1 kg = 2.2 lb); then multiply it by 12 if you're sedentary, 15 if you're moderately active and up to 22 if you're extremely active. That's about the number of calories it took to maintain your weight pre-pregnancy, and that's the number you'll be adding your 200 extra calories to. Because the rate at which calories are burned varies from person to person, even in pregnancy, calorie requirements vary too, so the figure you arrive at is just an estimate – don't count on it. Remember, the best indicator of whether you're getting the right number of calories or too many or too few: your weight gain. See Chapter 6 for more.

Every day, try to have about three servings of the following foods (or any combination equal to three servings). If you're using dairy sources for protein, don't forget to give yourself credit for calcium, too (credit works both ways, so count the protein in your calcium foods).

720 ml (3 x 240-ml glasses) of cow's or goat's milk or buttermilk

85 g hard cheese (check out the freeze-dried varieties, too)

225 g cottage cheese

250 g Greek or skyr yogurt

750 g regular yogurt

4 eggs

115 g cooked fresh fish (see page 72 for information on safe fish eating during pregnancy)

115 g cooked shellfish

100 g tinned tuna or sardines

115 g skinless chicken, turkey, duck or other poultry

115 g lean beef, lamb, veal, pork or buffalo (bison)

Have queasiness and aversions pushed meat and other animal products off the menu? Or are you vegan? There are plenty of protein sources beyond the animal kingdom. Many of the following also net a serving of complex carbs, and some add significant amounts of calcium or omega-3s:

Beans and Legumes
(half protein servings)

175–200 g cooked beans, lentils, split peas (dhal) or chickpeas

175 g cooked soya beans (or edamame)

55 g legume pasta

Visual Reality

Do your eyes deceive you when you're judging the serving of food on your plate? Chances are they do. Most Westerners, used to super-sized fast-food portions, extra-large beverage containers and all-you-can-eat buffets, are eating two to three times the recommended serving amount per food item. A plateful of spaghetti at a restaurant, for instance, can be closer to three servings of grains than it is to one. The hefty double burger weighs in at two protein servings, even before you add the cheese and bacon. Having a side salad as part of your lunch? You'll be helping yourself to several servings of vegetables. So before you dig into your Daily Dozen, here's a visual reality check:

- A serving of meat, poultry or fish (115 g) is equivalent to the size of a deck of cards.

- A serving of fruit or vegetables is roughly about the size of a standard light bulb.

- A serving of pasta (28 g) would fill an ice-cream scoop.

- A serving of butter or oil (1 tablespoon) would just cover the tip of your thumb.

In other words, you may find that your requirements aren't quite as filling as you thought – or that you're filling them far faster than you might expect. Not sure how much is in a serving of a particular food you're eating? Check the food label on the packet – you may find all your serving-size questions answered right there.

Pass the Peanuts

A peanut butter-and-jam sandwich is a quick-and-easy-to-assemble lunch. And the good news for those who crave this lunchtime staple: researchers have found that eating peanuts while pregnant not only doesn't trigger peanut and other allergies in babies-to-be, but may actually prevent them. So as long as you're not personally allergic to peanuts, there's no need to pass on the peanut butter – and maybe more reason than ever to reach for it. Same goes for nuts and nut butters of all kinds. If you're not allergic, you're good to go nuts when you're expecting.

If you have a history of allergies, ask your healthcare provider whether you should restrict your pregnancy diet in any way. The recommendations may be slightly different for you.

---

55 g soy pasta

115 g peas

40 g peanuts or peanut butter

70 g miso

115 g tofu

85 g tempeh

350 ml soya milk

95 g vegetarian 'beef mince'

1–2 vegetarian 'sausages' or 'burgers'

Grains
(*half protein servings*)

85 g (before cooking) wholewheat pasta or high-protein pasta

The Scoop on Protein Supplements

H oping to scoop up your protein requirement in a supplement? Supplement makers may have crowded the field, but nature – the first producer of protein – is still the best provider of this baby-building nutrient, and there are a few reasons why. First, supplements often contain a whopping amount of protein in a concentrated form, easily giving you too much of a good thing. Secondly, supplements usually come packaged with more than just protein. They may also contain ingredients (such as sugar substitutes, herbs and enzymes) that may not be pregnancy-appropriate, or they may be fortified with megadoses of vitamins and minerals that can push your intake beyond what's considered pregnancy-safe. That can apply to all types of protein supplements (whey, pea, chickpea and so on) and all forms (bars, powders and shake mixes). Another point to consider when thinking about turning specifically to whey protein bars, powders,and shake mixes: whey protein is made from cow's milk, which means it's not the way to go if you're lactose intolerant or have a milk allergy.

It's probably best to get most of your protein the way nature intended: in foods that come by their protein naturally, instead of through fortification. Want to shake up your protein intake? Skip the mix and blend a shake with protein-rich Greek yogurt.

Not Feeling the Milk?

If milk leaves a sour taste in your mouth, no need to drink it straight up – or even at all. You can cash in on calcium by eating cheese or yogurt or sipping calcium-fortified juice or other dairy-free beverages. Or by blending milk into soups, sauces or smoothies. Or subbing milk for the water in your morning porridge (you'll never know it's there, but your bones will). It's not your mouth that milk leaves sour, but your tummy? You, too, have options. If you're lactose intolerant or think you might be, simply sub lactose-free dairy (and see page 148). Not the lactose that's doing your tummy in, but the protein in cow's milk? Reach for A2 milk (available online), which comes from cows that naturally produce only the A2 protein and not the A1 that causes sensitivity in some people (see page 149 for more).

---

70 g oat bran

90 g (uncooked) oats or 235 g porridge

Approximately 170 g wholegrain ready-to-eat cereal

85 g (uncooked) couscous, bulgar wheat, buckwheat, farro, amaranth, freekeh, quinoa

4 slices wholegrain bread

Approximately 2–3 wholegrain pittas

Approximately 2 wholegrain muffins

Nuts and seeds
(*half protein servings*)

85 g nuts, such as walnuts, pecans and almonds

3–5 tablespoons nut butter

55 g sunflower, sesame or pumpkin seeds

Calcium: four servings daily. Make no bones about it – calcium intake is crucial during pregnancy, not only for your baby's bones (approximately 200 mg of calcium per day is deposited into your baby's skeleton during the last trimester of pregnancy), but also for yours. Women begin to lose bone mass in their thirties, and they'll lose it faster if calcium is drained from their own bones to help build baby's. Getting the right amount of calcium daily (especially during pregnancy) will keep your bones healthy and help prevent osteoporosis later in life. Getting enough calcium is also believed to lower the risk of developing pre-eclampsia. So it's clear that calcium does a mum-to-be's body (and her baby's) good.

Milk is the most well-known source of calcium, and a very efficient one, too. So if you 'got milk', and you love drinking it, great – you'll have no problem

CHEW ON THIS. In ancient Rome, pregnant women were advised that if they wanted their baby to be born with dark eyes, they should eat mice often. While a mouse might be an interesting protein choice (if you're a pregnant snake, that is), this is clearly a case where you wouldn't want to do as the Romans did – even if you did happen to be living in Rome.

Milking the Dairy-Free Alternatives

Cruising the dairy aisle, but you'd prefer to sport an alternative-milk moustache? Whether your reason for staying away from traditional sources of milk (cow's, goat's) are philosophical (you're vegan or concerned about dairy farming's impact on the planet) or physical (you're allergic to dairy or are lactose intolerant), you're in luck. The number of dairy-free 'milks' on supermarket shelves (and at coffee shops) is booming – which means there's no need to have your cereal dry or your coffee black ... or to chase your biscuits down with orange juice. But how do these milk alternatives stack up against the real thing? Results vary depending on variety, but also on brand. None mimic milk in flavour (some would argue that's a plus), or in naturally occurring nutrition (especially when it comes to protein and calcium), or even in texture (most aren't as creamy), but some perform better than others. Here's a quick introduction to some of the options:

Soya milk. Of all the milk alternatives, soya milk is considered the most similar to cow's milk. Its taste is subtle and bean-like, its texture is creamy and it contains comparable amounts of protein and calcium (though it comes by its calcium through fortification). It may also be fortified with vitamins B_2, B_{12} and D and iodine – check the label. Though the evidence is limited, some experts recommend restricting the amount of unfermented soya products (such as soya milk) during pregnancy because they contain isoflavones – chemicals that mimic the hormone oestrogen in the body.

Almond milk. With a slightly sweet and subtle nutty taste, almond milk gets top ratings because of its versatility. It's also often fortified with calcium, vitamins B_2, B_{12}, D and E (check the label for specifics), raising its nutritional profile, but it is far lower in protein than cow's milk or soya milk. Choose those that are fortified with calcium and vitamin D.

Coconut milk. Usually labelled as 'coconut milk drink', this milk alternative (it's different from the coconut milk that comes in tins, which is high in fat and calories and is used to replace cream, not milk) has a sweet coconut flavour that's almost tropical. Some brands are fortified with calcium (though less than other milk alternatives), vitamin D, vitamin B_{12} and other vitamins. Something you won't find in a coconut milk beverage: protein.

Rice milk. Low in fat and protein but high in calories, rice milk has a texture similar to skimmed milk with a

meeting your calcium requirement. If your tummy can tolerate milk, but you can't stand its taste, also no problem – it's easily disguised. It can be downed in delicious milkshakes, smoothies, soups, skimmed milk decaf lattes or reduced-fat chocolate milk. It can be eaten in hot or cold cereal, too. No tolerance for lactose? No problem. Milk and dairy products of all varieties (including cheese, cottage cheese, yogurt, ice cream and cream cheese) come in lactose-free form.

Just not that into milk? Calcium is supplied by many other dairy sources, from yogurt to cheese. For vegans (or others who prefer not to take their calcium in dairy form), there's no shortage of dairy-free sources.

barely there rice flavour. Rice milk is the safest option for those with allergies or intolerances to dairy, soya or nuts. But, because rice contains low levels of arsenic, it's best to limit the amount of rice milk you consume in general, and especially when you're expecting.

Cashew milk. Like almond milk, this nut-based milk alternative is sweet with a faint nutty flavour. Though cashew milk contains about one-third of the calories of cow's milk and half the fat, it's actually creamier than cow's milk, making it a great alternative for 'cream' sauces. Look for ones that are fortified with calcium and vitamin D.

Pea milk. Derived from yellow pea protein, creamy-textured pea milk has a similar amount of protein and twice as much calcium as cow's milk. Pea milk boosted with sunflower oil or algal oil also contains omega-3 fatty acids. Some are also fortified with vitamin B_{12}. Pea milk is allergy-friendly, too, since it's not made from nuts or soya.

Hemp milk. High in omega-3 and omega-6 fatty acids, hemp milk is thin with a hint of grassy flavour. Most brands have thickeners in them and a funky taste. Hemp milk contains a similar amount of fat to cow's milk, but around half the calories and protein. See the box on page 76 for caveats about hemp when you're pregnant.

Oat milk. Like hemp milk, oat milk is a plant-based dairy-free milk. It has a creamy texture and oaty flavour, but less than a third of the protein in full-fat milk. Look for ones that are fortified with calcium, vitamin D, vitamin B_{12} and other vitamins. If you have a gluten intolerance, check the label to ensure it's gluten-free.

And if that's not enough alt-milk options for you, not to worry. Scan the shop shelves these days and you'll find a host of others, from flax milk (made from flax or linseeds) to hazelnut milk. Not all provide the same amount of nutrients (like the all-important baby-building calcium and vitamin D), so be sure to check labels before you toss them into your shopping trolley.

A few other potential pitfalls in the alt-milk department: First, while cow's milk comes by its sweetness naturally in the form of lactose, many milk alternatives can be loaded with added sugars, so consider opting for the unsweetened kinds. Secondly, some alt-milks contain thickeners (carrageenan) and other additives (gellan gum), so scan labels before choosing brands with unneeded extras. You'll also want to choose milk alternatives that are as close as possible nutritionally to calcium-rich cow's milk, looking for those that contain important mum-to-be nutrients. Be sure to shake before using, because the added nutrients sink to the bottom.

Too much caffeine, salt or fizzy drinks (or more accurately, the phosphorus fizzy drinks contain) can interfere with calcium absorption, a good reason to order your latte half-caf. Alcohol, diuretic tablets and laxatives can do the same, but those aren't recommended during pregnancy anyway. Since a lot of dietary fibre can take calcium down the chute before it can be absorbed, try not to take the bulk of your fibre with the bulk of your calcium. (For instance, if you're counting on that calcium in your milk, you might not want to dunk bran muffins in it.)

Choose four servings daily from the following list of calcium-rich foods. And don't forget that many of the dairy

Divide, Combine and Conquer

Can't drain the whole glass of milk? Had your fill halfway through your serving of yogurt? Just because they don't add up to a full serving doesn't mean they can't be added to your daily total. When a full serving is just too much, combine a half (or a third or a quarter) servings together instead. For instance, that one egg (a quarter of a protein serving) plus a slice of whole-grain toast (a quarter protein serving) plus 120 ml of soya milk (a half protein serving) equals a full protein serving – and you don't even have to eat them all in the same sitting (just in the same day). Divide, combine and conquer – and you'll have to do a lot less eating to finish up your Daily Dozen.

sources (and the seafood ones) also provide protein and that some of the diary-free provide vitamin C and vitamin A:

240 ml cow's or goat's milk or buttermilk

250 g yogurt

250 g Greek or skyr yogurt

160 g kefir

28 g hard cheese (check the freeze-dried varieties, too)

240 ml calcium-fortified drinks (juice, soya, nut and other plant-based milk; check labels for varieties that have 30 per cent or more of the RI for calcium)

Shake It Up, Baby

Much of the calcium in calcium-fortified beverages (juice, soya milk, almond milk and calcium-added milk) tends to settle at the bottom of a container – good if you're getting the last sip, not so good if you're getting the first. To make sure the calcium is evenly distributed from first sip to last, shake these beverages thoroughly before each use.

335 g cottage cheese

85 g tinned sardines with bones

115 g canned salmon with bones

125 g ricotta cheese

Tofu (check the label, some tofu is higher in calcium)

Other calcium sources

Sesame seeds

Leafy green vegetables, such as kale or spring greens

Pak choi

Spinach

Edamame

Beans

Almonds or almond butter

Dried figs

Broccoli

Vitamin C: three servings daily. Because the body doesn't store vitamin C, you and baby will need a fresh supply every day. Easy enough, since vitamin C comes naturally in a wide variety of tasty packages. Effective ones, as well, since many vitamin C-listers play on the vitamin A team, too.

Can't stop at three servings of C? Help yourself to extra servings. Choose from the following (listed in order from highest to lowest vitamin C content):

Guava

Red, yellow, green or orange pepper

Kiwi fruit

Orange

Papaya

Broccoli

Kohlrabi

Parsley

Pineapple

Grapefruit

Brussels sprouts

Broccoli slaw

Daikon (Chinese radish)

Mango

Sugar snap peas

Peas

Strawberries

Cantaloupe

Tangerine

Coleslaw mix

White or red cabbage

Cauliflower

Pak choi

Leafy green vegetables, such as kale, spring greens or turnip tops

Swede

Honeydew

Blackberries or raspberries

Plantain

Count 'Em Once, Count 'Em Twice

Sometimes, you'll even be able to count them thrice. Many of your favourite foods may fill more than one Daily Dozen requirement in each serving. Case in delicious point: a slice of cantaloupe fills a vitamin A plus a C. Same goes for a tangerine. Broccoli covers A and C with a calcium bonus. Greek yogurt delivers calcium and protein. So don't forget to give yourself credit where credit is due. Count them once, count them twice.

Tomato

Sweet potato, baked in skin

Okra

Vitamin A: three to four servings daily. These A-plus powerhouses are the superstars of the produce section – serving up whopping quantities of vitamin A. It comes in the form of phytochemicals called carotenoids, including alpha-carotene, beta-carotene, lutein,

CHEW ON THIS. Here are a couple of old wives' tales that may well have been generated by old vegetarians: Chinese folklore maintains that a woman should avoid eating both rabbit and chicken during her pregnancy – or else her baby will be born with a hoarse voice. Eating squid and crab are also discouraged, according to Chinese tradition. Squid, so the tale goes, is believed to cause the uterus to 'stick' during delivery, and eating crab will result in a mischievous child.

If You're a Vegetarian or a Vegan

Got a beef with beef (or chicken, fish, eggs or dairy)? No worries. Vegetarians of just about all varieties, including vegans, can have pregnancies and babies that are at least as healthy as those of carnivores . . . or even healthier. So no need to swap your all-veggie burger for an all-beef patty, or even to add cheese to it. But because diets without animal products tend to be low in fat and high in fibre, you may find it hard to pile on enough pounds. If so, increase the weight shortfall by adding more fat servings to your diet, eating smaller amounts more often, and choosing foods that are particularly dense in both calories and nutrition (think avocados, nuts and nut butters, seeds, beans, peas and dried fruit).

Vegetarian mums easily score more of some nutrients (most B vitamins, folate, vitamins A and C, and more) from their grain and veggie-rich diet than pregnant meat eaters typically do. But without a little extra effort, it's also possible to fall short on a few important baby-building blocks, including:

- Protein. Vegetarians who include eggs and milk products in their diet usually have little trouble getting enough protein, but vegans may find it a stretch. If you're a vegan, net your protein share by eating protein-rich grains, beans, peas and lentils (and pastas made from them), and tofu and other soya products.

- Vitamin B_{12}. Since vitamin B_{12} is found only in foods that come from animals, vegans will have to look elsewhere for their B_{12}. A supplement can pick up the slack (ask your healthcare provider if you need more than what's provided in your antenatal vitamin), but you can also get an extra shot of this vital vitamin from fortified soya and other plant milks, fortified cereals, nutritional yeast and fortified meat substitutes.

zeaxanthin and beta-cryptoxanthin – all important in the making of a baby. To get the best mix of these phytochemicals, add a good mix of yellow and green vegetables into your diet each day.

And there are more good reasons to make green and deep yellow your Team Baby colours. The greens and deep yellows are also excellent suppliers of vitamin E, riboflavin, B_6, folate, magnesium and a host of other essential minerals – plus a bonus of fibre.

Maybe you've never been the type to volunteer for vegetables or choose a side salad over chips. Or maybe green describes how you've been feeling these days, not so much what you feel like eating. No need for kale coercion or to cosy up to spring greens (that is, unless you're up for the challenge). Instead, turn to soothing shades of yellow and orange: carrots, sweet potatoes, butternut squash, pumpkin. Or get sneaky with yourself, cleverly concealing very finely chopped veggies in your spaghetti sauce, meat loaf, lasagne, casseroles and soups. Or skip the vegetables altogether for now and get fruity. Cantaloupe and mango can be sweet revenge if you're feeling bitter about broccoli, filling requirements for vitamin A and vitamin C just as well as any green can. Or sip a vegetable or veggie-fruit juice or smoothie.

Try to have at least three to four servings from the following fruits and veggies every day, ideally including at

- Iron. It's not easy for anyone (except big red-meat eaters) to get enough iron from their diets, especially during pregnancy when iron's in high demand. For those who stick to plant foods, it's next to impossible. If you're a vegetarian – and especially if you're a vegan – you'll need to be extra diligent about taking your healthcare provider-recommended iron supplement. If you haven't been recommended one, ask.

- Calcium. For vegetarians who eat dairy products, cashing in on calcium is easy (just say cheese! Milk! Yogurt!). For vegans, getting enough calcium may be a taller order, but it's definitely not out of reach. Though dairy products are the most well-known sources of calcium, they're not the only ones. Calcium-fortified almond, other nut and plant-based milks and calcium-fortified juices, for instance, offer as much calcium as milk, ounce for ounce – making any

a perfect vegan source of this essential mineral. Other dairy-free sources of calcium include dark green leafy vegetables, sesame seeds, almonds and calcium-fortified soya products. Still, adding a calcium supplement is probably good insurance for pregnant vegans. Ask your healthcare provider for a recommendation, preferably one that adds vitamin D (see below) and magnesium to the mix.

- Vitamin D. Since there are few dietary sources of this vitamin available on plant-based diets, vegans will have to depend on their supplements (or fortified dairy-free milk alternatives or mushrooms) to provide them with all they need of this very valuable vitamin. Also look for breads and cereals that are fortified with it. Your best bet: ask your healthcare provider about testing your vitamin D levels and recommending a supplement if needed.

least one green and one yellow. Mix up your prep, too, if you can – eating some raw, some cooked. Bear in mind that in the case of many, you'll also be filling your vitamin C in the same serving:

Carrot

Sweet potato or yam

Pumpkin

Salad greens, such as romaine, rocket, red or green oak leaf lettuce

Cantaloupe

Spinach

Parsley

Red pepper

Green leafy vegetables, such as chard, kale or spring greens

Apricot

Pink or ruby red grapefruit

CHEW ON THIS. Here's an ancient custom that has modern applications, particularly for pregnant women: it was customary for the Romans to precede their banquets with refreshing salads, which they believed enhanced the appetite. Here's one that may not: in Elizabethan times, dried lettuce juice was used to aid sleep.

An Apple
(and Two Carrots and a Portion of Broccoli) a Day

For salad bar buffs and fruit fanatics, filling the various produce requirements of pregnancy may be a job they can't wait to sink their teeth into. But for those who've struggled to manage even an apple a day, packing in all that produce may seem daunting. It can also be a challenge for the easily bored (with steamed broccoli, tossed salad, that piece of fresh fruit). Here are some tips for fitting more fruits and vegetables into anyone's day:

- Top pancakes or waffles with sliced berries instead of syrup.

- Add mashed banana or blueberries to pancake batter.

- Whip up some fruit smoothies and drinks (see the recipes starting on page 342).

- Add peaches, bananas, strawberries or blueberries to your cereal. Or pop freeze-dried fruit right out of the bag and into your mouth.

- Add mushrooms, peppers, broccoli or tomato to your omelette (see page 193).

- Make friends with cauliflower rice – sautéed, it makes a super side or a delicious bed for just about any main dish. Baked, it also works well as a pizza base.

- Stuff a baked sweet potato with broccoli or mushrooms and cheese.

- Grab a packet of sweet potato, courgette or butternut squash 'noodles' or make your own with a spiraliser – then sauté and sauce as you'd prepare pasta.

- Toss kale leaves with olive oil, salt and pepper, and then roast until crispy. Bingo – it's kale crisps! Or just open a packet of kale crisps.

- Bake carrot muffins (see page 206).

- Add chopped dried apricots into anything you're baking.

- Grill vegetables on skewers. Fruit, too.

- Add carrots, tomatoes, peppers, mangoes or strawberries to your salad.

- Make pesto out of parsley and toss with brown rice or wholegrain pasta.

- Add lettuce and tomatoes to your sandwiches.

Pak choi	Prune
Persimmon	Tangerine
Mango	Red cabbage
Vegetable juice	Okra
Tomato	Green beans
Butternut or other squash	Broccoli
Papaya	Plum

- Layer spinach, avocado and porto-bello mushroom into your grilled cheese.

- Toss cauliflower, broccoli, squash, mushrooms or really any vegetable into your lasagne. Want to go extra veggie? Use sliced aubergine instead of lasagne sheets.

- Stir grated carrot into your meat loaf mix.

- Create a burrito bowl out of kale, avocado, salsa verde, seasoned black beans, cherry tomatoes and brown rice.

- Add fresh vegetables to low-salt tinned soups.

- Add pumpkin purée, diced red peppers, finely chopped carrot, parsley or kale to your tomato sauce – sauté first and you'll never notice them.

- Toss wedges of sweet potatoes with olive oil, salt and pepper, and roast for sweet potato chips.

- Top chicken or seafood with a mango salsa (see page 296).

- Add peas, red peppers, asparagus, squash or other colourful vegetables (roasted or raw) to quinoa, farro or brown rice.

- Put nutrition – and dinner – on the fast track by stirring up a veggie-filled stir-fry.

- Add dried fruit to stuffing.

- Pop some Brussels sprouts into an air fryer with a spray of olive oil and some salt. Add to the top of your salad for crunch, or eat as a snack.

- Blend a bowl of gazpacho (see page 226) or carrot soup (see page 224).

- Sauté mirepoix (diced carrots, onions and celery), add any kind of roasted vegetables (butternut squash, broccoli, mushrooms, cauliflower), cover with stock and simmer until soft. Blend until smooth for a delicious soup.

- Dip baby carrots, broccoli, cauliflower, green beans or peppers in salsa, hummus or guacamole.

- Stuff walnuts, raisins and cinnamon into an apple and bake or microwave for a sweet snack or dessert.

- Toss pomegranate seeds into a salad of kale, shaved Brussels sprouts and red cabbage.

- Have a virgin Bloody Mary (tomato or vegetable juice and spices, minus the vodka) as a pre-dinner mocktail.

Nectarine

Yellow peach

Celery

Other fruits and vegetables: one to two servings daily. So they're not the A-list or the C-list – but they dabble well in a variety of well-known nutrients, with some excelling in emerging categories, too. From that apple a day (full of fibre) to blueberries (abundant in antioxidants) and bananas (packed with potassium), you'll get more than you'd expect from these other fruits and vegetables.

Aim for one to two servings of the following delicious choices every day:

Apple

Apple purée

The Truth About Grain

Yes, you know that wholegrains are a healthier choice than refined grains. But do you know why? Understanding how white bread gets its colour (or lack of it) may help you see why wholegrains take the cake nutritionally. All grains start out whole (that's the way nature grows them). It's during their processing into refined bread, buns, cereals, pasta and white rice that the nutritious parts of the grains are removed (including the vitamin-and-mineral-packed germ and the fibre-packed bran). Just how much difference does a wholegrain make? Compare brown flour to white flour: brown flour contains four times more fibre, two times more copper, six times more magnesium, three times more potassium, two times more selenium, four times more zinc and 20 times more vitamin E than white flour. That's a pretty convincing profile.

Though enrichment of refined grain (as required by law) tosses back in a handful of the vitamins and minerals found naturally in wholegrains, it leaves out about 20 other nutrients (likely even more, including ones that haven't yet been discovered – that's how good nature is). Also missing: that naturally occurring fibre. In other words, nature's recipe for grainy goodness will probably never be duplicated.

Is white always wrong and brown always right? Not necessarily. Colour doesn't always tell the whole story when it comes to wholegrains. A brown bread can get its wholesome-looking hue from colouring, not just from wholegrain flour. Names may deceive you too: The label 'wheat' on a loaf of bread tells you only the type of grain it's baked with, not whether it's a wholegrain. To make sure you're getting the whole wheat and nothing but the whole wheat, read the label and the ingredients carefully (see page 58 for more).

Apple juice

Banana

Blueberries

Cherries

Cranberries

CHEW ON THIS. Here's another old wives' tale to help you figure out if you're carrying a boy or a girl: eat a clove of raw garlic. If the smell of garlic seeps out of your pores, it's a boy. If no garlic smell is detected at all, it's a girl. There's a 50 per cent chance this method will work, of course, but probably a much higher chance that it will leave you with heartburn.

Figs

White peach

Pear

Pomegranate juice

Pomegranate seeds

Rhubarb

Dates

Grapes or raisins

Avocado

Water chestnuts

Beetroot

Sweetcorn

Cucumber

Aubergine

Iceberg lettuce

Mushrooms

Onion

Parsnip

Turnip

Courgette

Radishes

Radicchio

Wholegrains and legumes: six or more servings daily. These days, it isn't easy being grains. Once valued as the staff of life – the most important link on the human food chain, a dietary staple around the world and throughout history, and yes, the breakfast of champions – bread, cereal, rice and pasta have been shelved by a generation of carbophobes. Unfair to carbs, unnecessary for those who love them (and really, who doesn't?). The truth is, while refined grains don't stack up, wholegrains of all kinds (and in all forms), as well as legumes (also called pulses), should be a healthy mainstay of just about every diet, especially every pregnancy diet. These complex carbohydrates contain a wealth of vitamins, particularly vitamin E and the B vitamins so essential for every part of your baby's developing body. They're rich in trace minerals such as zinc, selenium, chromium and magnesium. Full of constipation-fighting fibre. And for many queasy mums-to-be, their starchy, bland goodness is just the ticket to comfort. For some, maybe the only ticket.

Go for the wholegrain varieties of these whenever you can (see the box on the previous page for all the reasons why; see the box on page 48 for a list of great grains to choose from). Choose from the following (serving sizes vary, so check labels):

100 g cooked brown, other wholegrain or wild rice

100 g cooked quinoa, farro, barley, bulgar wheat, buckwheat groats (kasha), wholegrain couscous, spelt, wheatberries or other cooked wholegrains (see box, page 48)

75 g cooked wholegrain or legume-based pasta

115 g cooked oat porridge or other wholegrain hot cereal

85 g wholegrain, ready-to-eat cereal

30 g granola

1 slice brown or other wholegrain bread

Wholegrain corn or flour tortilla (1 small or ½ large)

Wholegrain wrap

Wholegrain pitta (1 small or ½ large)*

½ wholegrain muffin or bagel

Wholegrain crackers or crispbreads

Wholegrain corn or bean tortilla chips

Brown-rice cakes or crackers

15 g popcorn

25 g oats

60 g wholegrain polenta (non-degerminated)

30 g wholegrain flour

2 tablespoons ground linseeds (flaxseeds) or chia seeds

85–100 g cooked beans, lentils or split peas (dahl)

100 g cooked edamame (soybeans)

Toasted chickpeas, soya beans, lentils, or other beans and legumes

Great Grains

Looking for a change of wholegrain pace? Here are a few to look for, either on their own or in combos with other grains in bakes or cereals or in ready-to-cook form. They're all loaded with vitamins and minerals:

Amaranth has a nutty flavour and sticky texture and is rich in protein, iron, calcium, B vitamins and fibre. It's a nutritious gluten-free substitute.

Barley is a delicious stand-in for rice in salads and side dishes. Opt for hulled barley (it's wholegrain) over pearled (refined) – just plan for extra cooking time. Wholegrain barley flour can also sub for plain flour in most recipes.

Buckwheat isn't actually a grain – it's a seed that cooks and eats like a nutty grain. It also doesn't have any relation to wheat, so it's gluten-free. Use buckwheat groats (also called kasha) as a cooked cereal or side dish (see Three-in-One Pilau, page 341). You can also use buckwheat flour in a variety of bakes.

Bulgar wheat is a wholegrain made from dried, cracked wheat. It's best known for its starring role in Mediterranean dishes such as tabbouleh, but can also substitute for rice or couscous in pilaus, stews, casseroles, soups and stuffings – or for oats as a

wholegrain cereal. Bonus: it cooks quickly.

Sweetcorn is the only cereal grain native to the Americas. Unfortunately, most corn-based products today are stripped of their wholegrain goodness (aka degerminated). Look for bakes that contain non-degerminated or wholegrain corn, or for wholegrain polenta when you're baking cornbread, stirring up polenta or breading chicken or fish.

Farro has been a crowd-pleasing grain at Italian tables for centuries – and is now available at a shop near you. Its chewy texture stands up to soups, stews and salads, as a bed for just about any meat, fish or poultry, in a starring role in a pilau, or as a satisfying hot cereal.

Kamut (also called khorasan) is a high-protein ancient grain that was once a Pharaoh fan favourite – one taste and you'll likely be a fan too. Its toothsome chew and nutty, slightly sweet taste holds their own in salads, stuffing and side dishes of all kinds (sub it for the bulgar wheat in tabbouleh). Or cook it up for breakfast.

Millet is another wholegrain that's actually a seed. It's crunchy and mild-tasting, plus it's gluten-free. Look for it

Iron-rich foods: some daily. Your body will be working overtime to generate enough red blood cells to keep up with the demands of baby making while trying to keep you from developing iron-deficiency anaemia. Pumping up your blood supply will require pumping up your iron intake. Since it's hard to fill the pregnancy requirement for this must-have mineral through diet alone,

your healthcare provider will likely recommend that you take a daily supplement of iron (in addition to what's in your regular antenatal), beginning at week 20 and continuing through the rest of pregnancy. To maximise iron absorption, take your supplement with a vitamin C food or drink. On the flip side, chasing down your iron supplement with milk or other calcium-rich

in cereals and baked goods. While millet can be served like rice or quinoa in salads, pilau, as a stuffing (try it in Red Pepper Stuffed with Millet Pilau), or in side dishes, it's not the easiest grain to DIY – so check the packet instructions before committing.

Oats are, of course, well-known for their breakfast potential (in both hot and cold cereals), though perhaps are best loved for their biscuits. They're naturally high in fibre, and may help regulate both blood sugar and blood pressure, giving the humble bowl of porridge some impressive health credentials. Look for porridge oats (pass by the instant when you can), or wholegrain oat flour. Have time on your hands? Cook up an extra batch of slow-cooked coarse pinhead oats – Irish or Scotch are especially chewy and satisfying. Oats are considered gluten-free but there are some caveats for some with coeliac disease (see page 150).

Quinoa (KEEN-wah), has a unique fluffy texture and a delicate taste, but it's a heavyweight when it comes to nutrients, especially protein. It's also a quick cook and can be used in pilaus, salads, soups or in any recipe that calls for rice or another grain. It plays well with other grains too (see Three in One Pilau, page 341).

Rice clearly needs no introduction, but its many wholegrain forms may. Since white rice has been stripped of fibre and nutrients, explore rice varieties that haven't been milled – you'll be surprised at how many options you'll discover beyond the basic brown, including brown basmati, red rice, purple rice, black rice and wild rice (this chewy grain isn't actually a rice at all, but a grass). Use wholegrain rice of all varieties just as you would use white rice – just plan to add a little extra simmer time.

Spelt is an ancient grain that's undergone a culinary renaissance. Its nutty taste and chewy texture makes it an intriguing alternative to more common varieties of wheat – plus it's higher in protein. Use hulled spelt as a cooked grain, rolled spelt as a cereal, and spelt flour for pancakes, waffles or just about anything you're baking.

Wheatberries have a crunchy chew and a nutty, slightly sweet taste, but they adapt deliciously to both sweet and savoury recipes. High in protein and fibre, they can be added to hot cereal, pilaus, soups, stuffing, stews, breads, muffins and other bakes. They're yummy in salads too. Wheat flour comes from wheatberries that are milled and ground. Because wheatberries are hard, they take some time to cook, but soaking speeds that process.

foods (or with antacids that contain calcium such as Rennie or Gaviscon) may block iron absorption. Ditto high-fibre foods.

While iron comes from both the animal and plant kingdoms, it's much more absorbable when it comes from an animal source (that steak) than when it comes from a plant source (those beans). Good news if you're a meat eater, not such good news if you're a vegetarian or are meat-averse at the moment.

These foods are naturally high in iron:

Beef

Poultry

Cooked clams, oysters, mussels and prawns

Salt Sense

Classic cravings have you reaching for the pickle jar – and then emptying it, down to the last sip of zesty juice? Your body may actually be doing you a favour with those salty cravings: propelling you to drink more liquids. An adequate sodium intake is required to accommodate pregnancy's higher fluid volume, and overly restricting salt intake can disrupt that delicate fluid balance. What's more, contrary to popular belief, it's not the sodium that makes you puffy during pregnancy – it's the hormones. A certain amount of swelling is your body's way of ensuring it has enough fluids on board for baby making, and that's healthy and normal (if not so swell from a comfort perspective).

So go ahead and get busy with those pickles. Give yourself a fair shake from the salt shaker (doing it to taste, instead of routinely, will naturally moderate what you shake). Just remember that many of the fast and processed foods that give sodium a bad name actually earn their less-than-wholesome reputation for other reasons (they're full of fat, sugar and questionable chemicals, they're low in nutrients and fibre). Those are definitely worth limiting or skipping. Also remember that, especially as you close in on the end of pregnancy, too much salt can lead to too much swelling – and a lot more discomfort than you'll probably care to experience. There's no need to hold off on the pickles or the pickle juice – just moderate where you can, and don't sweat the rest.

How much salt is too much? Adults should consume no more than 6 g of salt a day, the amount in 1 teaspoon. However, sometimes food labels list the amount of sodium instead of salt. With 2.4 g of sodium equalling 6 g of salt, you'll need to do some maths to know your daily intake of salt. To convert sodium to salt, multiply the amount of sodium by 2.5: 2 g of sodium equals 5 g of salt, for instance. And remember sodium or salt is listed for every 100 g of the product. For more on reading food labels, see the box on page 58.

Sardines

Cooked dried beans

Soya beans (edamame) and soya products

Barley, bulgar wheat, quinoa

Pumpkin seeds

Jerusalem artichokes

Spinach, kale, spring greens and turnip tops

Seaweed

Dried fruit

Fat and high-fat foods: about four servings daily (more if you're having trouble gaining weight, less if you're gaining too fast). Here's a fact about fat: most people get more fat than they need without even trying – and many get more than they need even when they're trying (really, really hard) not to. After all, when stacked against other nutritional requirements, fat comes in relatively small packages (when it comes to oil or butter, for instance, just a tablespoon per serving).

But here's another fact about fat: your body needs it, especially when you're pregnant. Essential fatty acids are – wait for it – essential for a baby's growth and development. Especially important in the last month of pregnancy and first few months of breast-feeding are omega-3 fatty acids, since this form of fat is needed for optimal brain development (see below).

The foods listed below are composed completely (or mostly) of fat. Though they won't be the only source of fat in your diet (you'll get extra fat from dairy products, nuts, avocado, meat, poultry and more), they're the only ones you'll need to keep track of. Keeping track will be easier if you keep an eye open for the many places fat ends up (the mayo on your chicken salad sandwich, the oil in your salad dressing, the butter on your bun).

If you're gaining weight too quickly, you can cut back by one or two fat servings. You might also want to consider cutting way back on foods that are prepared with a lot of fat (anything fried or swimming in a pool of butter). If you're gaining weight too slowly, you may want to add a fat serving – as well as some extra high-fat foods (preferably nutritious ones such as nuts and avocados). One serving equals about a tablespoon of the following:

Oil, such as vegetable, olive, rapeseed, avocado, walnut and sesame

Butter

Mayonnaise

Regular salad dressing

Peanut, almond or other nut butter

Omega-3 fatty acids: some daily. Here's a fat you can really feel good about eating, particularly while you're eating for two: omega-3 polyunsaturated fatty acids (such as DHA). Touted for a variety of general health

Fatten Up Your Salad

Fat-phobics, it's time to confront your fears. And to start drizzling fats on your salads and steamed vegetables. Turns out that a little fat actually brings out the best in broccoli (or romaine or carrots). Though it's tempting to save yourself a few calories by pouring on the fat-free dressings or opting for a virtuous squeeze of lemon, research has shown that sparing the fat spoils the nutrients. Scientists have found that many of the vital dietary properties in vegetables (such as alpha-carotene, beta-carotene or lycopene) aren't well absorbed without a side of fat. So add some real dressing to your salad, dip for your carrots, oil to your stir-fry – or just a handful of nuts or a few slices of avocado to any veggie dish. Just remember as you drizzle and douse, sauté and stir-fry, that a little fat goes a long way – say, a tablespoon (not three or four) of dressing on your lettuce.

benefits, DHA is a major component of the brain and retina and is needed for proper brain growth and eye development in foetuses and young babies. Getting enough of this vital baby brain fuel in your diet is especially important during the last trimester (when your baby's brain grows at a phenomenal pace) and during breastfeeding (the DHA content of a baby's brain triples during the first three months of life).

Other potential perks? Getting enough DHA during pregnancy may reduce the chances of baby being born too early or being born at a low birthweight. And what's good for the expected is also good for the expecting.

Didn't Make the List?

Can't find your favourite fruit, grain or protein source on these food lists? Just because a food isn't listed doesn't mean it isn't worth a place in your diet. For reasons of space (and so you don't have to spend nine months flipping through pages to find the food you're looking for), only more common foods and drinks are listed in this chapter. If your inquiring mind wants to know more, you can search the British Nutrition Foundation's website at www.nutrition.org.uk.

Luckily, DHA is found in plenty of foods you probably already eat – and like to eat:

Salmon and other higher-fat fish such as sardines

Tinned light tuna

Walnuts and walnut oil

Brazil nuts

Seeds (pumpkin, sunflower, chia, and linseed/flax)

Seaweed

DHA-rich eggs (often called omega-3 eggs)

Omega-3 fortified milk alternatives and juice

Grass-fed beef, buffalo and lamb

Crab and prawns

Free-range or omega-3 chicken

You can also ask your healthcare provider about pregnancy-safe mercury-free DHA supplements (many antenatal supplements contain up to 200 to 300 mg of DHA already). Not a fan of the fishy aftertaste (and the fishy burps) some DHA supplements leave behind? There are vegetarian and vegan alternatives that are fish-free.

Fluids: at least ten 240-ml glasses daily. Water – essential for almost every function in your body – is especially essential during pregnancy, when there's another little body on board. That little body will need water to build cells, for its developing circulatory system, for the delivery of nutrients and for the excretion of wastes. Your body, too, will require more fluids during pregnancy, to help combat constipation, prevent dry skin, regulate body temperature and reduce the risk of urinary tract infection. And because water also helps your body flush out waste products, drinking enough can actually keep you from retaining too much fluid (aka swelling). These are all good reasons to aim for at least ten 240-ml glasses of fluid daily. You may need more during hot weather, if you're working out a lot or if you've been vomiting a lot. How will you know you're getting enough liquid in? When enough is coming out, in the form of pale or clear urine. Urine that's dark or scant means you need to step up your fluid intake.

When tallying your fluid intake, remember to also count fluids that don't come from the tap (or your water bottle). Milk (which is two-thirds water), juice, soups and stocks also figure. Fruits and vegetables count, too – five typical servings equal about two servings of fluid, with some (such as watermelon, cucumber and lettuce, which are all about 95 per cent water) outperforming on fluids. Count sparkling water, as well as decaffeinated coffee or tea, but don't count caffeinated beverages, since they act as diuretics, causing calcium and other key

Water, Water Everywhere

Never been a big drinker – of water? Here are some tips to help you get in the water habit:

- Carry a refillable water bottle with you wherever you go. Drink while you're in the car, on social media, waiting in line at the supermarket or riding the commuter train.

- Fill a 700-ml container with water and keep it with you all day, on the job or at home. You'll need to fill it only one more time to get just over half of your fluid requirement. Top it off with some servings of fruit, a salad, a bowl of soup, a glass of almond milk – and you've met your goal (plus covered a few other Daily Dozen bases).

- Aim to drink one glass of water every 2 hours during the day.

- Use larger glasses or mugs, so you'll drink more at each sitting.

- When eating out, down a glass of water before you leave for the restaurant. And down another one at the table while you're waiting for your food.

- Blend up a breakfast smoothie to start your day juiced on fluids – you'll score extra fluids from the ice and the juicy fruit you use.

- Remember to look for water, water everywhere in the produce department too. You'll find plenty of fluids in watermelon (obviously), other melons, lettuce, cucumbers, celery, tomatoes, strawberries, grapefruit, and oranges.

---

pregnancy nutrients to be washed out of your system before they can be thoroughly absorbed.

Are frequent trips to the toilet tempting you to cut back on fluids? Don't let them. All that wee is serving a vital (if annoying) purpose: flushing waste products from your system and your baby's.

Antenatal vitamin supplements: a pregnancy formula taken daily. Sometimes, despite your best intentions and your best efforts (you did try to eat that bowl of cereal between trips to the toilet to throw up), your diet may be lacking in a vitamin one day, a mineral or two another day.

That's where an antenatal vitamin-mineral supplement comes in. Not to stand in for a healthy diet (a supplement can't, since it doesn't provide many of the nutrients a healthy pregnancy needs and a healthy pregnancy diet contains, from calories and fibre to phytonutrients and certain vital minerals), but to fill in the nutritional blanks when what you eat comes up short. Not so you can intentionally let your diet slide, but for those days (and early months) when it inevitably does slide, maybe because you're too busy to eat well or you're too sick to eat well. To keep you covered on nutrients that are just plain hard to get enough of from diet alone such as iron (and for vegans, calcium, vitamin D and vitamin B_{12}). Or on ones that are so vital to baby's development that extra insurance makes extra sense, especially folic acid. Studies show that women who take antenatal vitamins before and during pregnancy dramatically

---

Take Your Iron with a Side of C

Chances are your healthcare provider might recommend another tablet midway through your pregnancy – an iron supplement – to be taken in addition to your regular antenatal supplement. It's to refill those stores of red blood cells needed as your blood volume increases. Try to avoid eating or drinking something high in calcium when you take your iron supplement, since calcium interferes with iron absorption. Instead, accompany your iron with food or drink high in vitamin C, which will aid in iron absorption.

---

lower the risks of having babies with spina bifida and cleft palate (probably because of the folic acid content of the supplements).

The formula you take should be specially designed for pregnancy. Ask your healthcare provider to recommend an over-the-counter one (if you're worried about the cost, ask about the Healthy Start scheme), or select one yourself that contains the vitamins and minerals in roughly the same dosages as these:

- At least 400 mcg of folic acid

- 250 mcg of calcium. If you're not getting enough calcium in your diet, you will need additional supplementation to reach the 700 mg needed during pregnancy. Don't take an iron supplement at the same time as or within 2 hours of a supplement containing more than 250 mg of calcium, since it interferes with iron absorption.

- 30 mg of iron

- 50 to 80 mg of vitamin C

- 15 mg of zinc

- 2 mg of copper

- 2 mg of vitamin B_6

- At least 10 mcg (400 IU as D_3) of vitamin D

- Approximately the RNI for thiamin (0.9 mg), riboflavin (1.4 mg), niacin (13 mg) and vitamin B_{12} (1.5 mcg). Antenatal supplements may contain higher amounts of these nutrients, but those higher doses aren't considered harmful.

- 150 mcg of iodine (not all antenatals contain iodine or this amount of it)

- Some formulas may also contain beta-carotene, vitamin E, magnesium, selenium, fluoride, biotin, choline, phosphorous, pantothenic acid, extra B_6 and ginger (to combat queasiness) and/or DHA

CHEW ON THIS. Pregnancy superstitions run the gamut from possibly plausible to downright peculiar. Definitely falling into the latter category is this one: pregnant women centuries ago were told that if they didn't drink enough water, their babies would be born dirty. (Care for some soap with that glass of water?) While there's clearly no truth to this tale, there is some obvious wisdom behind the advice: getting enough water is important during pregnancy, even if you're not superstitious.

Bar None?

They fit neatly in a handbag, glove compartment, desk drawer, even your pocket. Many are loaded with protein, fibre, vitamins and minerals, and are filling enough to keep you going when you're on the run. But do nutrition bars set a high enough bar when it comes to pregnancy nutrition? Do they really have what it takes to serve as a healthy snack, never mind a healthy meal replacement?

Well, that depends. If you check the labels, some nutrition bars definitely stack up better than others. When shopping the bar section, look for ones that are made with real food such as oats and other grains, nuts and seeds, eggs, and fruit. Look for little or no added sugar (some bars rival chocolate bars in the sugar department), and bypass bars sweetened the artificial way ('sugar alcohols' on the nutrition label will clue you in). A little fortification is fine, a lot is unnecessary (especially if you're already taking an antenatal supplement, plus eating a healthy diet).

If you're perusing a protein bar, check to see where the protein comes from: eggs? Grains, nuts and seeds? Or some lab-synthesised protein? Remember, too, that it's possible to pack too much protein, especially if you're eating protein bars and shakes on top of an already protein-rich diet. Avoid bars or jerky made from meat, poultry or fish since there is the possibility of bacterial contamination.

Now that you know which nutrition bars to reach for, how often should you reach for them? While snacking on one occasionally (or even daily) is fine, especially when you're on the go, using them to regularly replace real food in your diet isn't. Use them for a quick and convenient lift, but not as a meal. And add on when you can: when you grab a bar, also grab a piece of fresh fruit. And look beyond the bar too, for other nonperishable snacks that are easy to drop into your handbag such as nuts and seeds, and freeze-dried fruit and vegetables.

If you're a queasy mum, the best time to take an antenatal is when you're best able to keep it down – and that's typically at night, with dinner or a bedtime snack (of course, your results may vary – so go with what works for you). See the tips on page 112 for more on taking vitamins while combating morning sickness. Even if your stomach's not particularly sensitive, it makes sense to take the supplement with a meal or snack that contains some fat – some oil, some peanut butter, some nuts or avocado – to help you absorb those fat-soluble vitamins (A, D, E and K). And make sure you chase it with plenty of fluids to help it dissolve well. Wondering if more vitamins, minerals and other nutrients might be more beneficial to your body, your pregnancy and your baby? Scarf down as many as you care to in food form (double up on veggies, fruit, salad), but don't take any extras in supplement form without your healthcare provider's approval. Some nutrients, such as vitamins A and D, are toxic in doses higher than those found in antenatal vitamins. And since some supplements may contain herbs that aren't known to be safe in pregnancy, be sure to scan the ingredients (or run them past your healthcare provider) before choosing a brand.

Good Enough Is Good Enough

Here's some straight talk about a pregnancy diet. There are plenty of reasons why eating well is good for you and good for your baby. But eating well enough, especially when that's the best you can do right now, is also good . . . really good. Eat a mostly balanced diet most of the time, with an eye to a nice mix of fruits, vegetables, wholegrains, healthy fats and protein, and don't stress about the rest of the time. Reach for the nutritional sky, by all means, but don't give up if you reach for the brownie you were craving instead. Look at each day as a new opportunity to aim higher, not as a reason to put yourself down over yesterday's fast-food frenzy. Blend yourself a smoothie, build yourself a salad or cut up some cantaloupe . . . and move on.

CHAPTER 4

Selecting Well to Eat Well

W hether you're browsing groceries online, braving the supermarket, shopping at the local corner shop or foraging at the farmers market, chances are you have options – likely a dizzying array of options and a whole lot of competing packets, each promising to deliver on taste and nutrition. Happily, more and more of the products vying for your attention are healthy ones – which means that filling your trolley (and your tummy) with the best foods for you and your baby is easier than ever. Another plus to all those options: eating well doesn't have to be monotonous (at least once morning sickness has returned your appetite and released your taste buds from cracker captivity). Here's to choosing well to eat well.

Shopping for Two

H opefully you've got your comfy shoes on (or your comfy joggers on if you're shopping online), because it's time to fill your fridge, freezer, store cupboard, snack containers, handbag, gym bag, glove compartment and office drawer or locker with all the food you'll need to eat well. But even if you're just doing the supermarket sprint on the way home from a long day on the job, it'll help to keep these shopping dos and don'ts in mind as you fill a trolley.

- Do make a list. How long a list depends on how often you'll be doing your food shopping – and how many meals and snacks you're planning to create from the list. If you're extra-organised and motivated, writing down your menus for the week and generating the list from there (or letting an app generate it from recipes you choose) is ideal – it'll keep you focused and on track nutritionally. Plus, it'll help avoid those otherwise

Reading Food Labels

How does a product stand out in a sea of similar products? With a label, of course. A label will tell you just about everything you need to know about a product before you decide to drop it into your trolley – that is, if you know where on the label to look. Front and centre? Not so much. That's where you'll find the pretty pictures and the enticing descriptions – but not where you'll find a lot of real food facts. That's because manufacturers, for the most part, design their labels (no surprise) to sell products, not inform consumers – at least, beyond what regulations require. To do this, they highlight in big print the hype they'd like you to notice ('great taste!', 'wholesome!', 'made with natural ingredients!', 'no cholesterol!') and bury the details they'd rather you overlook on the side or back of the pack in small print. Here are some clues to bear in mind when you're playing label detective:

Ingredients list. You'll find out a lot about a product just by skimming this list – and you may often be surprised at what you find. All ingredients in a product must be listed on the packaging in order of predominance, with the first ingredient the most plentiful (by weight) and the last the least. So a fruit bar that lists 'sugar' and 'fructose-glucose syrup' before 'mixed berry purée' clearly has a lot more sugar than it does fruit. A bread that boasts 'multigrain' doesn't necessarily mean wholegrain: 'wheat flour' may be the main ingredient on the ingredients list with a smaller portion of wholegrains added.

You should also scan the list for ingredients the manufacturer is not likely to brag about elsewhere on the label such as starchy fillers and artificial preservatives, colourings and flavourings.

Serving size. What's in a serving? The nutrition information provided on the back of the packaging is based on 100 g or 100 ml of the product – this is mandatory – but a portion can also be voluntarily included (such as half a pizza or one biscuit). Get that product home, and the size of the serving can vary a whole lot, depending on who's dishing it out and who's eating it. So if the label says that a serving of pasta is 180 g cooked, but you eat 270 g, remember that all the numbers will go up (including the calories) – in this case, by 50 per cent. And if you serve yourself only 90 g, you'll have to halve the nutrient numbers promised on the label.

Nutrition information. If you're looking for nutrition facts, turn to the back or side of the packaging. The 'Nutrition' panel gives an idea of the nutritional profile of the product you're thinking about buying. It's mandatory to list how much energy (kcal or calories), fat, saturates (saturated fat), carbohydrates, sugars, fibre, protein and salt per 100 mg/ml of the food. Vitamins and minerals can be included if they are contained in significant amounts. Manufacturers can

inevitable food fails (like forgetting milk for your cereal, handy snacks to take to work or anything to eat for dinner) – all more likely as you add forgetfulness to your list of pregnancy symptoms. But even if you shop one day at a time, a list to hand will prevent you getting sucked into the shopper's twilight zone – wandering the aisles aimlessly looking for inspiration and finding it in a huge tub of mint chocolate chip. For best results, organise

voluntarily tell you the percentage of the RI (recommended intake) of these nutrients provided in a portion.

When looking at the front of the packaging, you might find a colour-coded traffic-light panel. It's designed to give you quick at-a-glance nutritional information, with green and ambers being good but reds a sign to cut back. However, since the portion size is the manufacturer's recommendation, it may be on the small size to have healthier numbers – and it won't be so healthy if you eat larger portions.

Now, this may seem like a lot more than you need to know about a product – and probably a lot more than you know what to do with. But the point of reading nutrition labels isn't so that you can calculate grams or add up percentages. After all, the Pregnancy Diet already ensures that you're getting the amounts of nutrients you need, without doing the maths – not to mention that the RI for pregnancy may be different from that listed on the label. It's to figure out whether the product you're picking up is worth dropping into your trolley.

The big type. Is the big type on a label just hype? It depends on the words being highlighted. Go online and you may come across some dubious claims on products sold in other countries, but for food products sold in the UK manufacturers are not permitted to make claims or otherwise imply that a food can treat or prevent a medical condition or disease. And words that describe a food's nutrient content such as 'light', 'low-fat' and 'high-fibre' are

regulated by the government to ensure they're accurate. However, even if a product is 'low-fat', it could be packed with sugar, refined grains and artificial colours and flavours. Here are some other tricks of the label trade:

- 'Fortified with 6 vitamins and iron' looks impressive, especially in that extra-large print. And for the most part, fortification with vitamins and minerals is a good thing. But fortification alone does not make a food healthy – especially if it's just tossing some vitamins and minerals into a food that's weak in nutrition to begin with. Just about all processed food, after all, is fortified.

- Think 'reduced-fat' and 'low-fat' are the same thing? Think again: 'low-fat' means there's a maximum of 3 g of fat per 100 g of the product. However, 'reduced-fat' refers to a product that is 25 per cent lower in fat than the standard product – but that isn't so helpful if the standard version is high in fat.

- 'No preservatives' or 'no artificial flavours' tells you only what isn't in a product. To find out what is in it (for instance, artificial colours), you'll have to read on.

- If you don't see 'sugar' in the ingredients list, the product doesn't have sugar, right? That's not necessarily true: there are other forms of sugar (many ending in -ose) and these may be listed as sucrose, glucose, fructose, maltose, honey, palm sugar, hydrolysed starch and syrup.

your lists by department or aisle – that way you won't end up visiting the produce section three times in the same visit or making a last-minute dash back to retrieve an item when you're already at the till.

- Do stick to the list. Supermarkets, even virtual ones, are full of temptations. And advertising and marketing ploys. And sales that entice you to buy what you don't need and maybe shouldn't have – or just more than you need or can use. Resist with your list. Also consider that coupons (or discount apps) can interfere with your healthy eating plans if you don't choose foods that come not just with savings but also with nutritional redemption.

- Do think outside the box. Yes, you've come equipped with your list – but don't let that stop you from picking up a healthy food that's new to you. A baby vegetable you've never seen, an exotic tropical fruit, an intriguing

grain to add to your pilau, a seed to snack on.

- Don't shop when you're about to drop. When you can avoid it, try not to schedule in big-time marketing when you're on your last legs (and possibly swollen ankles) of the day.

- Don't go hungry. Have a snack before you go shopping. A growling tummy will lead you away from the list – and down the snack aisle – every time.

Selecting for Two

You're motivated to eat well, you're ready to get started on the Pregnancy Diet and you're keen to select the best foods for your health and your baby's. Here's what to bear in mind as you do your choosing.

Meat and Poultry

Not sure which cuts of meat and poultry make the cut? Aim for the leanest cuts of beef, pork and lamb – look for the words 'lean' or 'extra lean', and select cuts with the least amount of visible fat (marbling). That's not only because less fat means fewer calories, but because fat is where any chemicals an animal ingests accumulate (this isn't a concern when it comes to organically raised animals; keep reading). Beef labelled as 'matured' has been hung for the specified number of days, which tenderises the meat and makes it more flavoursome. As a rule of thumb, anything labelled 'sirloin', 'fillet' or 'round' is lean. Silverside and topside are also lean cuts. When selecting lean or extra-lean beef mince, also check the percentage of fat and choose the lowest

fat percentage when you can. You'll pay more for less fat, but the meat will cook down less, leaving you with more meat by weight. Chicken or turkey on the menu? Reach for breasts, preferably skinless (or remove the skin, which is 85 per cent fat, before cooking – or, if that's not possible, before eating). Or choose chicken or turkey breast mince, instead of the minced dark meat.

When it's available and your budget permits, consider buying meat and poultry that has been raised organically. The label 'organic' or a green leaf logo on animal products means that the animals were fed organic food and not given antibiotics, growth hormones or other drugs – a definite plus, since the antibiotics, hormones, pesticides and chemicals you consume through your diet are shared with your baby both in the uterus and through breast milk. It makes even more sense to reach for organic when you're buying a fattier cut of meat or poultry (a marbled steak, chicken thighs, pork shoulder). Though an organic beef short rib will still contain as many calories as a short rib from a conventionally raised cow, it won't contain all the chemicals that may be stored in a conventionally raised animal's fat.

Bear in mind that organic beef doesn't mean it's exclusively grass-fed (and grass-fed isn't always organic – the grass the animals grazed on, for instance, may have been treated with pesticides or other chemicals). Regardless, grass-fed cows (organic or not) not only have a vegetarian diet, but they also have to work for it, resulting in leaner, lower-calorie meat. What's more, grass-fed beef is higher in omega-3 fatty acids, vitamin E and beta-carotene than grain-fed cattle – all excellent reasons to reach for the traditional grass-fed. Not sure if your meat is grass-fed? No need to stress: even though there are more nutrients in grass-fed than in other meats, the difference is small. One serving (115 g) of grass-fed top sirloin contains about 65–100 mg of omega-3 fats, while grain-fed beef has about 30–50 mg of omega-3s per serving. A difference, yes, but not a significant one – especially when you consider that a 115-g serving of salmon has over 1,000 mg of that baby-brain-boosting nutrient. So by all means, choose grass-fed when you can – which shouldn't be too hard in the UK – but don't worry if you can't find it or can't afford it. You could consider buying local, directly from the farm or a farmers market: the middle-man is cut out so prizes may be more affordable.

Something else to consider when selecting meat and poultry: animal welfare. Officially, a 'free-range' label on chicken indicates that the birds have access to the outdoors and are less likely to be contaminated with chemicals. A bonus: free-range chicken is usually less fatty and more tasty than intensely reared birds. Free-range can also apply to pigs (though it's not a regulated term) if they can go outdoors for at least part of their lives: If the product is labelled 'outdoor bred', the pigs are bred outdoors, but after weaning they are brought indoors for fattening; if the product is labelled 'outdoor reared', the pigs get to spend about half of their life outdoors.

Keeping cattle and sheep in pastures is the standard in the UK, but the US practice of concentrated animal feeding operations (CAFOs), in which cattle are fattened on grains indoors, has been on the increase. The old-fashioned methods for rearing cattle are now sometimes given trendy labels such as 'pasture-raised', where the animals spend time outdoors feeding on grass in the pasture, and 'grass-fed', where animals are fed a diet that consists mostly of grass, not grains. 'Pasture promise' indicates that the animals have been fed on grass outdoors for six months and are fed grass or hay during the winter.

Want to keep tabs on what your dinner ate for dinner or how it was treated? Check the labelling. A 'Red Tractor' label ensures good food safety and hygiene standards and provides traceability to the farm where the animal was reared – and if there is also a Union Jack, it means the farm was in the UK. However, a Red Tractor label doesn't mean better care for the animals. If you're concerned about better animal welfare, look for the 'RSPCA Assured' stamp on beef, pork, chicken and turkey. Whether free-range, organic, indoor or outdoor farms, it indicates that the animals are fairly treated and humanely slaughtered.

Fish

Loaded with baby-brain-boosting omega-3 fats, vitamins D and B_{12}, and a host of healthy minerals, fish should ideally make the menu cut at least two times a week when you're expecting (assuming you're a fish fan and you're not feeling too green around the gills to eat it). But what should you look for when you're in the market for fish? That depends on what you're fishing for. When selecting fresh fish, use your senses – especially your pregnancy-sensitive nose, which will quickly warn you if something's fishy (it should smell like an ocean breeze, not like a bait box). Fresh fish should look fresh, and if it's whole, it should have moist gills, shiny skin and clear, bright eyes. Fillets should also be shiny, not dull, and the flesh should spring back without leaving an indentation when pressed lightly with a finger. Hopefully the fish will be labelled as 'fresh' or 'previously frozen', but if it isn't, just ask. Fish that was quickly frozen after being caught and then thawed carefully may actually be fresher than fish that was caught, stored and shipped fresh. If the fish was previously frozen, don't refreeze it once you get home (you can freeze fish that has never been frozen). Buying fish that's already frozen? Just make sure you keep it frozen until you're ready to use it (thaw in the fridge before preparing). For a list of pregnancy-safe fish to choose and fish to avoid, see page 72.

Should you go wild (that is, caught in its natural habitat, whether that's an ocean, river or lake) or farm-raised (raised in a large tank)? That's not an easy call. Wild fish (wild salmon, for instance) may be lower in calories and higher in minerals, though farmed fish usually has an edge on omega-3s (because of fortified feed). Wild fish may also contain fewer contaminants than farmed, but either can contain mercury (which is why you should stick to low-mercury fish). Where the fish is sourced from (which farm, which ocean) can also impact the level of contaminants, since some countries are more lax than others when it comes to regulation of both farms and natural bodies of water. It can also impact the nutrients it contains (fish are what they eat).

If debates about which fish to buy don't mean much to you, either because farmed is the only option at your market

or because you can't afford to go wild, just remember this: any fish (as long as it's a safe fish) is better than no fish at all.

Wondering whether you should buy organic fish? Legally, it's not possible to label fish caught or harvested in the wild as organic because there's no way to know its history. However, there are fish farms in the UK that provide organic – and sustainably sourced – fish.

Eggs

Like your eggs any style? There's plenty to like: they're inexpensive, versatile and packed with protein, and they're a solid source of nutrients from vitamin A, B_{12} and D to selenium and zinc. But did you know that some eggs also provide more baby-brain-nourishing DHA than others? That's right. DHA eggs, more often called omega-3 eggs, come from chickens fed a diet containing sources of omega-3s, such as linseeds or marine algae. You'll also find plenty to crow about when it comes to free-range eggs (even ones not marked 'omega-3 eggs'). Compared with conventional eggs, they're higher in DHA, have more vitamins A and D, and double the vitamin E. So if you're looking to make a good egg better, look for 'omega-3' or 'free-range' on the box.

Wondering what the numbers on the egg mean?

- 0 – 'Organic': a maximum of six hens per metre indoors, plus access to outdoor space and pasture, with supplemental organic food.

- 1 – 'Free-range': as well as space within a barn (see below), the hens have access to the outdoors.

- 2 – 'Barn': no cages are allowed, hens can perch and there's a maximum of nine hens per metre in a barn.

- 3 – 'Caged': hens are kept in a cage.

Dairy

When selecting dairy, you'll score as much protein and calcium for fewer calories when you opt for semi-skimmed or skimmed milk or reduced-fat cheese. If your budget allows – and it's readily available at your supermarket – choose organic dairy products over conventional for a couple of reasons. First, because organically raised cows (and goats and sheep) are never given antibiotics or hormones, the milk they produce won't contain them (though most conventional milk won't contain them either; keep reading). Secondly, organic dairy products contain more omega-3 fatty acids than conventional dairy. That's because all organic milk comes from animals that are grass-fed to some extent, with the rest of their feed grown without chemical fertilisers, pesticides or genetically modified products. Milk that comes from 100 per cent grass-fed animals may be even richer in omega-3s.

Can't find – or can't afford – organic dairy? The good news is that the Food Standards Agency requires milk to be checked for antibiotic residue (any milk that contains it can't be sold). Additionally, most milk is pasteurised, which means it is treated by heat to kill off bacteria (see the box on this page). The milk you take from the chiller cabinet in the supermarket will always be pasteurised, but it is possible to buy untreated raw milk from cows, sheep, goats and even buffalo and horses directly from farmers. However, any dairy products you drink during pregnancy should always be pasteurised, for safety's sake (see the box on this page).

Other labels to consider: lactose-free if you're sensitive to the lactose in milk (see the box on page 37), and A2 milk if you have an intolerance to a certain protein in cow's milk (see page 149).

Pasteurised, Please

Pasteurisation may be the best thing that ever happened to a glass of milk (or a wedge of cheese), but it shouldn't stop at dairy products. Eggs in some countries are pasteurised to eliminate the risk of salmonella, but due to different farming practices, it is not necessary in the UK unless the eggs are used commercially. Juices sold with a longer shelf life are also pasteurised (to eliminate *E. coli* and other harmful bacteria). Check the label of commercially packaged juices to see if they are pasteurised before you buy. Not sure if a juice is pasteurised or pretty sure it isn't (say, because it's freshly squeezed at the juice bar)? Don't drink it if you're pregnant. Ditto for smoothies made with juice, unless you're sure it's pasteurised. Fresh coconuts cut open right in front of you and served with a straw are fine to drink since the coconut water is sterile and well protected inside the hard coconut shell. Look for pasteurised cider vinegar too. (Just bear in mind that if you're turning to cider vinegar because you've heard claims that it will heal what ails you – from morning sickness to gestational diabetes – those claims have not been backed up by science.)

Wondering about the label 'flash-pasteurised'? It's a faster yet just as effective pasteurisation process that kills bacteria while preserving flavour. And how about juicing you do at home? That's all good (and yummy, and nutritious) – as long as you've thoroughly washed the produce before juicing.

Looking for dairy-free milks? See the box on page 38 for a list of options. There are also dairy-free cheeses.

A Fresh Approach to Dried

When it comes to picking the most nutritious foods, nothing compares with fresh, right? Maybe not. Freeze-dried fruits, vegetables and even cheese pack a nutritional punch equal to the fresh varieties. The freeze-drying process removes nearly all the water content of a food (around 98 per cent), leaving it crunchy, more intensely flavoured and – key when you're snacking on the run or at your desk – not perishable. No spoiling, no need for refrigeration, and no preparation or cooking necessary. Open the packet, open your mouth and start popping everything from strawberries to mango, broccoli to carrots, Cheddar to mozzarella.

Wondering how much freeze-dried fruit differs from traditionally dried? A lot, actually. First, freeze-dried is crunchy, while dried (aka dehydrated) is chewy. Dried fruit is higher in calories than freeze-dried, and often lower in nutrients (the dehydration process requires the use of heat, which can strip foods of naturally occurring nutrients, especially heat-sensitive ones such as vitamin C). There may be sugar added to some dried fruits (particularly tropical fruits such as pineapple, plus cherries, cranberries and other berries), as well as preservatives and oil. Even dried fruit that doesn't contain added sugar may be more likely to contribute to tooth decay and gum troubles (that's because it's so sticky).

Craving something crispy and salty? Seeking a snack you can take anywhere, including to bed? Freeze-dried cheese (available online and in some health-food shops) provides protein, calcium and a satisfying, nutritious alternative to that bag of crisps. And, unlike fresh cheese, you can keep it in your gym bag or your car without worrying about refrigeration. Looking for a blood-sugar-sustaining or quease-easing combo of protein and complex carbs you can tote for emergency snacking? Pack a bag of freeze-dried cheese and a bag of freeze-dried fruit, and you're good to go . . . anywhere, anytime.

Fruits and Vegetables

Green means go. And when it comes to fruits and vegetables, so does red, yellow, blue, orange and purple. When selecting fresh fruits and vegetables, pick the most ripe, richly coloured and fragrant options. And try to think seasonally – although most fruits and vegetables are available year-round, produce will be more flavourful, more nutritious and probably cost less in season.

Check these rainbow hot hues in the produce aisle:

- Red. Red is the colour of lycopene, one of nature's super-star phytonutrients. Tomatoes, both raw and cooked (though cooking pumps up their nutritional content), are a great source. So, too, are ruby red (or pink) grapefruit, watermelon, persimmon and guava. Another reason to see (and eat) red is the high antioxidant content of red fruit favourites such as strawberries, cranberries, cherries and pomegranates.

- Orange and yellow. Fruits and vegetables that are orange or yellow are usually rich in baby-friendly vitamin A (or, more precisely, beta-carotene). Colour your world with winter squash (from butternut to kabocha to delicata), carrots, sweet potatoes, apricots, yellow peaches, cantaloupes,

The Biotech Boom

Heard that you should avoid genetically modified foods, but not sure why – or even what they are? Here are a few fast facts. Genetically modified organisms (GMO) are plants that have had their DNA modified. It's not technically a new process – farmers have been finessing their crops for thousands of years, breeding them to be hardier, tastier, more adaptable and more resistant to pests – but this far higher level of crop engineering has definitely become a far higher tech process, as well as a far bigger business. Not to mention, a major source of controversy among consumers and consumer groups concerned about the safety of genetically modfied (GM) foods.

What are the benefits of GM crops – or at least the potential benefits? Crops that are designed to acquire more desirable traits, such as the ability to grow faster and less expensively under harsher weather conditions, stay fresher longer, be more nutritious, or resist pests or disease without (again, potentially) the use of as many pesticides. These days, anything from sweetcorn to plums, potatoes to rice, can be genetically modified in the United States (the practice is banned in Europe, but there are experiments of growing GM crops in the UK), with soya beans being by far the most commonly grown GM crop.

So is this biotech boom a boon or a bane, or somewhere in between, especially from where you're sitting – pregnant and legitimately concerned about the food you eat and share with your baby? From the research so far – and there has been a lot of research done – it appears that GM crops are not harmful. The consensus of the vast majority of scientists (including, among others, those in the American Medical Association, the World Health Organization and the National Academy of Sciences) is that such biotechnological advances are safe, and that their responsible development may ultimately result in a healthier population and planet. So there's a significant upside to the GM boom long-term, they say, and no particular downside in the meantime. That is, as long as consumers choose healthy GM products (those huge crops of soya beans often end up in less healthy foods). Still, many consumer groups remain critical of GM crops, insisting that there are too many unanswered questions about how these changes in our food supply will impact our health.

Feel better about staying GM-free? The European Union requires that imported products containing GMOs are labelled as such, so avoiding GMs is as easy as avoiding foods with a GM label. You can also look for foods labelled 'GM-free'. Or choose organic products, which even in the United States are required to be GM-free.

mangoes, papayas, pumpkins, and yellow and orange peppers. Other oranges and yellows, such as oranges, tangerines, lemons and pineapples, are also high in vitamin C.

■ Green. Some dark green varieties of produce are excellent sources of carotenoids (lutein and zeaxanthin) that may help reduce the risk of slow foetal growth and premature delivery. These carotenoids also play a role in the healthy development of vision and the nervous system. Leafy green vegetables help you score some baby-friendly folate (folic acid), too. Besides lettuces, stock up on spinach, kale, chard, broccoli, artichokes,

When Organic Makes a Difference

Can't always spring for organic produce, or can't always find it at your supermarket? Knowing when organic makes a difference and when it doesn't can help prioritise your purchases:

- Certain produce carries higher levels of pesticide than others, even after washing. So it's best to buy organic strawberries, spinach, kale, nectarines, peaches, apples, pears, grapes, cherries, tomatoes, celery and potatoes.

- Other fruits and vegetables usually don't contain pesticide residue, so it's safe to buy them conventionally grown. They include cantaloupe, honeydew, pineapples, kiwi fruit, avocados, sweetcorn, peas, onions, papayas, aubergine, asparagus, cabbage, cauliflower, broccoli and mushrooms.

green peas, green beans, Brussels sprouts, green peppers, courgettes, okra, avocados, honeydew, green grapes, kiwi fruit and parsley.

- Blue. The antioxidant anthocyanin makes the blueberry blue and is a powerful cancer fighter. Clearly, you won't find it in those boxes of Froot Loops – that blue (and pink, and yellow, and green) comes by its colour in an entirely different way.

- Purple. Purple (or red) grapes contain lutein and zeaxanthin; plums, prunes, blackberries and purple cabbage are also rich in antioxidants. Beetroot is rich in the antioxidant betacyanin. And acai (pronounced ah-sa-EE) berries – nicknamed 'purple gold' (think

of them as somewhere between a grape and a blueberry) – get their purple colour from good-for-you phytonutrients, including polysterols and anthocyanins. In fact, acai packs more antioxidants than cranberries, raspberries, blackberries, strawberries or blueberries (but eat acai in moderation and don't take it in supplement form, since its safety in pregnancy hasn't been studied). Other purple produce to colour your world with: purple asparagus, purple carrots, purple figs, purple cauliflower, purple Brussels sprouts, purple peppers, purple potatoes and purple sweet potatoes.

- White. They're not exactly colourful, but don't overlook paler fruits and vegetables. Garlic, onions, shallots, spring onions and leeks contain compounds that protect DNA. Cauliflower contains a hearty dose of vitamin C, manganese and phytonutrients (including antioxidants). And chicory, mushrooms (particularly wild varieties), celery and pears are rich in flavonoids (another phytonutrient) that protect cell membranes. You can't go wrong with that, baby!

What about organic? Is the heftier price tag that comes with the organic designation worth it? Does organic produce have an edge nutritionally? The latest research indicates that organic crops do not have higher levels of most vitamins compared with conventionally grown produce, though they do have substantially higher concentrations of antioxidants and phytonutrients. But let's face it – most people don't buy organic fruits and vegetables for their nutritional content, especially when that content doesn't always offer significant differences. They shop for organic produce because of what it doesn't contain: pesticides and chemicals . . . a definite plus, since the pesticides and chemicals

Spotting Organic

It's easy to spot an organic product – just look for the word 'organic' on the packaging or sticker. There is often also a logo if the supplier follows a specific organisation's rules. The words 'Organic Soil Association' (the largest UK organisation) appears in their logo (there are Celtic and Welsh versions).The EU 'green leaf' logo is on organic food sold by or to EU countries.

you consume through your diet are shared with your baby both in the uterus and through breast milk. And while taste isn't usually directly impacted by how produce is grown, organic fruits and vegetables are usually fresher than conventional when they hit the market. That's because they're more perishable and must be rushed to the market within days (conventional produce can tough it out during long stays in warehouses).

With that in mind, if organic products are available locally and you can afford the premium price, make it your choice – just keep in mind as you load up your shopping trolley that organic produce will have a much shorter shelf life than conventional. If price is an object, pick organic selectively (see the box on the previous page). And remember: while organic produce won't be contaminated with pesticides, it could – like any produce – be contaminated with bacteria. That's why thorough washing is a step you shouldn't skip just because you've sprung for organic. In other words, no nibbling on those farmers market blueberries before they've been brought home for a thorough rinse. And of course washing or peeling conventional produce can eliminate or greatly decrease pesticide residue. Remember,

too, that what you eat overall matters more than whether you're eating conventional or organic foods. The benefits of eating more (even conventional) fruits and vegetables will outweigh the possible risks from pesticide exposure.

For more information on the UK's organic food labelling rules see www.gov.uk/guidance/organic-food-labelling-rules. Wondering about genetically modified produce? See the box on page 65 for the lowdown.

Wholegrains

Finding wholegrain wheat bread in the bakery department is as easy as scanning the shelf for bread and buns labelled 'wheat', right? Not exactly. Wheat (or oat, or sweetcorn) specifies only the type of grain, not whether it's whole. Instead, look for the 'wholemeal' banner on the packaging (or 'brown'), and also make sure that the first ingredient is 'wholemeal wheat flour'. Take a closer look when you see a product tagged 'multigrain' or 'granary' – this lets you know only that it contains multiple grains, not necessarily wholegrains. Some breads also include seeds, but even these don't necessarily include wholegrains. Check the ingredients list to see whether all (or any) of the featured grains are actually wholegrain.

The same rules apply to cereals and other grain products as well. Read up on your favourite cereals to ensure that the 'oat' cereal you're buying is made from 'wholegrain oats', not just 'oats'.

The following glossary should help you in the screening process:

- 'Wheat flour', 'fortified wheat flour' or 'white flour' isn't wholegrain wheat. It means the flour is made by grinding wheat and typically does not contain the bran or germ, only the endosperm. It must, by law, be enriched with some of the nutrients

Prefer White?

Not a wholehearted fan of wholemeal bread? Wheat flours in the UK are ground from white wheat, a grain that has a mild, sweet taste, made all the more milder in white bread if it's been refined. However, there may be something on the supermarket aisles just for you. Some bread manufacturers have produced white loaves that include either a percentage of wholemeal flour or that have added wheatgerm. So if you're a staunch white bread fan, try compromising by choosing these loaves – they offer some of the better nutritional benefits found in regular wholemeal bread but with that just-like-white taste. Baking your own? Trying adding some wholemeal flour or wheatgerm to boost the nutrtional value of your white bread.

that have been lost during the refining process.

- 'Wholemeal' is flour in which the whole wheat is ground, so you get the nutrients from all three parts of wheat: the endosperm, germ and bran. Look, too, for whole oat, whole barley and whole rye flour for a whole lot of naturally occurring nutrition.

- 'Wholemeal bread' can be used on a label only if all the flour used in the bread is wholemeal flour.

- 'Milled' (for instance, 'milled corn') sounds promisingly wholesome, but is actually often a sign that the grain is refined.

- 'Stoneground flour' describes merely how the wheat grain (without the bran or germ) was milled. Whether it was ground by stones or machines, it's still refined if it doesn't specify 'whole'.

- 'Wheatgerm' can appear on a label only if at least 10 per cent of the dry ingredients includes wheatgerm.

Pasta That Packs in Protein

Back off, beef. Step aside, poultry and pork. There's a new protein source in town: pasta made from legumes (pulses). Made from chickpeas, lentils, black beans and more, and available in a variety of shapes – from spaghetti to penne – these pastas are super-high in protein, fibre and iron, lower in carbohydrates (making them the perfect pasta for diabetics or those at risk for gestational diabetes), and often gluten-free. The texture is a little different from grain-based pasta, but it's close enough to pass (just make sure you don't overcook it). Toss a legume-based linguine with a pasta sauce, penne with broccoli and cheese, or (if you're feeling the meat love after all) spaghetti with meatballs.

Looking for rice that's nice and high in protein, plus grain-free? Look to chickpea rice (you'll find it in the rice aisle in health-food shops).

CHAPTER 5

Shelved for Two

....

N ow you know what to eat when you're expecting. But what about all the foods and drinks you shouldn't be consuming . . . or should be limiting? The ones that are off-limits entirely? The ones that are considered safe when they're cooked but are red-lighted when raw? The ones that are questionable, and the ones you have questions about? Happily, most foods and drinks can find their place on a mum-to-be's menu. But it's always best to play it safe when you're playing for two, so you'll also need to know which foods and beverages should be shelved during your nine months and which can safely appear on your table in moderation. This chapter will clue you in on what should be off the menu when you're expecting.

What to Limit When You're Expecting

B racing for the bad news about your morning coffee? Or your tea for two? Or maybe concerns about chemicals in your pregnancy diet have you second-guessing your Splenda, passing up ingredients you can't pronounce or fearing fish? There's really more good news than you might think: many of the foods and drinks you love (but may be worrying about consuming now that you're expecting) are safe to consume, especially in moderation. Here's the lowdown on what to limit.

Coffee

M aybe you're the type who can't get through the day without a cup of coffee by your side (in a bottomless mug). Maybe a cup or two will see you through, at least on most days. Maybe it's not the pick-me-up you need, but the creamy deliciousness of that caramel macchiato that you crave . . . at least twice a day. Or maybe you're somewhere in between. No matter where you land on the caffeine map – or if you're all over

Caffeine Counts

You'd be surprised at how quickly the caffeine adds up even when coffee's not on the menu. Caffeine hides not only in coffee, but also in caffeinated soft drinks (too many Diet Cokes are a pregnancy don't), coffee ice cream and yogurt, many varieties of tea, energy bars and drinks, and chocolate (the darker the chocolate, the more caffeine it packs). Here's the approximate amount of caffeine you can expect to find in some of your favourites:

- 1 cup brewed coffee (240 ml) = 135 mg
- 1 cup instant coffee = 95 mg
- 1 cup decaf coffee = 5 to 30 mg
- 1 shot espresso (or any drink made with 1 shot) = 90 mg
- 1 cup tea = 40 to 60 mg (green tea has less caffeine than black tea)
- 1 cup matcha = 70 mg
- 1 can cola (350 ml) = about 35 mg
- 1 can diet cola = 45 mg
- 1 can energy drink = 50 to 350 mg
- 28 g milk chocolate = 6 mg
- 28 g dark chocolate = 20 mg
- 240 ml chocolate milk = 5 mg
- 65 g coffee ice cream = 20 to 40 mg

the map, depending on the day you're having or how much sleep you got the night before – you're probably wondering if you'll have to cut out coffee altogether now that you're expecting.

Well, java lovers (and cravers of caffeine in other forms), get ready to rejoice – in moderation. Most evidence suggests that drinking up to about 200 mg of caffeine a day is perfectly safe for your little bean. What does that break down to exactly? Possibly not as much as you'd hope – about 350 ml of brewed coffee (two small cups or one 'tall') or about two shots of espresso. Drink more, however, and there's less cause for celebration. Heavy caffeine intake (more than five cups of coffee a day) has been linked to miscarriage.

Other reasons to stick to the recommended limit? For one, too much caffeine can irritate your bladder, which may step up the number of those already-too-frequent trips you make to the toilet and possibly lead to urinary

tract infections. It can also irritate your emotions – exacerbating normal pregnancy mood swings and preventing you getting the rest you need (especially when you drink it after noon). As if all that's not enough, caffeine interferes with your body's ability to absorb iron that both you and your baby need. And here's a potential downside to high consumption of caffeine that you probably wouldn't expect: research has found that an intake of 300 mg or more per day may be linked to a baby growing too big and too fast during his or her first year, and to an increased risk of being overweight throughout the toddler years and beyond.

The conclusion: there's no need to cut coffee out of your life entirely when you're expecting (unless you really want to) – as long as you stick to the recommended 200 mg per day. One to two cups of coffee doesn't satisfy? You can stretch the two into three or more by adding more milk to each cup

Energy in a Can?

Looking for a pick-me-up now that pregnancy fatigue's got you down? Wondering whether a jolt from one of the many energy drinks lining supermarket shelves may be just the ticket? Well, think (and read the labels) before you drink. Though a jolt-in-a-can energy drink might pick you up briefly, that blood-sugar high will be followed by a free-falling crash, leaving you dragging more than ever. Plus, many canned energy drinks may contain dietary supplements that aren't safe for pregnancy use, as well as a whopping amount of caffeine. So pass on the cans, and seek your energy boost the natural way instead (see page 125).

(you'll get a calcium bonus) or by ordering decaf every so often. Need tips for cutting back on caffeine? See *What to Expect When You're Expecting.*

Prefer to get your caffeine kick from an endless stream of Diet Coke? See the box on the opposite page for a caffeine breakdown of your favourite beverage.

Herbal Tea

Had an extra long day? Feel like curling up on the sofa with a good book and a steaming cup of herbal tea? Before you reach for those herbal tea leaves, it's wise to read them – or at least the packaging they come in. The effects of herbs in pregnancy have not been well researched, and until more is known, the advice is that pregnant (and breastfeeding) women should use herbal teas with caution. Another reason why it's smart to proceed with caution when contemplating a cup of herbal tea? Because herbal products manufactured outside the UK may not be regulated, some herbal blends may contain contaminants or ingredients that aren't listed on the label. Some brews that sound like they're fruit- or spice-based (with names like 'Lemon Ginger' or 'Orange Spice') may actually be blended with herbs (another case for being a careful label reader).

How can you tell if you're brewing up trouble with your tea? It's actually not that easy, even if you're a label reader. While some herbal teas are probably safe in moderate doses, there's no scientific consensus on which ones are, which ones aren't and what 'moderate' means. You can ask your healthcare provider for

Herbs You Don't Have to Curb

Think no-go when you think herbs during pregnancy? That depends on what kind of herbs you're thinking. Medicinal herbs (like all drugs) should not be taken (or in the case of herbal tea, drunk) without the advice of a healthcare provider who knows that you're pregnant. Parsley, sage, rosemary and thyme? They – along with other culinary herbs, from that basil and dill to that coriander and mint – are entirely safe to eat. And they add not only flavour, but also nutrients. Basil, for instance, packs in vitamin A, vitamin K, lutein and zeaxanthin, among other essential vitamins and minerals. So chop some fresh basil and parsley into your spaghetti sauce, toss your cucumbers with coriander and mint, stuff your chicken breasts with sage, and go rosemary, baby.

a list of which teas to enjoy and which to avoid, or you can play it extra safe by sticking to regular (black) tea that comes flavoured, or adding any of the following to boiling water or regular tea: slices of fruit (lemon, orange, apple, pear); fruit juice; mint leaves; cinnamon; nutmeg; cloves; or ginger (an effective calmer of queasy tummies). And (of course) never brew up homemade tea from a plant growing in your garden unless you're absolutely certain what it is and that it's safe for use during pregnancy.

Keen for an easier labour, or impatient for one that's overdue to begin with? Then you may have heard that raspberry leaf or black or blue cohosh can fast-track your trip to the birthing room. See the box on page 141 to find out if there's truth to that tea tale.

Green Tea

It's long been touted for its health benefits. But the jury's still out on whether green tea gets the green light during pregnancy. That's because green tea can decrease the effectiveness of folic acid, that vital pregnancy vitamin. If you're a green-tea drinker, drink it in moderation, and ask your healthcare provider for a specific recommendation.

Matcha – ground green tea leaves in a powder form – is known for its antioxidants and anti-inflammatory properties. It can be used to make tea, sprinkled into smoothies, or mixed into biscuits and other bakes. But again, because green tea in large amounts can decrease the effectiveness of folic acid, and because you're using the leaves themselves (instead of merely steeping green-tea leaves in water and then discarding), causing you to consume a larger dose of the active ingredients of green tea, you'll want to drink matcha in moderation when you're pregnant.

Another reason to moderate your matcha: One 240-ml cup of matcha has about 70 mg of caffeine, a little over one-third of the daily limit for caffeine intake during pregnancy.

Fish

It's an excellent source of lean protein, baby-brain-boosting omega-3 fats, and vitamins D and B_{12}, plus a host of healthy minerals, from iron and iodine to selenium and zinc – all good reasons to keep fish (and other seafood) on your pregnancy menu, or even to consider adding it if you've never been a fish fan before. In fact, experts agree that pregnant and breastfeeding women should aim to eat two portions of fish a week, one of which should be an oily fish. You can safely eat cooked or smoked fish, cooked shellfish, cold pre-cooked prawns and, if the fish was previously frozen, raw or lightly cooked fish in sushi. But avoid raw shellfish, which may have bacteria, viruses or toxins that can give you food poisoning.

So go fish, by all means. But when you're casting your net at the seafood department, be sure to fish selectively, sticking to those varieties that are lower in mercury – a chemical that in large, accumulated doses may be harmful to a foetus's developing nervous system. For this reason, the NHS recommends eating no more that two portions of oily fish within a week and no more than two tuna steaks (about 140 g cooked or 170 g raw) a week or four 140-g (drained weight) tins of tuna a week. Tuna is not considered an oily fish, so you can eat two portions of oily fish along with the recommended amount of tuna.

According to recommended guidelines from the UK and the USA (in case you plan to travel there), during pregnancy and lactation, you should:

> **CHEW ON THIS.** In Nigeria, lore has it that eating snails during pregnancy can make your baby sluggish. In other words, that escargot may end up being more like escar-not-go. Sounds fishy.

EAT UP *(two servings per week)*

- Anchovy
- Butterfish
- Catfish
- Clams
- Cod
- Crab
- Crawfish
- Eel
- Gurnard
- Haddock
- Hake
- Herring
- Kippers
- Langoustine
- Lobster
- Mackerel (but not king mackerel)
- Mullet
- Oyster
- Perch (freshwater and ocean)
- Pickerel
- Pilchards
- Plaice/flounder
- Pollack/pollock
- Prawns/shrimp
- Salmon
- Sardines
- Scallops
- Sea bass
- Shad
- Skate
- Smelt
- Sole
- Squid
- Tilapia
- Trout (freshwater)
- Tuna, tinned
- Whitefish
- Whiting

EAT IN MODERATION
(no more than one serving a week)

- Bluefish
- Buffalofish
- Carp
- Chilean sea bass/Patagonian toothfish
- Grouper
- Halibut
- Mahi-mahi/dolphinfish
- Monkfish
- Rockfish
- Sablefish
- Sheepshead
- Snapper
- Striped ocean bass
- Atlantic tilefish
- Weakfish/sea trout

- White croaker/Pacific croaker
- Fish caught recreationally: limit to one serving a week and don't eat other fish that week

AVOID ENTIRELY

- Bigeye tuna steaks
- King mackerel
- Marlin
- Orange roughy (overseas)
- Raw shellfish
- Shark
- Swordfish
- Tilefish (from the Gulf of Mexico)

Sugar Substitutes

Hoping to spare those empty sugar calories by choosing an artificial sweetener? Sugar substitutes are a mixed bag when you're expecting – not only when it comes to their composition (some are straight-up chemical compounds, others are derived from natural sources but processed in a lab), but also to their calorie content and the way they're metabolised. Though most are considered safe, others should probably be consumed with a side of caution. Here's what's known about the most popular sugar substitutes so far:

Sucralose (Splenda). Made from sugar, but chemically converted to a form that's not absorbable by the body, sucralose appears to be the best bet safety-wise for pregnant women seeking sweetness with no calories and little aftertaste. Sweeten your coffee, tea, yogurt and smoothies with it if you want, or use foods and drinks presweetened with it. It's also stable for cooking and baking (unlike aspartame), making that sugar-free chocolate cake less pipe dream, more possibility.

Still, moderation is probably smart, even with sucralose.

Aspartame (Equal, NutraSweet). The research jury's still out on this zero-calorie artificial sweetener. Many in the medical profession consider it harmless and will okay light or moderate use in pregnancy. However it's recommended that mums-to-be limit consumption. A packet or two of the blue stuff now and then, a can of Diet Coke every once in a while – no problem. Just avoid consuming aspartame in large amounts during pregnancy. Women with PKU – phenylketonuria – must limit their intake of phenylalanine and are generally advised not to use aspartame.

Saccharin (Sweet'N Low). While saccharin has been deemed safe, some studies suggest that this zero-calorie artificial sweetener reaches the placenta and that when it does, it's slow to leave. For that reason, you might want to stay away from the pink packets – or pick them up only occasionally. Don't worry, however, about saccharin you had before finding out that you're pregnant, since the risks, if any, are extremely slight.

Acesulfame-K (Sunett). This artificial sweetener, 200 times sweeter than sugar, is approved for use in bakes, gelatin desserts, chewing gum and soft drinks. It's considered okay to use in moderation during pregnancy, but since few studies have been done to prove its safety, ask your healthcare provider for guidelines before gobbling the stuff up.

Sorbitol. This 'sugar alcohol' is found naturally in many fruits and berries, but its life as a commercial sweetener usually begins as corn syrup that undergoes chemical conversion in the lab. With half the sweetness of sugar (but more calories than most sugar substitutes), it is used in a wide range of foods and beverages and is safe for use in pregnancy in moderate amounts. But it does present a problem in large doses: too much can cause bloating, painful wind and diarrhoea – a digestive trio no pregnant woman needs.

Mannitol. Less sweet than sugar, mannitol is another form of sugar alcohol that is poorly absorbed by the body. Like sorbitol, it contains fewer calories than sugar but more than most sugar substitutes. Mannitol is also considered safe in modest amounts, but large quantities can cause diarrhoea.

Xylitol. A sugar alcohol derived from plants, xylitol can be found in chewing gum, toothpaste, sweets and some foods. Considered safe during pregnancy in moderate amounts, it has 40 per cent fewer calories than sugar (still 10 calories per teaspoon) and has been shown to prevent tooth decay – a good reason to chew xylitol-sweetened gum after meals and snacks when you can't brush.

Erythritol (Swerve). This sweetener is a fermented sugar alcohol that's found in grapes and pears. It has nearly zero calories, is about 70 per cent as sweet as table sugar and can be used in cooking and baking. Studies have shown that this sweetener, like xylitol, also prevents tooth decay. Erythritol is probably safe when you're expecting, but check with your healthcare provider before you reach for it, since there is limited data on its use during pregnancy.

Stevia (SweetLeaf, Truvia). This zero-calorie sweetener is made from erythritol and the leaf of the stevia plant. Though it's far sweeter than sugar (so you'll have to adjust the amount you use in cooking and baking), it can have a bitter aftertaste. Stevia is believed to be safe during pregnancy, but check with

your healthcare provider before you dip deeply (again, there's little data on it).

There are plenty of natural sugar substitutes hitting the market (and your coffee) as well. Monk-fruit sweetener (sometimes found in blends with erythritol), BochaSweet, allulose, lactose, Whey Low, agave and many others are probably safe for use during pregnancy (most are derived from fruits or vegetables), but it doesn't hurt to ask your healthcare provider for the green light . . . just in case. And asking your doctor or dietitian about these sweeteners (and others) is also wise if you have gestational diabetes. Some (such as allulose) are calorie-free, while others (such as agave) contain even more calories than sugar.

Some Health Foods

Are health foods extra healthy when you're expecting – and super foods extra super? Most probably are – but as in so many other departments, it's smart to proceed with caution down the health-food aisle, browsing this list before you browse those shelves:

Linseeds. There seems to be a health benefit for everyone in linseeds (also called flaxseeds) and products made from them, with research linking consumption to a lower risk of diabetes, heart disease and cancer. And their high level of baby-friendly omega-3 fatty acids makes linseeds sound like a natural for expectant mums, too – and they probably are. But because they're also a source of phytoestrogens (an oestrogen-like substance found naturally in some plants), some healthcare providers recommend limiting the amount of linseeds expectant mums consume in oil, seed or supplement form. Others say moderate amounts (up to 4 to 6 tablespoons per

Safe Right from the Tap?

Some would say it's the best drink in the house (or the restaurant), especially because it's free. But is tap water safe to drink when you're expecting? Most often, it is. Still, water safety varies from community to community, home to home – and can even vary because of storms or other natural disasters (for instance, flooding can contaminate drinking water), a lapse in oversight or lax maintenance. To find out if you should be drinking the water that flows from your tap (or your community's taps, including those in your favourite restaurants), contact your local water supplier. If there is a possibility that your home or your community's water supply is unsafe (because of pipe deterioration, a contaminated water source, proximity to a waste disposal area, or because of odd taste or colour), ask your water supplier to test it – they should take a sample of your water and analyse it for you. Or contact your local council for advice.

If testing reveals that your water contains unsafe contaminants – or if your community has been alerted to system-wide issues – invest in a filter (the kind you get depends on what's in your water) or use bottled water or purified water delivery for drinking and cooking (keep reading for more on bottled water safety). Some potential contaminants: bacteria, microorganisms, chemical or industrial runoff and pesticides.

Of most concern when you're expecting – and when there are little ones drinking the water in your home and community – is lead, which can leach from lead pipes or be present in the water supply even if your pipes aren't made from lead. High levels of lead in your body can cause serious problems during pregnancy such as premature birth, low birthweight and

---

day) of linseeds blended in a smoothie or spooned into cereal, are safe and healthy during pregnancy. Unsure whether to reach for linseeds or in what amounts? Ask your healthcare provider.

Hemp. Hemp seeds, hemp food products and hemp seed oil in moderation (one to two servings a day) are probably safe for expectant mums – and a good source of protein, fibre and fatty acids. But since hemp's use during pregnancy has not been well studied, it makes sense to avoid it in large concentrations (as in a supplement). See the box on page 39 for info on hemp milk.

Chia. Chia seeds are an excellent source of fibre, omega-3 fatty acids, protein, calcium and iron – but while a sprinkle on a salad, yogurt or cereal, or in a smoothie is likely a safe and nutritious bet, ask your healthcare provider before you chow down on large amounts of chia. Its safety in pregnancy hasn't been studied.

Spirulina. The pregnancy safety of spirulina (a natural algae powder that's high in protein and calcium and a good source of antioxidants, B vitamins and other nutrients) also hasn't been established, leading some healthcare providers to suggest that mums-to-be limit or even avoid using this nutrient-packed powder. It's also sometimes contaminated with toxins, including heavy metals, as well as harmful bacteria – another reason to avoid it during pregnancy. Ditto for spirulina's close relative chlorella.

miscarriage. Lead will also cross the placenta and can impact the healthy development of your baby's brain and nervous system. Lead exposure during pregnancy and childhood has also been associated with reduced cognitive function, lower IQ and increased attention-related behavioural problems. If testing shows lead in your water, switch to bottled water or water that comes from a filtration system certified to reduce or eliminate lead for cooking, drinking and brushing your teeth. If you use water from a borehole on your property, the Environmental Health Department or your local authority are responsible for testing your water, which may be done for free or at cost. You do not have to tell your local authority if you have a private supply of water, but doing so will mean they can contact you if there's a pollution risk.

While there's no harm from the small amount of chlorine that's in your tap water (it acts as a disinfectant), the right kind of filter will remove chlorine before it reaches your cup. If your water smells and/or tastes like chlorine, boiling it or letting it stand, uncovered, for 24 hours will allow much of the chemical to evaporate.

Are you always better off – and safer – opening a bottle of water than turning on the tap? The reality is that bottled waters vary a lot too, depending on if it is natural mineral water or from a spring, with some brands containing more impurities than tap water, and some actually coming directly from a municipal supply before being purified. Also bear in mind that bottled water may contain lower levels of fluoride (fluoride levels will be on the label), a mineral that's vital for growing teeth (your baby's). Also look for bottles labelled 'BPA-free' that don't contain BPA, which is banned in baby bottles but may still be in plastic bottles. Avoid distilled water, since the distillation process removes all beneficial minerals.

Raw cacao powder. Made by cold-pressing unroasted cacao beans, raw cacao is high in antioxidants and minerals. Don't confuse it with cocoa powder, which is cacao that's been roasted at high temperatures, effectively killing all the natural enzymes found in the cacao bean. But is mixing it into your morning smoothie or nibbling on cacao nibs safe during pregnancy? While dark chocolate is safe – and even beneficial – during pregnancy, it's less clear whether raw cacao, which contains much higher levels of caffeine and theobromine (a stimulant), is also safe. The jury is still out, but most experts would suggest a path of moderation when it comes to nibbling on those nibs – especially because roasting cacao beans is what destroys harmful bacteria, leaving the raw version susceptible to bacteria and other types of contamination.

Wheatgrass. Wheatgrass doesn't get a pregnancy pass – not only because there's no proof that it's safe during pregnancy, but because it can be contaminated with bacteria.

Maca. Maca powder may be touted as a fertility enhancer, but without any studies to show its safety during pregnancy, experts say it's best to avoid when you're expecting.

Moringa. This purported super food comes from a plant native to Africa and India. It's packed with nutrients, but because it acts as a natural form of birth control and may cause the uterus to contract (which could lead to miscarriage), moringa in all forms should be avoided completely during pregnancy.

Already tossed back a few wheatgrass shots or sucked down some spirulina shakes? Not to worry – the potential risks (besides bacterial infection, but you'd know if you'd developed one of those) haven't been proved, and probably wouldn't apply to average intake anyway.

Some Chemicals

Do you usually run for cover at the mention of the word 'chemical'? If so, you might want to sit back down and continue reading. Not every food that lists chemicals on its ingredients list is necessarily bad (or dangerous) for you, just as not every food that doesn't list any is automatically safe and healthy.

But first, a chemistry lesson. All foods, from garden-variety tomatoes to laboratory-variety tomato-flavoured sauces, are made of chemicals. A just-picked, organically grown strawberry, for instance, is composed of (among other chemicals) pelargonidin 3-glucoside, citric acid, malic acid, ellagic acid, auxin, methyl butanoate, ethyl butanoate, butyl ethanoate, methyl hexanoate, ethyl hexanoate, (Z)-3-hexenol, hexanal, (E)-2-hexenal and (Z)-3-hexenal. How's that for a chemical profile?

Chemical additives found in processed foods are synthesised in the lab from a variety of organic and inorganic

materials, or extracted from completely natural sources (sodium caseinate from milk, lecithin from soya beans). Some are suspected of being harmful (those that are indisputably proved to be harmful are taken off the market). But the good news is that more are believed to be harmless – and some are even beneficial such as the chemical ascorbic acid, otherwise known as vitamin C. From what is known right now, potential risk to a developing foetus from chemical additives in the average diet is extremely remote.

Still, many processed foods are far from nutritious – and typically, the greater the number of unpronounceable additives a product contains, the less wholesome it is. Bear that in mind when selecting processed foods. Whenever possible, cook from scratch with fresh ingredients, or use frozen or organic ready-prepared foods. You'll avoid many questionable additives found in processed foods, and your meals will be more nutritious, too. Whenever you have a choice (and clearly you won't always), choose foods that are free of artificial additives (colourings, flavourings and preservatives). Read labels to screen for foods that are either additive-free or use natural additives (a Cheddar cheese cracker that gets its orange hue from annatto instead of red dye no. 40, and its flavour from real cheese instead of artificial cheese flavouring). For a listing of questionable and safe additives, go to www.food.gov.uk/business-guidance/approved-additives-and-e-numbers.

What to Omit When You're Expecting

It's only nine months, but when you're kept apart from your favourite foods and drinks, it can seem like forever (and

at least a day). Even when you know that your sacrifice is in the name of a safe pregnancy played extra safe. Even

Wine in Dinner?

Hungry for some coq au vin or beer-braised short ribs, but not sure whether the pregnancy alcohol ban carries over from the bar to the cooker? Feast away, within reason. Although alcohol does not cook out completely when you add it to a stew or baked dish (the amount of alcohol that actually cooks off depends on how long the food has been cooked; keep reading), the alcohol that remains will not add up to much in the context of a single serving. So unless you're planning to sip almost a litre of sauced sauce, you've got nothing to worry about. To be safe, stick to recipes that require cooking times of at least half an hour, avoiding those that expose the alcohol to only passing heat (such as flambéed cherries), or choose alcohol substitutions in your recipes instead (see the box on page 80).

IF YOU BAKE OR SIMMER FOR	THE AMOUNT OF ALCOHOL REMAINING IS
15 minutes	40 per cent
30 minutes	35 per cent
1 hour	25 per cent
1½ hours	20 per cent
2 hours	10 per cent
2½ hours	5 per cent

when you're all in (if not super happy about) giving up what you shouldn't have. Hopefully, you won't find too many of your favourites on this list of foods and drinks that are shelved when you're expecting, but chances are (sorry!) you'll find a few.

Alcohol

Wine with dinner? Cocktail before-hand? Beer at the barbecue? As you probably already know, total tee-totalling during pregnancy is recommended not only by doctors, midwives and all health organisations, but also by the UK government (in the form of labels plastered on all containers of wine, beer and other alcoholic beverages). And for good reason. Alcohol crosses the placenta in concentrations almost identical to those in the mother's blood – which means she shares each drink with her baby, and due to baby's tiny size, a higher share proportionately. What's more, it takes a foetus twice as long to eliminate the alcohol from its system. Drinking heavily throughout pregnancy or binge drinking (having four or more drinks at a time, even occasionally) can result not only in serious complications of pregnancy, but in foetal alcohol syndrome. This condition produces babies who are born small for gestational age, with facial deformities and with brain damage (which later shows up as tremors, motor development problems, attention deficits, learning disabilities, lower IQ and possibly other mental deficiencies). But even drinking moderately throughout pregnancy can increase the risk of miscarriage and stillbirth, as well as the risk of developmental and behavioural problems in a child.

Since no 'safe' limit of alcohol consumption has been determined – and even occasional light drinking hasn't been completely cleared – you're definitely safest staying on the wagon during your nine months.

Standing in for the Sauce

Is your kitchen an alcohol-free zone now that you're expecting? Here are some ways to stir comparable flavour into your favourite recipes, without the sauce:

INSTEAD OF	TRY
Amaretto (2 tablespoons)	Almond extract (½ teaspoon)
Beer	Ginger ale or chicken stock
Brandy	Pressed apple juice, apricot juice
Calvados	Pressed apple juice
Champagne	Ginger ale or sparkling white grape juice
Cognac	Peach, apricot or pear juice
Dry red wine	Grape or cranberry juice (cut the sweetness with red wine vinegar), or beef stock
Framboise	Raspberry juice
Cassis	Cherry, blueberry or pomegranate juice
Frangelico	Hazelnut or almond extract
Grand Marnier	Orange juice or orange marmalade
Kirsch	Raspberry or cherry juice or pressed apple juice
Port wine (or sweet sherry)	Grape or pomegranate juice
Rum	White grape juice or pineapple juice
Sake	Seasoned rice vinegar
Sherry or bourbon	Vanilla extract or orange or pineapple juice
Vermouth (sweet)	Apple or grape juice
Vermouth (dry)	White grape juice mixed with white wine vinegar
White wine	Chicken stock, diluted cider vinegar or white wine vinegar

Which doesn't mean that you should worry about the wine, beer or cocktails you drank before you found out you were expecting. What it does mean is that you should give up alcohol the moment you know you're pregnant (in the best of all possible pregnancy scenarios, you'd give it up when you first start trying to conceive). If you decide to take a very occasional celebratory sip or two, do so with food, which slows the absorption of alcohol into the system. For tips on giving up alcohol, see *What to Expect When You're Expecting*.

Raw Fish and Seafood

You probably knew this was coming – and if you're a raw seafood fan, you've probably already sighed deeply (maybe even cried a little) over the loss of your sushi and oyster bar privileges. Off the menu during pregnancy according to the NHS and leading medical authorities: all raw or rare fish – unless first frozen – and seafood. That includes sashimi and sushi rolls that contain raw fish, fish tartare, carpaccio or crudo, raw oysters, clams and other seafood, as well as any fish or seafood that's served 'seared' or 'rare' but not cooked through (as salmon, tuna and scallops often are). Why this rule? It's to protect pregnant women from bacteria, viruses, parasites and other microscopic organisms that can cause infections, from food poisoning to hepatitis, if they're not killed by thorough cooking (and yes, anyone can get sick from eating raw fish or seafood, but pregnant women are at extra risk when they do). Marinating fish and seafood (say, in ceviche or poke) or dipping it in even the hottest of hot sauce doesn't kill those organisms, so those preps don't offer protection. Even pregnancy-safe varieties of fish (see page 72) should be cooked until they easily flake with a fork and reach the appropriate temperature (63°C). Seafood should be cooked through and firm.

Smoked and Cured Fish

Refrigerated smoked seafood – such as salmon, trout, whitefish, cod, tuna or mackerel – most often labelled as 'kippers', 'smoked', 'nova-style', 'lox' or 'jerky' – are also off the menu when you're expecting, because they can harbor the pregnancy-dangerous bacteria Listeria. Ditto, salt-cured fish (aka gravlax), pickled fish or cured fish that isn't

Champagne Dreams and Caviar Wishes

Champagne is definitely off the menu when you're expecting, but what about caviar? As with raw fish, there's a risk that caviar may be contaminated with Listeria. You can avoid that risk by choosing pasteurised caviar.

cooked or heated to a high enough temperature to kill Listeria (63°C). Happily, you can cook away bacterial risk in a piping-hot casserole, quiche or omelette. You can also safely serve up tinned or bottled shelf-stable smoked fish and seafood, as well as fish that's cooked thoroughly to the proper temperature while it is being smoked (grilled or baked with smoke chips or on a wood plank).

Unpasteurised/Raw Dairy Products

Pasteurisation is a form of food processing that's actually good for you and your baby, safely destroying bacteria in dairy products and some juices without destroying nutrients. And it comes in handy when it comes to certain soft cheeses – fresh mozzarella, feta, Brie, blue cheese, Camembert, soft Mexican-style cheese – since these can be contaminated with Listeria, a dangerous bacteria (see the box on the following page). If you see a hunk of cheese that doesn't say 'pasteurised' on the label, pass it by. All varieties of cheese are pasteurised if sold in UK supermarkets or shops – raw dairy produce is only allowed to be sold directly from the farmer in the UK. If you're not sure if

Listeria Alert

What's this you hear about eating your sandwich meats hot now that you're pregnant? And skipping the locally produced cheese in your salad (unless you're positive it's pasteurised)? And cooking your smoked fish? These pregnancy diet restrictions may seem random – and unfair – but they're actually designed to protect you and your unborn baby from Listeria, a harmful bacteria that can cause listeriosis. This serious illness is particularly dangerous for pregnant women, for a couple of reasons. One, because expectant mums are about 20 times more likely than other healthy adults to contract listeriosis, due to the normal immune suppression of pregnancy. And two, because listeriosis can lead to premature delivery, miscarriage or serious illness in a developing baby. And, unlike other bacteria, Listeria enters the bloodstream directly and can get to the baby quickly. Though the overall risk of contracting listeriosis is extremely low – even in pregnancy – the potential of it causing problems in pregnancy is higher, which is why you should avoid unpasteurised juice, unpasteurised dairy, raw or undercooked meat, fish, shellfish, poultry or eggs, unheated sandwich meats or smoked fish, and unwashed raw vegetables and salad.

For more information on what's to eat during pregnancy, ask your healthcare provider or visit www.nhs. uk/conditions/pregnancy-and-baby/ healthy-pregnancy-diet/.

a soft cheese is pasteurised when travelling, don't eat it unless it's cooked until bubbling. All pasteurised dairy products are safe to eat when you're expecting – including mozzarella, feta, blue or Brie. Processed cheeses, cream cheese, cottage cheese and yogurt are also safe – if not made from raw milk. What about hard cheeses such as Parmesan? Due to their much lower moisture content, hard cheeses are far less likely to be contaminated with Listeria, even if made with raw milk. Still, with so many pasteurised cheeses available, why take any risk?

Raw Eggs

Feeling uneasy about your runny egg yolks? Wondering whether it's safe to poach a taste of your partner's eggs Benedict at brunch? You'd been wise to be wary in the past, when raw and undercooked eggs could be contaminated with salmonella. Today, as long as there's a British Lion stamp on the eggs, you can safely eat eggs, even if raw or partially cooked, including ready-prepared foods made with raw egg. Restaurants should also be using British Lion stamped eggs in their recipes, too – but to be safe get the all-clear from the kitchen before sampling the house Caesar or hollandaise.

If eggs do not have a British Lion stamp – because they're from a local farm or your own chickens or because you're travelling overseas – it's best to eat only fully cooked eggs and avoid eating them in all forms raw and runny: soft poached, fried with runny yolks, soft boiled. Skip raw eggs in salad dressings (try one of the Caesar salad dressing recipes on page 263 instead of a traditional one). And don't eat homemade foods that contain raw eggs, including ice cream, mayonnaise, hollandaise, eggnog, biscuit dough and cake batter – even if it's finger-licking good. Same for whipped-up desserts that won't be cooked (like mousse). Also avoid eggs

Try These Instead

What happens if your pregnancy cravings get in the way of sensible and safe eating? Not to worry. There are many ways to safely satisfy those yearnings – even when they're for foods you're supposed to be steering clear of. Try these sensible substitutions:

INSTEAD OF	TRY
Sushi with raw fish	Rolls made with cooked fish or vegetables
Raw shellfish	Steamed or boiled shellfish
Swordfish	Roasted or grilled halibut
Deli turkey	Fresh roasted turkey
Salad dressing with raw eggs	Substitute mayo or avocado or use pasteurised eggs in the dressing
Raw sprouts	Shaved carrots or cucumbers
Ready-prepared freshly squeezed juice (unpasteurised)	Juice squeezed or juiced at home

from ducks, geese and quails unless they are completely cooked with solid whites and yolks.

Raw or Rare Meats

Sorry, rare-meat lovers – it's time to change your order to well-done (with no traces of pink or blood). That's because undercooked meats can harbour microorganisms that can make you sick. Any raw meat, including tartare and carpaccio, is considered unsafe during pregnancy. Smoked meat is also considered unsafe (see below). See page 183 for more info on safe meat prep.

Cold Meats

Ready-to-eat doesn't always mean safe-to-eat when you're expecting. Case in point: all cold cured meats – salami, sausages, prosciutto,

pepperoni, chorizo and paté – and other charcuterie should be heated until steaming. That's to protect against the dangerous bacteria Listeria. Same goes for ready-to-eat sausage rolls (they're not ready for you to eat until you heat them up) and all types of smoked or cured (not cooked) meats. Even meat jerky may expose you to harmful bacteria unless it's heated first. Not loving the idea of hot sandwich meats or steaming jerky? Nobody does – but it's safer than going cold (smoked) turkey and risking infection. Fresh roasted meat (such as that fresh roasted turkey, fresh roast beef or pork loin) is safe to eat cold.

Another reason to steer clear of smoked or cured meats such as bacon, ham, cured pork, sausage, dried beef, luncheon meats, salami and hot dogs (as well as smoked fish): they often contain nitrates. Nitrates are used as a preservative in processed meats (actually keeping the amount of bacteria down). But

Now You Tell Me

Does this chapter have you stressed about all the things you'd have done differently if only you'd have known? Like sucking down that sake (and that huge plate of sashimi) two days before the pregnancy test came back positive? Ordering a cold meat-filled baguette before reading the section on cold meat risks? Tossing down a Caesar salad before realising the dressing was made with raw eggs?

Relax. Most women have at least a few expectant encounters with food or drink that isn't considered fit for pregnant consumption (especially before they find out they're expecting) – some have many. In the vast (very, very vast) majority of cases, there's no harm done. For instance, sushi and sashimi only rarely contain organisms that cause illness, ditto cold meats. So use this chapter as a guide to making your pregnancy diet as safe as you can make it from now on – but don't use it to drive yourself crazy about the food and drink that's already behind you.

they can be converted in your stomach to nitrites or nitrosamines, powerful carcinogens – something you don't want at any time during your life, and especially not when you're pregnant.

Raw Sprouts

Raw sprouts (including alfalfa, clover, radish and mung bean sprouts) may look pretty (and pretty healthy) on top of your salad or stuffed into your wrap,

but what's not pretty is the bacteria they may harbour. Sprouts have sometimes been linked to outbreaks of *E. coli*, Listeria and salmonella and, unfortunately, should be avoided when you're pregnant. So no sprouts for your little sprout when you're expecting. That is, unless you cook them through (and from a taste and texture perspective, hot sprouts aren't so hot). And while you're playing it safe on your salad or sandwich, it makes sense to stay away from microgreens, too, which may be cross-contaminated.

Raw Juice

Before you waddle up to the juice bar or apple juice stand – consider this: raw (unpasteurised) juice or drinks or smoothies made from it can be contaminated with bacteria such as Listeria (see the box on page 82) and should be off the menu when you're expecting. Make sure all the freshly made juice you drink is juice you squeezed or juiced yourself from washed produce.

Kombucha

Seems like everybody's sipping kombucha these days, but it's probably best for pregnant women to take a pass on this health-food trend. Kombucha, a fermented drink made with tea, sugar, bacteria and yeast, can cause stomach upset in some new drinkers, something no mum-to-be needs more of. Unpasteurised kombucha (particularly home-brewed varieties) can be contaminated with harmful bacteria. What's more, some kombuchas contain alcohol (clearly a no-go when you're expecting).

CHAPTER 6

Gaining for Two: Baby and You

M aybe you've spent half your life trying to lose weight – chasing a goal that you've never managed to reach. Or you've been happily hovering at about the same weight for years, give or take a few holiday pounds. Or you've yo-yoed your way up and down the scales, and have a wardrobe full of jean sizes to prove it. Or maybe you've always wished you could add a little more to your frame, especially around your bottom. Maybe you're at peace with your weight, maybe you fluctuate between embracing it and battling it.

Whatever your relationship with your weight, there's one thing for sure: it's time for change. Your weight, wherever it is, will likely be on the upswing now that you're expecting. A healthy weight gain is a key ingredient in the making of a healthy pregnancy and a healthy baby. So get ready to get gaining for two . . . baby and you.

How Much to Gain?

Are you fully over the moon at finally having a fully legit reason to pile on the pounds (you're pregnant!)? Or are you a bit unnerved at the thought of watching the numbers on the scales creep upward, even though you know they're supposed to? Or maybe you've never been a scale watcher, and plan to take pregnancy weight gain equally in your stride. You're probably still wondering just how much weight you should plan on gaining over the next nine months. After all, you've heard of women gaining as few as 9 kg and as many as 30 kg . . . or even more. What's the right gain plan for you?

Calculating Your BMI

Weight alone doesn't tell the whole story – for a better base-line assessment, your healthcare provider will also take a look at body mass index, or BMI. Your BMI is a calculation of your weight in relation to your height. When used alone it doesn't give a full picture of your actual body fat amount or overall fitness, but BMI is often used as a starting point for determining if a person is underweight, average weight, overweight or obese. Doctors and midwives use the measurement as the basis when monitoring your weight gain during pregnancy.

You can calculate your BMI using this formula in imperial: weight (in pounds) ÷ height (in inches squared)^2 × 703. (But remember 1 st = 14 lb and 1 ft = 12 in).

For example, a woman who is 5 ft 5 tall and weighs 10 st 5 lb will have a BMI of 24.1, based on the following equation:

First, figure out the inches:
5 feet 5 inches = 65 inches

Next, square 65 (multiply it by itself):
65 × 65 = 4,225 inches

Then divide the weight by the inches:
145 ÷ 4,225 = 0.0343

And multiply the result by 703:
0.0343 × 703 = 24.1

BMI (kg/m^2)	18	19	20	21	22	23	24	25	26	27	
Height (in)	Weight (lb)										
58	87	91	96	100	105	110	115	119	124	129	
59	90	94	99	104	109	114	119	124	128	133	
60	93	97	102	107	112	118	123	128	133	138	
61	96	100	106	111	116	122	127	132	137	143	
62	99	104	109	115	120	126	131	136	142	147	
63	102	107	113	118	124	130	135	141	146	152	
64	105	110	116	122	128	134	140	145	151	157	
65	109	114	120	126	132	138	144	150	156	162	
66	112	118	124	130	136	142	148	155	161	167	
67	115	121	127	134	140	146	153	159	166	172	
68	119	125	131	138	144	151	158	164	171	177	
69	122	128	135	142	149	155	162	169	176	182	
70	126	132	139	146	153	160	167	174	181	188	
71	130	136	143	150	157	165	172	179	186	193	
72	133	140	147	154	162	169	177	184	191	199	
73	137	144	151	159	166	174	182	189	197	204	
74	141	148	155	163	171	179	186	194	202	210	
75	145	152	160	168	176	184	192	200	208	216	
76	148	156	164	172	180	189	197	205	213	221	

Prefer metric? The formula is: weight (in kg) ÷ height (in m²).

Once you've calculated your BMI (or just check the imperial chart below), you can determine the category you fall into:

- If your BMI is less than 18.5, you're considered underweight.

- If your BMI is between 18.5 and 24.9, you're considered average weight.

- If your BMI is between 25 and 29.9, you're considered overweight.

- If your BMI is greater than 30, you're considered obese.

28	29	30	35	40
134	138	143	167	191
138	143	148	173	198
143	148	153	179	204
148	153	158	185	211
153	158	164	191	218
158	163	169	197	225
163	169	174	204	232
168	174	180	210	240
173	179	186	216	247
178	185	191	223	255
184	190	197	230	262
189	196	203	236	270
195	202	207	243	278
200	208	215	250	286
206	213	221	258	294
212	219	227	265	302
218	225	233	272	311
224	232	240	279	319
230	238	246	287	328

Since every pregnant woman – and every pregnancy – is different, one answer to that question doesn't fit all. Just how much weight you should put on during pregnancy depends on a number of factors, including your height and your weight before you conceived. Your healthcare provider may recommend an ideal weight gain, possibly based on your body mass index (BMI, see the box on these pages).

- If your BMI is average – or close enough – you'll probably be advised to gain between 25 and 35 lb (11–16 kg), the weight-gain total recommended for an average-weight pregnant woman.

- If your BMI is well below average, meaning that you're considerably underweight, you may be advised to gain a little – or a lot – extra, about 28–40 lb (13–18 kg), to compensate for the fat stores you don't have.

- If your BMI classifies you as overweight, you may be advised to gain between 15 and 25 lb (7–11 kg), because you'll have some extra fat stores to tap into.

- If you're obese, you may be told to limit your gain to about 11–20 lb (5–9 kg), or perhaps less. This may help you prevent some of the pregnancy complications related to obesity such as gestational diabetes or having a too-big baby.

- Got twins (or more) on board? The weight recommendations differ for you. See page 101 for more.

Ideal recommendations aside, how much you actually gain – and how quickly you gain it – will depend on your metabolism, a bit on genetics, your level of activity and, of course, how many calories you consume. Take in more calories than your body needs to fuel baby making and other activities (like exercise), and you'll likely gain more than recommended. Take in too few calories (or burn too many through exercise), and you'll gain less weight than you should. More about those weight-gain equations – and how to help get yours to add up in your favour and your baby's – later.

Gaining Weight at the Right Rate

Now you know about how much weight you should plan to gain over the next nine months. But how quickly should you plan to gain it? A little at a time? In bigger chunks? Does it really matter how fast or slowly you pack on the pounds if you end up packing on just the right number?

Actually, it does matter. Slow and steady wins the pregnancy weight-gain race hands down, and here's why. For your baby, who's constantly growing, a continuous supply of nutrients and energy guarantees the fuel necessary for that epic growth. Not surprisingly, the bigger baby gets, the more fuel your baby-making factory will require. So while a skimpy first trimester weight gain (or even a loss, if mum's having trouble eating or keeping food down) won't slow down a still teensy-tiny baby's growth, gaining too little weight in the second and third trimesters might not meet a bigger baby's growing needs.

But it's not just your baby who stands to gain from a well-paced weight gain – you do, too. Your body will have an easier time adjusting to the extra pounds if they're added gradually – which could mean, among other perks, less strain, fewer aches and pains, and possibly even fewer stretch marks (after

Recommended Rate of Weight Gain

BMI	Average Weekly Weight Gain per Week During Second and Third Trimester	Total Weight Gain
Underweight (BMI less than 18.5)	Slightly more than 1 lb (450 g) per week	28–40 lb (13–18 kg)
Normal weight (BMI 18.5 to 24.9)	Approximately 1 lb (450 g) per week	25–35 lb (11–16 kg)
Overweight (BMI 25 to 29.9)	Approximately 10½ oz (300 g) per week	15–25 lb (7–11 kg)
Obese (BMI greater than 30)	Approximately 8 oz (225 g) per week	11–20 lb (5–9 kg)

Weight Check Dos and Don'ts

DO follow your practitioner's recommendation for weight gain. It'll be tailored to your individual needs.

DO check with your healthcare provider if you gain more than 3 lb (1.4 kg) in any one week in the second trimester or if you gain more than 2 lb (900 g) in any week in the third trimester, especially if it doesn't seem related to overeating. Too much sudden and unexplained weight gain can indicate a pregnancy problem, such as pre-eclampsia.

DO check with your healthcare provider if you gain no weight for more than two weeks in a row during months 4 through 8. Also check in if you lose a significant amount of weight at any time during your pregnancy (don't worry if it's just a few pounds). While a little weight loss isn't uncommon in the first trimester (especially if you've been vomiting up a lot), a greater than 5 per cent weight loss can signal hyperemesis gravidarum (severe nausea and vomiting during pregnancy) or other pregnancy complications.

DON'T try to lose weight or try to keep yourself from gaining weight (unless your doctor has advised you to), either by undercutting needed calories or overdoing exercise. A healthy pregnancy and a healthy baby require a healthy weight gain.

DON'T obsess about the numbers. Keep an eye on your weight gain to make sure you're hitting your healthcare provider-recommended weight-gain goal, but don't lose sight of your most important goal: nourishing your growing baby. Remember, if your doctor or midwife is content with your weight gain, you should be, too.

---

all, gradual weight gain allows skin to keep pace, so that stretching is gradual and less likely to leave as many marks). A slow and steady gain may also lead to a somewhat speedier post-delivery return to your pre-pregnancy shape.

Bear in mind that a steady pace doesn't mean spreading your recommended weight gain evenly over 40 weeks of pregnancy. Early on in the pregnancy game, with baby as light as a grain of rice, weight gain can be light, too – about 2–4 lb (0.9–1.8 kg) in the first trimester usually gets the job done. In fact, gaining nothing at all (or even losing some pounds because of nagging nausea and frequent vomiting) won't impact baby's development or eventual base line. But as baby's (and pregnancy's) needs grow, so should mum. In the average pregnancy, weight gain should pick up to a rate of 1–1½ lb (450–675 g) per week in months 4 through 6 (for a total of about 12–14 lb/5.5–6 kg), then drop off again in the last three months to a pound or even less per week (for a total of about 8–10 lb/3.6–4.5 kg). In the home stretch of the ninth month, however, mum's weight gain typically tapers off. Some mums gain only a pound or two during the entire last month, while others even lose weight during the final weeks of pregnancy.

Will every mum-to-be follow this model formula precisely? Far from it. Some mums start off with a bang (adding 10 lb/4.5 kg or more in the first trimester, instead of just a few), then slow down to a more reasonable weight-gain rate as the weeks pass (and as they realise that they might be taking the phrase 'eating for two' just a little too literally). Others may be too queasy to add an ounce, but do a good job of catching up once meals start staying down. Even a woman who eats with an eye on the scales right from the start will find the numbers fluctuating a little (maybe it's an 8-oz/225-g gain one week in the second trimester, 1½ lb/675 g the next week). As long as your overall gain stays approximately on target, and your rate of gain averages out pretty close to the model formula (without any long lulls, huge dips or giant jumps), you're in good shape. Literally.

One reason why weight gain tends to fluctuate so much during pregnancy is that appetite fluctuates, too. Your hunger will come in peaks, valleys and plateaus, and so will your food intake. You'll have periods of below-average appetite (most common in the first few months, when nausea nips hunger in the bud, and again in the last month or two, when heartburn rules and tummy room starts to run out). And you'll have periods of above-average appetite (typically spurred on by baby's growth spurts). Mums-to-be often enter the 'hunger zone' somewhere around weeks 12 to 14 as the queasy cloud lifts, aversions clear up and appetite starts to soar. Follow those hunger pangs to the fridge – they're nature's way of ensuring you're eating enough to fuel your growing baby's needs.

Carrying more than one baby? You'll need to pack on more total pounds, and your rate of gain will reflect that. See page 101 for more.

The Downside of Too Little Weight Gain

Many mums-to-be sweat the numbers when the pounds are adding up too fast. But what if the numbers on the scales aren't moving up at all, or are even creeping down – is that cause for concern, too? It's not a worry in the first trimester, when it's common to lose weight (or not gain any at all). But weight loss or lack of weight gain that continues into the second and third trimesters is a red flag. In fact, the risks of gaining too little weight can outweigh the risks of gaining too much weight, and for an average-weight woman, there can be a significant downside to continued below-average weight gain. The risks include:

Preterm delivery. Mums-to-be who don't gain enough weight throughout pregnancy are at an increased risk of delivering too soon, especially if they came into pregnancy underweight or even average weight. Full-term babies are more likely to arrive healthy than premature babies, so gaining enough weight during pregnancy can pay not only in a more safely timed delivery, but in a healthier bundle at birth.

Low birthweight for baby. Gaining too little weight during pregnancy can keep your baby from gaining enough, restricting growth and sometimes resulting in a low birthweight (aka small for gestational age, or SGA). Very small babies are at an increased risk of complications and health problems at birth and beyond. Bear in mind, however, that not all cases of SGA are caused by a mum-to-be gaining too little weight – there are also genetic, environmental, foetal and health factors that can contribute to a low birthweight.

Working Through Weighty Issues

Does the thought of gaining weight during pregnancy (even if it's for the benefit of your baby-to-be) make you shudder – and then reach for the celery sticks instead of the cheese and biscuits? You're not alone. Many women – especially those who've experienced eating disorders (see the box on page 102) and/or body image issues, even mild ones – become unsettled, unnerved, anxious, even panicked at the thought of adding any pounds, anywhere, anytime. But now's the time to work through weight phobia (and any persistent body image issues) – before it can have a negative impact on your pregnancy and your growing baby. Remind yourself often: pregnancy weight is both healthy and beautiful. Also remember: you're not losing your body – you're gaining a healthy baby (and besides, your body is still yours, even as it's being used for the awesome purpose of nourishing a pregnancy, and later to breastfeed). And most important, remember who you're gaining weight for. Your gain is baby's gain – literally. As long as you stick pretty close to the recommended weight-gain guidelines, each and every ounce you put on has a purpose in pregnancy – nourishing that beautiful baby of yours. And that's something to celebrate.

The Downside of Too Much Weight Gain

It's clear why gaining too little weight while you're pregnant can hamper your baby's growth and development, as well as the health of your pregnancy. But piling on far too many pounds may present its own set of problems. Many of the problems are mummy-centric, affecting the mum-to-be, her health and her comfort (make that her discomfort), while putting her pregnancy at greater risk. Expectant mums who gain much more than the recommended amount of weight during pregnancy may be at risk for:

An uncomfortable pregnancy. Pregnancy complaints multiply with the pounds. Excessive weight gain can be a contributing factor to just about every discomfort of pregnancy, from backaches to fatigue, leg pain to varicose veins, heartburn to haemorrhoids, breathlessness to joint pain.

Labour and delivery complications. As a general (if not inevitable) rule, the heavier mum is before pregnancy and the heavier she gets during pregnancy, the heavier baby gets. Not surprisingly, bigger babies have a harder time exiting the traditional way than ones of average size, increasing the chance that a caesarean delivery may be necessary and increasing the chance of labour complications (such as excessive bleeding).

Weight that lasts. A woman who gains more weight than recommended during pregnancy tends to hold on to more

Where Does All the Weight Go?

With the average bundle of joy weighing in at about 7–8 lb (3–3.6 kg), there's definitely more to pregnancy weight gain than baby's weight. In fact, a lot more – for an average-weight woman, upwards of 28 lb (12.7 kg) more. All of these extra pounds (even the ones slated for places you may wish they weren't headed) serve one of two important purposes: baby making (during pregnancy) or baby feeding (after delivery). Adding to these main factors will be pounds allocated to baby-making materials (including the growing placenta), maternal fat stores (these are the ones your body will use to fuel baby's growth during pregnancy and produce breast milk after delivery), extra breast tissue (clearly earmarked for milk production), and the expanded blood volume pregnancy requires. And while baby will be a lightweight through most of the action, he or she will double in size during the last trimester (happily, you won't).

Although the numbers vary from mum to mum, this is how those pounds may add up:

Baby:	**7–8 lb (3–3.6 kg)**
Breast enlargement:	**1–3 lb (0.9–1.4 kg)**
Placenta:	**18 oz (500 g)**
Enlargement of uterus:	**2 lb (900 g)**
Amniotic fluid:	**2 lb (900 g)**
Your extra blood:	**3–4 lb (1.4–1.8 kg)**
Your body's extra fat:	**6–8 lb (2.7–3.6 kg)**
Your body's extra fluids:	**2–3 lb (0.9–1.4 kg)**
Average total weight:	**30 lb (13.6 kg)**

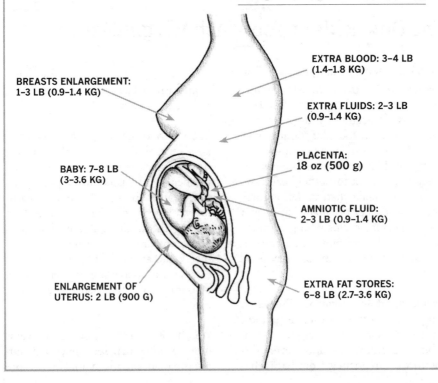

EXTRA BLOOD: 3–4 LB (1.4–1.8 KG)

BREASTS ENLARGEMENT: 1–3 LB (0.9–1.4 KG)

EXTRA FLUIDS: 2–3 LB (0.9–1.4 KG)

PLACENTA: 18 oz (500 g)

BABY: 7–8 LB (3–3.6 KG)

AMNIOTIC FLUID: 2–3 LB (0.9–1.4 KG)

ENLARGEMENT OF UTERUS: 2 LB (900 G)

EXTRA FAT STORES: 6–8 LB (2.7–3.6 KG)

weight afterwards – an average of 10–20 lb (4.5–9 kg) that she's not likely to shed. That extra weight may set her up for a variety of potential health problems later in life, including hypertension, diabetes, stroke and heart disease.

Complications in future pregnancies. You may not be thinking ahead to another pregnancy, but here's something to think about during this one. Gaining too much weight in a first pregnancy increases the chances of gaining too much weight in a subsequent pregnancy – again increasing the risks of complications. Another minus to adding on too many pounds in this pregnancy: data shows women in general are statistically likely to gain weight between pregnancies – a factor that adds risks (of gestational diabetes, pregnancy-induced hypertension, pre-eclampsia, caesarean delivery, preterm birth and more) to a next pregnancy.

When a mum who has already accumulated extra pounds from her previous pregnancy gains more weight between pregnancies, she's further increasing her risks of a complicated next pregnancy.

Complications for baby. Babies born to mums who have gained too much weight during pregnancy are at a higher risk of being born overweight (LGA, or large for gestational age). Having a bigger bundle of joy sounds like a good thing – but LGA puts a baby at risk for birth injuries such as shoulder dystocia (when baby's shoulders get stuck inside mum's pelvis during delivery) and collarbone fractures (from having a hard time making it out of the birth canal), as well as hypoglycaemia (low blood sugar), respiratory distress and low Apgar scores. Extra-large babies are also at increased risk of being overweight or obese and/or developing diabetes during childhood and beyond.

Weighing In

Let's face it. Many women have a complicated relationship with the scales – whether it's love/hate, all hate, or can't live with/can't live without. While some end up making peace with their scales (or at least de-escalating to something of a friend/enemy status), few become best friends with them. Even fewer actually look forward to stepping on their scales, whether in the privacy of their bathroom or in front of a healthcare provider. And for some women, the scales represent painful, very real struggles with body image and eating issues that can bubble up big-time during pregnancy, when vital weight gain has the scales' numbers edging up.

Fortunately, weighing yourself daily during pregnancy isn't necessary – or even the most effective way of tracking your pregnancy weight gain. Your weight can fluctuate too much from day to day, depending on how much you've eaten, how much water you've retained (from that pickle juice chaser, for instance), and whether you've moved your bowels (or how long it's been since you've pooed). And if you have a really uneasy relationship with your scales, stepping on them too often can sabotage your best intentions to gain the weight you should.

On the other hand, waiting too long between weigh-ins can also undermine

Plot Your Weight Gain

As you'll find out, keeping track of anything when you're expecting becomes a challenge. That's why it may help to write down your weight gain as you go (or input it digitally on the What to Expect app weight-gain tracker). Weigh yourself every week or two if you have scales at home (or use your monthly weight check from your antenatal appointment). Then plot your gain using this graph. First, locate the number of weeks along you are in your pregnancy at the bottom of the graph. Then find your weight gain in pounds along the left side of the graph. Make a dot where the pounds meet the weeks. Play 'connect the dots' to watch your curve as you add those beautiful pregnancy curves. Or let the What to Expect app do the tracking for you.

	First trimester	Second trimester	Third trimester

W E I G H T   G A I N

44
42
40
38
36
34
32
30
28
26
24
22
20
18
16
14
12
10
8
6
4
2
0
-2
-4

0 2 4 6 8 10 12 14 16 18 20 22 24 26 28 30 32 34 36 38 40 42

WEEKS

Eating for Two After Weight-Loss Surgery

Lost a lot of weight after bariatric surgery – and now you're gaining a baby? That's plenty of good news already, and there's even more to celebrate: your weight loss has increased your chances of having a healthy pregnancy and a healthy baby, plus decreased your risk for gestational diabetes, pre-eclampsia and having a too-big baby.

Still, there are some extra precautions you'll have to take as a mum-to-be who's had weight-loss surgery:

■ Watch your weight. Keeping an eye on the scales is nothing new to you – but since your weight-loss surgery, you've likely become accustomed to (and proud of!) watching the numbers go down. Now that you're growing a baby, those numbers will have to start inching up so you can reach (without overshooting) the weight-gain goal recommended by your healthcare provider. Bear in mind that there's an increased chance of having a too-small baby after bariatric surgery, but that gaining the right number of pounds can help ensure a healthy base line for your baby at birth. On the flip side, gaining too few pounds or too many can add unnecessary risks.

■ Get those vital vitamins. Something else you're used to since your bariatric surgery: taking vitamin supplements to fill in nutritional blanks left by restricted food intake and post-surgery malabsorption issues. Your antenatal vitamin is a good place to start when filling in those blanks, but you'll probably need even more iron, calcium, folic acid, vitamin A and especially vitamin B_{12} than a standard pregnancy formula can provide. Be sure to discuss your specific supplement needs with both your antenatal healthcare provider and your weight-loss consultant.

■ Focus on high-quality eating. Your stomach space has been downsized by your weight-loss surgery, making eating for two already somewhat more challenging – and more challenging still when your uterus and baby start to grow, crowding out your already small stomach. Since the quantity of food you can comfortably eat is limited, you'll need to focus on quality: foods that efficiently pack the most nutrients into the smallest volume (see page 27 for more).

those best weight-gain intentions. Step on the scales just once a month at your regular antenatal visits and you might find you've lost a pound when you should have gained 4 lb (1.8 kg) – or that you've gained 10 lb (4.5 kg) instead. Either scenario could throw your total off target, but could also spell extra risks if it's a trend that's not reversed.

That's why, at least for most pregnant women, a once-a-week (or once-every-other-week) weigh-in is the best way to go – so you can keep your eye on your weight gain without obsessing over it. If you feel compelled to step on the scales every day, record a week's worth of weigh-ins, then add them up and divide by 7 to calculate your average weight for the week. Compare that number to last week's base line to see how much you've gained week to week. This figure will give you a more accurate picture of your progress. And no matter how often you weigh yourself, make sure you do it at

Look the Other Way

If you're the type to obsess about your weight gain (and you know who you are), make a conscious effort not to. Don't weigh yourself every week. Don't plot your weight gain on the graph in this chapter or on an app. Don't even peek at the scales during your health checks – and ask the nurse not to say the number out loud. If your doctor or midwife is satisfied with your weight progress, you should be, too.

about the same time and under approximately the same conditions each day (before breakfast, for instance – naked, or with the same amount of clothing).

Also, remember: Your results (from scales to scales) may vary – so comparing your weight on your bathroom scales against your weight on the health provider's scales won't be helpful, and it could add up to unnecessary stress. Compare weights only on the same scales.

Bear in mind, too, that even weight gain that's right on target rarely comes in precisely packaged instalments (½ of a lb a day, 1 lb a week, 4 lb a month, 8 lb over two months). Instead, it'll average out over time: 2 lb (900 g) one week, 8 oz (225 g) the next week, 1 lb (450 g) the following and so on. Or in month 5, 3 lb (1.4 kg); month 6, 5 lb (2.3 kg). Don't forget either that there's a pretty wide range to aim for (in the case of average-weight women, a 10-lb/4.5-kg spread of 25–35 lb/11–16 kg), which allows even more weight-gain wiggle room.

If You're Gaining Too Fast

How can you tell if you're gaining too much or too fast? Some research suggests that the first trimester gain is key: if you find you've piled on more than 3 lb (1.4 kg) at that 12-week milestone (2 lb/900 g if you're overweight, 5 lb/2.3 kg if you're underweight), you may need to watch your eating (and your scales) more closely to keep those numbers from rising out of the recommended range. But even a mum-to-be who ends her first trimester with a considerably higher net – and many women do, often because nausea leads them to reach for box after box, bag after bag, and carton after carton of comforting carbs – can finish up her pregnancy well within healthy weight-gain limits. Which is why most healthcare providers won't worry about a slightly greater weight gain in the first trimester, especially if a mum-to-be is eating well.

If you and your healthcare provider do decide it's smart to slow down a weight gain that's been on the fast track, these tips can help:

- Curb your calories. Okay, you've probably heard this one before: too many calories in, too many pounds on. Though cutting calories to lose weight is never a good idea when you're pregnant, curbing calories to curb excess weight gain may be – particularly if your healthcare provider has recommended that you slow down your rate of gain. Apply some simple, calorie-cutting strategies, aimed at delivering the most nutrition for the fewest calories. Sub

Already Reached Your Limit?

Nowhere near the pregnancy finish line, but you've already reached your pregnancy weight-gain goal – and don't want to exceed it? Unfortunately, slamming the brakes on your weight gain now may not be a smart strategy. You may feel like you're finished growing, but your little one still has lots of growing to do – and needs a steady supply of calories and other nutrients to keep that growing going all the way to delivery day, courtesy of your womb service. Bear in mind, too, that while you're winding down pregnancy-wise (or at least starting to feel like you're over it), baby has plenty more to do to get ready for birth. Calcium is being laid down in those baby bones (which means you need to keep drinking that milk or eating that cheese and yogurt).

Baby's developing brain, eyes and nerves are working overtime – work that requires plenty of healthy fats, especially omega-3 fatty acids. Baby also has a number of pounds to add to his or her own base line – which means you do, too. Cut back too much on calories in the last weeks of pregnancy, and you could cut into baby's growth potential.

But that doesn't mean you can't slow down your weight gain some, especially since it's been on the fast track up until now. Ask your healthcare provider to come up with a revised weight-gain goal. And as you close in on the end of pregnancy, eat as efficiently as you can to ensure you're getting the most nutrients for the calories you take in (and follow the other tips on page 27).

---

fat-free milk, yogurt and cottage cheese for whole or reduced-fat, bake your chips, dole out 35 g of pistachios instead of munching straight from the bag (and possibly polishing it off), add fresh or freeze-dried strawberries to your cereal instead of raisins, take the skin off your chicken.

■ Cut that fat. Some fat is essential in your pregnancy diet, but too much can add those pounds faster than you can say 'Extra Value Meal'. Try eating one less serving (1 tablespoon) of fat to see if that puts the brakes on your runaway gain. If it doesn't, trim another serving. Bear in mind that fat takes a variety of forms besides straight-up oil, mayo, butter and dairy-free butter alternatives. Pay attention to sources that may slip by unnoticed (those in the salad dressing, the sautéed scampi, the fried eggs). One easy way to reduce

fat in cooking? Use nonstick cooking oil sprays or a sprayer filled with oil to spray instead of pour. Another way: choose low-fat preparations whenever you can (roast, bake, poach, steam or grill instead of fry).

■ Be a mindful eater. Can't figure out where all the pounds are coming from? Paying close attention to your eating may help you solve that weight-gain mystery. Eating while distracted (when you're working, catching up on social media, watching TV) can lead to eating more than you should, intended to or even notice. Like that bowl of Smarties you went deep into while you were deep in a client presentation (wait, wasn't everyone eating them?). Or that whole packet of crisps you polished off while checking your WTE app (when you really meant to stop at a handful). Instead of

Fighting the Fat with Fact

Myth: Foods that are labelled 'fat-free' are a better choice when you're trying not to gain too much weight.

Fact: Do fat-free biscuits sound too good to be true? That's because they often are. That fat-free banner may seem like an invitation to reach the bottom of the box or packet, but eater beware: being free of fat doesn't make a product free of calories. In fact, manufacturing a palatable product while taking out the fat typically requires adding other ingredients that can add up in calories but usually don't add up nutritionally. In fact, these products can score extra low on the nutrition scale. So watch portion size, and for a moderate weight gain, eat any processed foods – even the 'fat-free' ones – in moderation. Incidentally, the same can be said for many 'sugar-free' foods: what's free of sugar may be full of calories from a variety of other sources.

Myth: 'Low-carb' foods aren't fattening, so you can eat as many as you like.

Fact: Turns out there really is no such thing as a free lunch – or, in this case, a free bag of crisps, chocolate bar or cheesecake. Truth is, many products labelled 'low-carb' are highly processed, high in fat and high in calories – definitely not a dieter's dream come true. What's more, low-carb products aren't designed for pregnant women, who need carbs in their diet. Another reason to step away from the low-carb section of your market: many of the ingredients that stand in for carbs aren't pregnancy-friendly (such as sugar alcohols). So (low) carb your enthusiasm. Favour foods that are naturally low in carbs, not ones that are processed to fit that formula, and balance them with plenty of healthy carbs (such as wholegrains and legumes/pulses) and healthy fats.

distracted eating, try putting mindfulness on the menu – eyes on your meal (or your dining partner) instead of on a screen. And because eating on the run can also lead to overeating, brake for meals. Take a seat at the table (or the breakfast bar or your desk) even at snack time. Slowly savour your food (taking the time to actually taste what you're chewing – and while you're at it, taking your time with chewing), and you'll feel full and satisfied before you've overdone it.

■ Get active. There's more to the calories-in, pounds-on equation – that is, if you add exercise. Getting a minimum of 30 minutes a day of moderate exercise – as recommended for most pregnant women – will allow you to eat more calories while keeping your weight gain in check (that's the calories-out part of the equation). Plus, fitting in fitness is good for your body, your mood, your sleep and your overall pregnancy health. Your workout even offers baby benefits, especially in the brain development department, research shows. Ask your healthcare provider for exercise guidelines, and then consider going to the gym or pool, joining a pregnancy exercise class, tuning in to the *What to Expect When You're Expecting* pregnancy workout – or just taking a few brisk 10-minute walks a day. You'll find more fitness facts and workout ideas in *What to Expect When You're Expecting.*

Myth: Eating foods that are 'gluten-free' will keep you from gaining too much weight.

Fact: Hoping to catch the gluten-free express to avoid excess weight gain? Don't hop on just yet. Products labelled 'gluten-free' are a must for people with coeliac disease or gluten intolerance. But if you don't have either one, ditching gluten in an effort to keep your weight from escalating too fast isn't the best move. Sure, if you replace your lunchtime cheeseburger with a gluten-free grilled chicken salad, you'll be piling on fewer pounds – but that's because the salad is lower in calories than the cheeseburger, not because there's no gluten in the salad. If, on the other hand, you swap something healthy for a gluten-free version of the same – say, a bowl of wholegrain cereal for a bowl of processed gluten-free cereal – you're probably not saving yourself calories, but you probably are inadvertently skimping on nutrients. That's because processed gluten-free foods are often full of fillers (including fat, sugar and starches) added to compensate for loss of taste and texture when wholegrains are swapped out.

Processed gluten-free foods tend to have less fibre, fewer B vitamins and lower amounts of minerals than their gluten-containing counterparts. Which means that if you're cutting out gluten, you're also losing all the nutritional benefits found in foods with gluten – all without cutting any calories. Bottom line: if you're going to go gluten-free (or need to because of a health condition), stick to unprocessed GF foods. Bake your own GF bread and desserts using healthy gluten-free grains, focus on vitamin- and mineral-packed high-fibre, naturally gluten-free substitutes (brown rice, quinoa, buckwheat), and keep your diet high in healthy foods. For more on gluten-free diets, see page 150.

■ See your healthcare provider. If you're eating sensibly, getting plenty of exercise and still packing on weight too quickly, there may be a medical reason to consider (such as a hormonal imbalance). Sudden rapid weight gain (more than 3 lb/1.4 kg in a single week in the second trimester or 2 lb/900 g in a single a week in the third trimester), especially when accompanied by swelling of hands and face, headaches, blurring of vision or any combination of these, could be a sign of the serious pregnancy complication pre-eclampsia and should be reported to your healthcare provider right away.

If You're Gaining Too Slowly

Nagging nausea. Annoying aversions. Metal mouth that makes everything you eat taste like loose change, and bloat that leaves you feeling full when you're actually running on empty. There are plenty of reasons why your first trimester appetite might have taken a hit, or even a nosedive – and why gaining enough

When a Big Weight Loss Can Lead to a Big Weight Gain

Are you gaining too much weight, but can't figure out why? Unfair as it seems, overweight women who are chronic dieters or who lost a substantial amount of weight just before becoming pregnant may be prone to gaining too much weight during pregnancy, even if they don't overeat. Experts speculate that a body that's been through a recent major weight loss may feel 'starved' and overcompensate during pregnancy for that earlier loss of fat by piling on more pounds. Tell your healthcare provider or dietitian about any significant pre-pregnancy weight loss, and discuss a game plan for keeping your pregnancy weight gain on target.

weight may have become an unexpected struggle. (Wasn't that supposed to be the easy part of pregnancy?) Happily, there's nothing to worry about if your weight gain is still at a standstill as you end your first trimester, or even if it has dipped into the negative zone – after all, your baby (and baby's needs) are still relatively tiny. Once you graduate to the second trimester, though, it's time to start putting on the pounds. To get your weight gain going:

- Fatten up your diet. Since pure fat is the most concentrated source of food energy (aka calories), adding fat to your diet is usually the easiest way to pack on pounds. While any fat will get the job done from a calorie perspective, choosing healthy fats will help get it done nutritiously, too. So butter up your toast, by all means, but also try spreading peanut butter on your apple slices, adding nuts to your yogurt (make it full-fat yogurt while you're at it), adding avocado to everything and saying 'cheese' often.

- Don't be too efficient. For an expectant mum who's gaining weight too quickly, efficient eating is often the

answer – filling up on foods that supply the most nutrients for the fewest calories (those veggies, that salad). Gaining too slowly? Just flip the equation. Focus on foods that are dense in nutrients and calories, supplying more of both with every bite: nuts and seeds, avocados, cheese, beans, hearty wholegrains.

- Sneak in snacks. Snacking is a smart strategy for every mum-to-be, but it's wiser still if you're looking to jump-start your weight gain. Build snack breaks (one mid-morning, one mid-afternoon and one before bedtime) into your schedule. Make the snack substantial in calories (go nuts!), but not so filling that you end up sabotaging your appetite for your next meal.

- Slow down the burn. If you're working out too much or too hard, you may be burning calories you need to nourish your body and your baby – and to gain those pregnancy pounds. So cut back on strenuous workouts, and don't forget to replace calories you do burn so you're not running at a deficit. And speaking of slowing down, if a high-stress job plus a fast-paced

Boys Will Be Boys

Are you eating like a teenage boy? It could be you're carrying one – or at least a baby boy on his way to becoming a teenage boy. According to researchers, women pregnant with boys tend to eat 10 per cent more calories (approximately 200 calories), 8 per cent more protein, and more carbohydrates and fat per day than those carrying girls. And a boy bonus: piling on those extra calories doesn't necessarily mean you'll be piling on extra pounds. Boy-carrying mums-to-be don't gain more weight, on average, than girl-carrying ones do. These findings may explain, in part, why boys are typically heavier than girls at birth. It also suggests a fascinating antenatal premise: that the foetus sends signals to its mother that drive her appetite during pregnancy (as in 'Feed me, Mum – I'm hungry again!'). In other words, male foetuses require more calories for their optimal growth in the uterus, so they send their mums to the refrigerator more often. Interesting science and, perhaps, a glimpse of refrigerator raids to come during those teenage years?

schedule has you missing breakfast or working through lunch, schedule eating into your daily calendar (even if it means setting reminders).

- See your healthcare provider. This is important, especially if your slow weight gain doesn't seem related to undereating or doesn't change after you add extra calories. A thyroid condition or some other undiagnosed medical problem may be keeping you from achieving your weight-gain goals and needs prompt attention.

If You're Gaining for Multiples

More than one baby on board? Then your goal will be to gain weight faster than the typical expectant mum, right from the start – not only because you're housing two (or more) growing babies, but also because you're toting two placentas (unless your identical twins are sharing a large one). You'll also be carrying additional blood and fluid supplies, a larger (and heavier) uterus and more amniotic fluid.

Your recommended weight gain will, not surprisingly, be substantially higher than that for a single pregnancy. If you're carrying twins and your pre-pregnancy weight (and BMI) was normal, it's recommended that you gain 37–54 lb (17–24.5 kg). If you started pregnancy overweight, aim to gain 31–50 lb (14–22.7 kg). If you have triplets on board, your weight gain recommendations will be a little higher (your healthcare provider will give you a target number).

Problem is, gaining enough weight isn't always as easy as it seems when you've got two or more on board. That's especially true during the first trimester, when double the hormones can spell

Eating Disorders and Pregnancy

There isn't much research in the area of eating disorders and pregnancy, mostly because few women suffering from anorexia or bulimia become pregnant in the first place (these disorders often disrupt the menstrual cycle). But the studies that have been done suggest that having an active eating disorder during pregnancy can increase the risk of many complications, including miscarriage, pre-eclampsia, premature birth, caesarean delivery and postnatal depression. Taking laxatives, diuretics, appetite suppressants and other drugs during pregnancy is harmful, too, leading to multiple serious problems, including possible birth defects, if used regularly. Happily, the studies also suggest that mums-to-be who once suffered from eating disorders but have put those unhealthy habits behind them are just as likely to have a healthy baby as anyone else.

But what if you're no longer anorexic or bulimic, yet the thought of pregnancy weight gain has brought back some of those old feelings about your body image that you'd fought hard to overcome – and thought you'd shed forever? What if you're having trouble eating normally now that you're eating for two? Or if you're having a hard time distinguishing between morning sickness and bulimia? Or if you're hiding a return of your bulimia under the cover of morning sickness? Or you have signs of disordered eating: anxiety around specific foods, meal skipping, feelings of guilt and shame when you eat, a rigid approach to eating, self-esteem that's based on body shape and weight, preoccupation with food and weight, and/or using exercise to make up for bingeing?

Firstly, make sure you get the help you need as soon as possible. Start by telling your antenatal healthcare provider about your eating disorder – not only so he or she can help make sure it doesn't affect your baby or your pregnancy, but also so you'll get the supportive care you need to get healthy and stay healthy. Then ask for a referral to a therapist who is experienced in treating eating disorders. Professional counselling is always smart when you've been

double the morning sickness, making it difficult to get food down – and then keep it down. Eating tiny amounts of comforting (and, hopefully, sometimes nutritious) food throughout the day can help get you through those extra-queasy months. Aim for a 1-lb-(450-g)-a-week gain in the first trimester, but if you find you can't gain that much, or have trouble gaining any at all, relax. You can have fun catching up later (or not – read on). Just be sure to take your antenatal vitamin and stay doubly hydrated.

Your second trimester will probably be your most comfortable and the easiest for you to do some serious chowing down in, so use it as an opportunity to load up on the nutrition your babies need to grow. If you didn't gain any weight during the first trimester (or if you lost weight because of severe nausea and vomiting), your healthcare provider may want you to gain an average of 1½– 2 lb (675–900 g) per week starting now. If you've been gaining steadily through the first trimester, you can aim a little lower. Either way, that may seem like a lot of weight in a short time, and you're right – it is. But it's weight that's doubly important to gain. Supercharge

battling anorexia or bulimia, but it's really essential when you're trying to eat well for two. Seeing a registered dietitian may also be helpful in coming up with a healthy pregnancy eating plan you can feel good about. And look to support groups, too – made up of pregnant women and mums who are currently facing the same struggles or have faced them before. Search online, or ask your healthcare provider or therapist for a recommendation.

Secondly, try to put the dynamics of pregnancy weight gain and the normal body changes that go along with it in perspective (something your therapist and a support group can also help you do). Pregnancy curves and weight gain are healthy and beautiful – signs that you're growing a baby. And the right amount of weight (as recommended by your healthcare provider), gained at the right rate, on the right foods, is vital to your baby's growth and well-being in the uterus and beyond (some of the extra fat you lay down during pregnancy will be used after delivery to help you breastfeed your baby). Be prepared for – and talk to your therapist

about – the reality of what a healthy new-mum body looks and feels like after pregnancy and delivery: that you won't lose all the pregnancy pounds or inches overnight. That it takes nine months to gain pregnancy weight, and it can take at least that long to lose it. That the weight you'll still be wearing postnatal is not only normal, but necessary to fuel your recovery and to feed your baby. Don't try to minimise weight gain during pregnancy in an effort to avoid the postnatal body image struggles you may be anticipating (there's no reason to struggle if you know you're supposed to look that way postnatal). The most important thing to bear in mind: your baby's well-being depends on your well-being during pregnancy. If you're not well nourished, your baby won't be either.

If you can't stop bingeing, inducing vomiting, using diuretics or laxatives, or practising semi-starvation during pregnancy, discuss with your healthcare provider the possibility of hospitalisation until you get your disorder under control – which, with the right care and support, you absolutely can.

your eating plan with extra servings of protein, calcium, wholegrains and healthy fats. Heartburn and indigestion (again, both more likely to be more miserable in a mum-to-be of multiples) starting to cramp your eating style? Spread your nutrients out over six (or more) mini-meals.

As you head into the home stretch (the third trimester), you'll still need to continue your steady rate of gain. By 32 weeks, your babies may be just under 4 lb (1.8 kg) each on average, which won't leave much room for food in your crowded tummy. Still, even though you'll

The Long Road Back

Gaining the weight is (usually) the easy part. It's losing all that weight after the baby is born that's often hard. Bear in mind that it takes time – and that there shouldn't be too many shortcuts on that long road back, especially if you're breastfeeding. Check out Chapter 10 for tips on how to shed the pounds sensibly postnatal.

CHEW ON THIS. Going for a baby surprise? Or know your baby's sex but not yet telling – or not sharing with random strangers at the shops? Then you've probably been treated to any number of predictions based on any number of pregnancy legends, including this one: if the weight you've gained has headed straight to your bump, you're having a boy. If it's spread out all over your body (with special mention to those X-chromosome favourites: hips, buttocks and thighs), you're be feeling bulky already, your babies will have to bulk up quite a bit more – and they'll appreciate the nutrition a healthy diet provides. So focus on quality over quantity, and expect to taper down to carrying a girl, destined for curves of her own.

Guessing this isn't the most reliable way to predict your baby's sex? You're right. The fact is how you carry has far more to do with a variety of other factors (including your size, shape, genetics, diet and rate of weight gain) than it does with the sex of your unborn baby. Like all unscientific methods of predicting a baby's sex, this one has just about a 50 per cent chance of being correct.

be feeling bulky already, your babies will have to bulk up quite a bit more – and they'll appreciate the nutrition a healthy diet provides. So focus on quality over quantity, and expect to taper down to 1 lb (450 g) a week or less in month 8 and just 1 lb (450 g) or so total in month 9. (This makes more sense when you remember that most multiple pregnancies don't make it to 40 weeks.)

CHAPTER 7

Eating Well When You're Feeling Unwell

O h, the irony: the reason you want to eat healthy is that you're pregnant – and the reason you're having a hard time eating healthy is . . . that you're pregnant. Let's face it – between morning sickness, food aversions, constipation and indigestion, there are plenty of appetite-cramping pregnancy complaints that can come between a mum and her broccoli. Or that can push her buttons at breakfast time – and have her pushing the buttons on the vending machine 2 hours later. Or that can have her gagging over a glimpse of a raw chicken breast or a sniff of steamed spinach from several feet away.

A few lucky mums-to-be may breeze through pregnancy with healthy appetites for healthy foods for a full nine months. But most find that their tastes change and their tummies take a hit when they're expecting – especially in the first trimester (when cravings, aversions and morning sickness peak) and in the last trimester (when heartburn flares up and a growing baby encroaches on tummy space).

So, it's completely understandable if on some days (or most days) you're far more interested in feeling well than eating well – reaching for what helps ease the quease instead of what fills your calcium quota. Happily, however, many of the pregnancy symptoms that can dampen your appetite for healthy foods can actually be minimised by eating healthy foods – it's just a matter of finding the right ones. That way, everyone wins – you feel better and your body and your baby score the nutrients they need.

Morning Sickness

Do you heave at the sight of beef mince? Are you queasy just contemplating a bowl of your formerly favourite cereal (or even seeing the box on your cupboard shelf)? Are you looking greener than that salad you were planning to eat? Welcome to the first trimester of pregnancy, a time when, if you're like about 75 per cent of all pregnant women, morning sickness will change the way you look at food (not to mention the way you smell it, taste it, even think about it), taking a toll on both your tummy and your ability to fill it. Or, at least, to keep it filled.

As just about every veteran of morning sickness knows, the joker who coined this pregnancy symptom's name clearly never experienced it. Morning sickness isn't just for mornings – it's a round-the-clock, 24/7 sickness. Which is one reason why some experts have tried (with minimal success) to get a more accurate name trending: NVP, or nausea and vomiting of pregnancy.

Whatever you call it (besides miserable), there's no such thing as a textbook case. Morning sickness symptoms vary from mum to mum – and sometimes, from pregnancy to pregnancy in the same mum. Some may experience only occasional queasiness. Others may suffer through constant nausea and frequent bouts of vomiting, especially during the early weeks. While symptoms typically taper off by the end of the third or fourth month, a small percentage of women find the misery lingers – at least to some extent – into the ninth month. And even those who sail through that second trimester without a queasy moment may find it returns with a vengeance during the third trimester. It can even make its pregnancy debut in the third trimester (though late-pregnancy nausea and vomiting should always be checked by your healthcare visitor to rule out a complication).

Those who have spent weeks hovering over the toilet, avoiding onions (and people who eat them) like the plague, and subsisting on ginger ale and crackers may find it hard to believe that there's a silver lining to the cloud of morning sickness. But actually, there is. Since it's pregnancy hormones that trigger the nausea and vomiting of early pregnancy, morning sickness usually means that those hormones – which also help protect a pregnancy – are in good supply. Which is definitely not to say that morning sickness is a must-do for a healthy pregnancy (plenty of mums never have a queasy moment), just that morning sickness is usually a sign that pregnancy is proceeding normally. What's more, while you're certainly suffering, your baby almost certainly isn't. Even if you have a hard time keeping much of anything down, and even if you lose a little weight during the first trimester, your baby is able to weather morning sickness far better than you.

Of course, while all this good news about morning sickness probably makes you feel better about having it – it won't make you feel better while you have it. But, queasy fingers crossed, some of these tips will:

- Follow your nose. Your pregnant nose knows – everything. What your co-worker had for dinner last night. What your partner had for lunch. What your neighbours are cooking for breakfast (sausage again?). That's because the hormones of pregnancy sharpen the sense of smell, making for

The Six-Meal Solution

When heartburn, nausea, wind and other pregnancy symptoms make eating (and digesting) three meals a day seem like too much hard work, turn to the Six-Meal Solution instead. Eating half as much twice as often will keep your blood sugar steady, your appetite appeased and your digestive tract running more smoothly, providing relief from pregnancy tummy troubles. Dividing your meals will also help you conquer your nutritional requirements more easily.

There are two ways to tap into the Six-Meal Solution. One is to cut your usual three squares in half, so you're eating half of each meal every 2 to 3 hours. Or put traditional meals out to pasture for now (at least until you're feeling less green), and try grazing your way through your day. Opting for six mini-meals or six maxi-snacks will not only be gentler on your overtaxed tummy, but sustaining to your blood sugar – boosting energy, minimising mood swings and headaches, and helping you get a better night's sleep, among other benefits.

Here are some mini-meal suggestions (see page 138 for snack ideas):

- A small bowl of soup sprinkled with grated cheese, wholegrain crackers
- Half a peanut butter sandwich, a snack bag of freeze-dried fruit
- A muffin, a cheese wedge, a clementine
- Half a bagel and a scrambled egg
- 'Egg-in-a-hole' (egg fried in a hole made in a slice of bread), made crispy with a sprinkle of Parmesan
- A baked potato filled with Cheddar and broccoli
- A small bowl of wholegrain cereal with milk, half a banana
- A small salad topped with sunflower seeds and grated cheese

- A yogurt-and-fruit smoothie
- Sliced tomato and Emmental cheese melted in a small wholemeal pitta
- Half a grilled chicken breast wrapped in a wholegrain tortilla
- 250 g of yogurt topped with granola and blueberries
- 250 g Greek yogurt with chopped cucumber, spring onions, cherry tomatoes and a sprinkle of salt
- Two hard-boiled eggs, sliced in half and topped with flaky salt and cracked pepper or bagel' seasoning
- Baked sweet potato with butter and hot sauce
- Pasteurised mini mozzarella balls and roasted peppers (from a jar) on wooden skewers
- Sliced ripe tomato, lightly salted, on lightly buttered multigrain toast
- Bowl of porridge with strawberries and milk
- Wholegrain waffle with peanut butter and chopped strawberries (or blueberries)
- Quick quesadillas with grated cheese, beans and salsa, heated for a few minutes in a skillet or microwave
- Avocado toast (sliced avocado, lemon and olive oil on wholegrain toast)
- Breakfast muffin pizza (wholemeal muffin, pasta sauce, grated mozzarella, melted, black olives or another favourite topping optional)
- Vanilla Greek yogurt, dark chocolate chips, salted almonds
- Cottage cheese, sliced almonds, a drizzle of honey

a super-sensitive sniffer that's easily offended, heightening nausea. So go out of your way to avoid those now-sickening smells, at least as much as you can. Steer clear of cooking on the hob when the ingredients will make a stink as they're fried – say, onions, garlic, peppers. Or nix those ingredients altogether (substitute garlic granules for fresh garlic, or leave the onions out of the recipe). Favour microwave cooking, which minimises odours (especially if you cook in baking paper packets that enclose the aromas). Be mindful of odours when you pack a lunch so that opening it up later won't knock you off your feet. Choose restaurants with outdoor dining, weather allowing, and opt out of those where you can smell what's on the menu before you even walk in the door.

- Eat often. Empty tummies can brew up trouble. That's because when there's no food around to break down, digestive acids are left with only stomach lining to munch on – a process that produces nausea. To keep your tummy from running on empty, eat six mini-meals a day (see the box on the previous page). And sneak in plenty of between-meal snacks such as freeze-dried fruit, crunchy freeze-dried cheese, nuts or crackers.

- But don't eat too much. An overfilled tummy is just as likely to cry queasy as an empty one. During pregnancy, food travels at a snail's pace through your digestive tract so that nutrients are better absorbed. Cram in the chow, and you'll end up with more than your tummy can digest – something you'll end up regretting (and possibly, bring back up).

- Eat in bed. Before you settle down for the night, snuggle up with a snack that's high in both protein and carbs, such as a fruit-and-nut bar with milk, cheese and crackers, or half a peanut butter sandwich on wholemeal. A sustaining bedtime snack will sustain your blood-sugar levels during the night – helping you to not only sleep better, but (hopefully) wake up feeling better. Does morning sickness tend to creep in with dawn's early light? Open a bedside snack stand-stashed with crackers, dry cereal, freeze-dried fruit and cheese, or nuts, and get in the habit of having a nibble before you even swing your legs over the side of the bed. Let that early morning snack settle in before you attempt to start your day, and hopefully you won't start your day as sick as you were the day before.

- Stay ahead of the game. To kick morning sickness in the buttocks, nip it in the bud. Stay ahead of the nausea game by eating before those queasy waves hit (if your nausea is on a schedule), when food is more likely to go down and stay down. And, if you're really lucky, filling up (a little) before

> **CHEW ON THIS.** B.C. (before crackers), there were a variety of other morning sickness cures far more exotic than the humble cracker. For centuries, healers (and those who play them at home) have suggested ways for mums-to-be to combat morning sickness through diet. From wild yam to papaya, many of these cures have been passed down from generation to queasy generation as supposedly effective weapons in the fight against morning sickness. Ginger and fresh lemons are among those that have survived the test of time – and in the case of ginger, even some medical testing.

Thinking Outside the Cracker Box

Sick of choking down dry crackers every morning to combat your queasies? You've discovered, as so many morning-sick mums-to-be eventually do, that these savoury biscuits aren't always all they're cracked up to be – especially once you've crunched your way through boxes of them. While some mums find crackers comforting throughout their queasy weeks (or months), others find them tummy-turning from day one. Still others may find that comfort can turn to discomfort once crackers (or any food) become deeply associated with nausea and vomiting – and even the sight of a dry cracker starts the dry heaves. That's just sometimes how the cracker crumbles – and, if that's the case, it's time to kick them out of bed once and for all.

Where can you turn when you're thinking outside the box of crackers for bedside relief (or relief at your desk, or in your car)? Think of other foods that you can reach for and munch on easily – without having to drag yourself to the kitchen or the office fridge: dry cereal (no need to bring the box to bed – just keep a container handy), snack bags of popcorn or popcorn crisps, pretzels, salted or unsalted nuts, trail mix, all-fruit fruit snacks, freeze-dried fruit, freeze-dried cheese. Can't contemplate chewing anything? Keep pouches or individual servings of apple purée stashed within reach. And of course, don't forget the ginger – whether it's a ginger drink that doesn't need refrigerating, some gingernut biscuits or ginger chews.

an attack may actually help to ward it off. Caught in a vicious morning-sickness cycle (you're too queasy to eat, but when you don't eat, you get more queasy – making it hard to eat)? The best way to break out is to remember the three S's: slow, small, steady. Even if you're hungry, or in a hurry to get something in your stomach before you start feeling super sick again, don't gulp or gobble. Too much, too soon, and you'll pay the queasy cost. Instead, have a few sips of lemon water, ginger tea, cold smoothie or whatever liquid your tummy can tolerate. Alternate sips with a nibble of a solid you can stand – whether that's a chunk of cheese or a chunk of watermelon, a few almonds or a few pretzels . . . or yes, even a few of those crackers. Once you've let those sips and nibbles settle and coat your stomach, gradually move on to your

mini-meal or maxi-snack (hopefully one that contains the quease-easing combo of complex carbs and protein; keep reading). Or if that proves too tummy taxing, just keep the grazing going for now. And don't forget the steady part. To prevent that cycle from starting all over again, keep your blood sugar up and your tummy just a little bit full all day long (including just before you head to bed and as soon as you wake up in the morning).

- Concentrate on carbs. From the cliché cracker to the driest of dry toast, carbs often bring comfort to the queasy. When you can (that is, when your tender taste buds will cooperate), go for the grain when satisfying your craving for the bland and starchy – opt for wholegrain toast, pretzels, crackers and digestives. Another carb that's complex yet easy to get down: fruit.

Soothing Smoothies

Need something in your stomach besides water but can't stomach solids? Try a liquid that eats like a solid: a smoothie. Hydrating, soothing and packed with nutrients (more than many solid meals have, depending on which ingredients you're blending together), a fruit smoothie can be tummy coating without being tummy overloading. Use frozen fruit (berries, bananas, mangoes) instead of fresh, and you'll make your smoothie extra icy – and extra easy going down (the colder a food or drink, the less pronounced the smell or taste, usually a plus for sensitive pregnant palates). Experiment with the milk you use (coconut and almond make great dairy-free options), or blend with Greek yogurt (high in protein, a proven quease-reliever, especially when teamed with the complex carbs found in fruit). And don't pack away your blender after your morning sickness (hopefully) passes. Smoothies make a perfect energy-boosting pick-me-up or a power-packed breakfast-on-the-go anytime during your pregnancy and beyond (new mums, you may have heard, are always on the go). Ready to get blending? You'll find some smoothie ideas starting on page 345.

Not near a blender but need a little something smooth and refreshing? Chilled apple purée, fruit or yogurt pouches designed for little ones are also super-convenient and potentially comforting mum snacks, too.

Many mums find relief in fresh fruit, particularly when it's juicy (nature's way of ensuring fluid intake) and icy cold: watermelon, oranges (or those cute easy-peel seedless clementines), grapefruit, frozen grapes, frozen bananas, frozen mango chunks. Others prefer a chewy or crunchy approach to their fruit – raisins and dried apricots, or freeze-dried strawberries and bananas.

- Think protein. Though carbs are the first food group mums-to-be usually turn to when they're queasy, adding a little cheese (or another protein food, like almond butter) to those crackers can fight nausea even more effectively. Studies show that pregnant women experience less nausea when eating high-protein snacks – and that eating them in combo with complex carbs brings even more relief. So reach for any protein your tummy finds tolerable (a cheese stick or some crunchy freeze-dried cheese, some almonds, a pot of Greek yogurt, for instance). Peanut or almond butter (ready to pull out and spread on crackers or apple slices) may be an especially handy protein source.

- Stay off the fat track. If it's greasy and/or fried, your stomach will have a harder time digesting it. Those oils can also send your nervous system into overdrive, activating more nausea.

- Let your tastes take the wheel. If the sight, smell or even suggestion of a food makes you sick, don't eat it – no matter how healthy it is. Veer, instead, for foods that you find appealing, or at least inoffensive – even if they're not the healthiest food since sliced wholemeal bread. And remember what they say about variety being the key to good nutrition? Forget about it for now if only a few foods make the quease-easing cut. Once the morning sickness cloud has lifted, you'll be able to lift yourself out of your food rut.

- Be dense. In your food selections, that is. If half of everything you eat comes up, the half that stays down should (as much as possible) provide you with as many nutrients as possible. So choose foods that are packed densely with high-quality nutrients. Think wholegrains, nuts, peanut or almond butter, cheese, beans, avocados, sweet potatoes, dried or freeze-dried fruit, mangoes, melon.

- Take a fluid approach. Fluids are more important in the short term (aka your first trimester) than solids are, and they'll be more important still if you've been doing a lot of vomiting. So do your best to drink up and stay hydrated (you'll know you're lagging on liquids when your urine is dark – it should be clear). If even the thought of drinking glass after glass of water makes you gag, quench your quota with icy cold watermelon (150 g of watermelon cubes equals 120 ml of water), suck on ice chips, slurp some frozen juice ice lollies, chew on some cold, crunchy cucumber or celery. Flavouring your water with cucumber, lemon or watermelon slices, or a squeeze of lemon or lime juice (and sticking it in the freezer for a few minutes to get it as cold as possible) may make it more palatable, too. Switch to electrolyte water, which may replenish better than regular – or sip cold coconut water, which may be extra soothing and hydrating. Or icy almond milk. And if solids are not your friend, take a fluid approach to those, too, in the form of a fruit smoothie or a soup. Turn to the smoothie recipes starting on page 345 and the soup recipes starting on page 222.

Whatever Gets You Through the Day (and Night)

Morning sickness has cut your can-eat list to two foods? Or maybe just one? No worries. For now your only objectives are staying hydrated and keeping your head out of the toilet, at least as much as possible. So eat whatever gets you through the day (or night) – even if it's breakfast served for breakfast, lunch and dinner. Once morning sickness has passed, you'll have plenty of time to add variety back into your diet.

- Freeze the quease. Many women find that icy-cold or frozen fluids and foods are easier to get down. Try frozen grapes or bananas or mango, well-chilled fruit pots or fruit pouches (they may be marketed for tots – but they also hit the spot for those growing a tot). Or try sipping on icy-cold almond milk, also touted for its tummy-settling benefits (it works on heartburn, too). Another reason why you may want to chill out: cold foods don't come with as much of a smell or taste.

- Snap out of it with ginger. Score one for the ages – and an age-old solution to the age-old problem of tummy troubles. Ginger has been used for generations to settle stomachs, ease cramps, combat indigestion, nix nausea – and as it turns out, this is one remedy that has made it out of the home and into the medical books. Already scientifically proven to alleviate motion sickness, ginger can also be good for what ails a queasy mum, according to research. Take it in capsule form (sold in the supplement aisle, but ask your healthcare provider to recommend a safe dose, and check the label for other ingredients), make ginger tea by infusing ginger root in boiling water or using ginger teabags (again check labels for added ingredients that might not be pregnancy-safe), cook with ginger (in those biscuits, muffins or a soup) or turn to prepared ginger-based foods and beverages: gingernut biscuits, crystallised ginger, ginger boiled sweets, soft chews and lollipops, and real ginger ale. Even the smell of fresh ginger (cut open a knob and take a whiff) may quell the queasies.

■ Find the power in sour. You can also try another trick of the queasy trade: lemons. Many women find both the smell and taste of super tart and sour foods super comforting. So when life gives you morning sickness, try making lemon- or limeade (or a lemonade slushie). Or reaching for a grapefruit – the more mouth-puckering, the better. Or a jar of sauerkraut – or a bowl of hot-and-sour soup. Wondering if there's really any cred behind the pregnancy cliché of pickles? Pickles (or really anything pickled in vinegar, from mushrooms to carrots to chilli peppers) do comfort many queasy mums. And while the pickle jar is open, consider that some mums-to-be actually find sipping pickle juice incredibly (and surprisingly) soothing – and some swear by cubes of frozen pickle juice (freeze the juice in ice cube trays). Sour or peppermint-flavoured boiled sweets spell relief for others.

■ Take your vitamins. In general, women who get enough vitamins and minerals before they get pregnant (say, from taking an antenatal vitamin pre-conception) experience less morning sickness misery than those who come

into pregnancy vitamin deficient. The train has already left the pre-conception station? Taking your one-a-day antenatal supplement can decrease nausea symptoms once you're pregnant.

■ And keep them down. Wondering how that daily antenatal is supposed to relieve your morning sickness if you can't choke it down (or keep it from coming back up)? Pharmacy shelves are lined with antenatal supplements, and one's bound to be better tolerated by your tummy. Your healthcare provider can recommend some good options such as a coated one, one that has a slow-release formula or one that adds ginger. Ask about ones that come in powder form (you can sprinkle it into your smoothies or mix with water – just remember you'll have to drink the whole dose) or as gummies. Minimise the tummy troubles an antenatal may trigger by taking it with a meal or substantial snack. Taking it with dinner or a bedtime snack may provide the perfect timing, since you might be able to sleep through any queasiness it causes. If you find your antenatal vitamin doesn't agree with you no matter what time of day you take it and no matter what form or brand you use, ask your healthcare provider about prescribing one that has a greater amount of vitamin B_6 than a standard antenatal vitamin. (Research has shown that vitamin B_6 in moderate dosages – 30–75 mg per day – successfully relieves nausea for many mums-to-be.) Bonus if it also has a controlled formula that releases the vitamins in your body evenly throughout the day and contains no iron, which can upset the stomach. You probably won't need the added iron until mid-pregnancy, when mums start running low on stores – and by that time, you'll hopefully be out of the morning sickness woods. If not, your healthcare provider can recommend a formula that's easier on the stomach.

■ For a tough case, try a tough approach. Is your morning sickness significant enough that dietary changes aren't changing a thing? It's time to ask your healthcare provider about medication options. For information on prescription and over-the-counter medicines to help combat morning sickness, see *What to Expect When You're Expecting.*

If your nausea and vomiting are severe and unrelenting, you may be experiencing hyperemesis gravidarum, a pregnancy complication that requires prompt treatment. Treatment will include IV fluids as needed to combat dehydration, medications and sometimes hospitalisation. See your healthcare provider for advice, and see more about hyperemesis gravidarum in *What to Expect When You're Expecting.*

Food Cravings

Was that you foraging in the freezer for the slow-churned vanilla ice cream, and in the fridge for the sliced pickled chilli to sprinkle over it? Spending your whole lunch hour searching for a deli that would make you a peanut butter and pickle sandwich on raisin bread (then adding a layer of chocolate chips while no one was looking)? Embarrassing your partner at the buffet table during last week's cocktail party by dipping the grapes into mustard? Wishing you could find a pizza place that serves chocolate pudding – not for dessert, but to spread on your black-olive-and-anchovy pizza? Or a lunch place that serves breakfast all day – because it's the only meal you can stomach?

Welcome to the cravings club. More than three-quarters of all women experience food cravings at some point in their pregnancy, usually in the first trimester. The most commonly reported cravings (not surprisingly, many women prefer to keep their cravings to themselves rather than report them) are for sweet, sour, salty and spicy foods – often in combination, sometimes in unlikely combinations. Carbs top the cravings

chart (again, no surprise), as does fruit. But few mums-to-be actually go by the book when it comes to their pregnancy cravings, which can range from the peculiar (potato chips layered between waffles, topped with equal amounts of hot sauce and maple syrup) to the particular (an artisan brand of salt-and-vinegar potato crisps available only from a local gourmet food shop, dipped in an egg salad made only at a certain cafe, topped with a salsa available only at a single market that's 30 miles away), from the unexpected (raw red onion, eaten like an apple, or pecan pie topped with ketchup) to the obvious (a whole box of doughnuts), from the downright healthy (citrus fruit by the crateful, cheese by the wheel) to the downright dangerous (such as dirt or clay; see the box on page 116).

Can you blame your pregnancy cravings on pregnancy hormones? Of course you can – just as you can (justifiably) blame those monthly hormone-charged visits for your monthly visits to the House of Fudge. Except, supercharged, since the hormonal changes of pregnancy are far more dramatic than the premenstrual

Craving That? Try This Instead

From salty to sweet, starchy to crunchy, hot to cold, there's a nutritious yin for just about every food you have a yen for during pregnancy. Will it be easy to convince your inner chocoholic that fruit is just as sweet as fudge? To fill that doughnut hole in your heart with a bran muffin instead? Realistically, not always. But with a little creativity

– and some willpower – you may sometimes be able to secure a substitute that truly satisfies both body and soul. Accept substitutes often, and you may be surprised to find your tastes – and your cravings – adjusting accordingly, ultimately making that slice of melon as tempting as that slice of cake. Well, almost.

INSTEAD OF	TRY
Chocolate bar	Low-fat chocolate milk or hot chocolate
Frozen chocolate bars	Frozen bananas, dipped in chocolate
Cinnamon bun	Wholegrain cinnamon toast
Jam doughnut	Grilled peanut butter and jam sandwich
Chocolate doughnut	Grilled peanut butter and chocolate sandwich
Cake	Any of the nutritious and delicious biscuits and muffins in this book (recipes begin on page 352)
Sweets	Trail mix (made with dark chocolate chips)
	Dried or freeze-dried fruit, frozen grapes
Apple pie	Baked apple
	Peanut butter on apple slices, sprinkled with muscovado sugar, raisins and cinnamon, microwaved until gooey
Gummies	All-fruit snacks
Slushie	Apple purée, frozen until slushy; an icy smoothie (recipes start on page 345)
Ice cream	Frozen yogurt
Potato crisps	Soya, vegetable, grain, kale or bean crisps, baked cheese puffs or veggie puffs, wholegrain tortilla chips, air-popped popcorn (tossed with grated Parmesan cheese for extra flavour), pretzels, salted edamame, seaweed snacks, lentil snacks, toasted chickpea snacks
Potato chips	Baked sweet potato chips
Fizzy soft drink	Fruit juice mixed with sparkling water
Soured cream	Greek yogurt

CHEW ON THIS. Old wives, not surprisingly, have their share of theories about pregnancy food cravings. Here are a few tales:

- If you crave sweets, you're having a girl.

- If you crave meat or cheese, salt or spice, you're having a boy.

- If you crave something during pregnancy and don't get it, the baby will have a birthmark in the shape of the craving. (A good reason to give in to that chocolate-dipped dill pickle?)

variety. Possibly intensifying those cravings are a mum-to-be's intensified senses, especially a keener sense of taste and smell, also triggered by hormonal surges – which drive her away from some foods and have her (or her partner) driving at 2 a.m. to the nearest newsagent for others.

Another popular explanation for pregnancy cravings: you crave what your body needs. Crave salty foods? It may be your body's signal that it needs more sodium as it pumps up your blood volume. Or more fluid (if you listen to your body and break out the salted nuts, you'll get thirstier, sending you to grab a glass of water). Can't get enough grapefruit? Maybe it's your body's way of sending an SOS for vitamin C. Cheese on everything? Your body might be campaigning for calcium.

Can you bet on your body delivering accurate messages through your cravings? Sometimes probably yes, but sometimes maybe not. This biological messaging system probably worked best before humans started departing from the food chain and relying so much on fast-food chains – and, of course, before the invention of fast fast-food delivery

(your cravings delivered). With no apps and limited food choices, a pregnant cavewoman's craving for something sweet sent her foraging for berries full of vitamin C or picking fruit packed with vitamin A – a sign that she and her body had communicated well. Today, it's too easy for your body's signals to become scrambled – having you scrambling for the nearest tub of cookies-and-cream ice cream instead of the nearest punnet of berries. Far from a nutritional disaster, but definitely a disconnect.

Most likely, food cravings are a complex mix of physiological, psychological, behavioural and cultural factors – with a personal component tossed in (you crave the comforting foods of your childhood when you need that comfort most). Handling them, however, doesn't have to be so complicated. Here are some tips that might make your cravings easier (and healthier) for you to deal with:

- Cave when you crave. Pregnancy cravings are a powerful force of nature, and fending them off around the clock could take everything you've got – maybe more than you've got. So don't feel compelled to fight them, at least not all of the time. Remember, they're not likely to last – they're usually at their peak in the first trimester, when hormonal changes are also at their peak, and even when they do linger, they usually ease up in intensity. Caving to cravings occasionally (or even regularly) won't wreak nutritional havoc during that first trimester, when your baby's nutritional needs (like your baby) are tiny. Especially if you add a side of good sense (you submit to a single brownie, but not the whole tray). Plus, if you're trying to battle your cravings while you're battling morning sickness, nobody's going to end up a winner – catering to your cravings may be

Don't Eat This at Home (or Anywhere)

Most pregnancy cravings can be satisfied safely – even if they're for foods that aren't exactly nutritious. But sometimes pregnancy cravings take a turn for the inedible and the dangerous. Women who experience the eating disorder called pica crave the taste, smell and textures of nonfood items such as dirt, clay, soap, chalk, tar or ashes. Giving in to these (sometimes uncontrollable) cravings can be harmful to both mum and baby, and can even be fatal.

What triggers such a risky compulsion? It's believed that pica may be linked to an extreme deficiency in minerals, such as iron or calcium, or to general malnutrition. No matter what the cause, if you find yourself craving anything that isn't edible, don't give in (and if you have trouble controlling the urge to eat it or drink it, make sure you don't keep the substance in your home or anywhere you can access it). Call your healthcare provider for advice.

Another compulsion that might signal a nutritional deficiency (but isn't harmful, except to your teeth) is ice chewing. Research has shown that ice-cravers are more likely to be suffering from iron-deficiency anaemia. Though sucking ice chips to relieve nausea is perfectly fine (and a good way to stay hydrated if you've been vomiting) talk to your healthcare provider if you're constantly craving that icy crunch.

---

the only way you can get or keep anything down at all. And if you're craving something healthy – like mounds of melon – by all means, yield to your yearnings without limit. Go for that third serving of cantaloupe. Or that bowl of cereal for breakfast, lunch, dinner and snacks. Craving something that isn't a food at all, like dirt or laundry detergent? Don't give in, and do read the box above.

- Eat before you crave. You're more likely to give in to a less wholesome craving when you're running on empty, so (when possible) try to pre-empt cravings with sustaining meals and snacks. Eating breakfast Cheerios can avert a mid-morning croissant crisis, while breaking for a sensible sandwich can stop you from braking for an afternoon brownie binge.

- Seek substitutes. When you can, try to find (somewhat) nutritious foods that can fill in for the less wholesome ones you crave. If you're longing for potato crisps, reach for bean or wholegrain tortilla chips instead, which offer protein and fibre along with that salty crunch. Focused on potato chips? See if sweet potato will get the job done, but with a vitamin A bonus. Satisfy your sweet tooth with chocolate-dipped strawberries instead of chocolate-dipped biscuits – or at least give a nod to nutrition with a dark chocolate bar that's packed with nuts. (See the box on page 114 for more substitution ideas.)

- Think small. If you're craving chocolate, go for a snack-sized bar instead of a jumbo-sized one (freeze it first, and it'll satisfy even longer). If ice cream is what your heart desires, follow your heart to the freezer aisle, but choose a variety that builds in portion control (such as single-serving ice cream pots or lollies), so that a scoop doesn't lead to a tub.

Food Aversions

So, maybe it's the sight of chicken that suddenly has you running scared – and gagging – to the nearest toilet. Or your must-have fried eggs with a runny yolk are now making you unexpectedly queasy. Or the taste of that foamy, hot latte (the one that you could never start your day without) that's inexplicably leaving you cold. Or the smell of melting cheese (the smell that always melted your resolve to not go for another slice of pizza) that's currently giving your tummy a meltdown.

If pregnancy has you loathing the foods and drinks you've always loved, you've discovered the flip side of food cravings: food aversions. And, as with food cravings, you're in plentiful pregnant company – in fact, up to 85 per cent of expectant mums experience at least a single food aversion (many have multiple ones). Thought cravings were a compelling force of pregnant nature? Aversions can be even stronger. Confusing, too, since they can have you heaving over the sight, smell or even suggestion of foods you've always favoured.

Some researchers say that food aversions, like cravings, are related to your hormone levels: they peak when your hormones are in their greatest period of flux, during the first trimester (which explains why most – though not all – food aversions pass by the time you're midway through your pregnancy). They can also be closely tied to morning sickness – the sicker you are, the more likely you are to have aversions . . . and in turn, the sicker the aversions will probably make you feel.

Another popular premise parallels the your-body-craves-what-it-needs theory of food cravings, but in reverse: food aversions are nature's way

of steering you away from foods that might be harmful to your pregnancy or your baby. Which makes a lot of sense when you consider that two of the most common early pregnancy aversions are to alcohol and coffee – beverages that don't mix well with pregnancy (at all, in the case of alcohol, and in large quantities, in the case of coffee). Or when you think of other foods that newly expectant mums often shun, such as chicken, meat, fish and eggs. Nutritious, for sure – but in the days before refrigeration (and meat thermometers) made these animal-sourced foods a mostly safe bet, they were a risky proposition, a potential breeding ground for the kinds of parasites and microorganisms that could make anyone sick (particularly pregnant women, whose immune systems are naturally suppressed). Another wise (if outdated) example of how nature may have had mum's back, and her baby's, when coming up with food aversions.

Broccoli's turning you green? Kale has you cringing? Some scientists suggest that these common pregnancy aversions also have their roots in ancient times – when vegetables were foraged for, not shopped for in the produce aisles. The very plausible theory: an aversion to bitter, pungent flavours was nature's way of steering mums-to-be away from toxic plants that might poison their babies. These days, it's a lot safer to eat green – and foraging for them doesn't get any easier than going to your local market or opening an app. And while vegetable aversions have clearly outlived any protective purpose, the instinct to step away from the salad bar lingers on, especially in the first trimester.

Because food aversions are so closely connected with nausea and

Metal Mouth

Do even your favourite foods taste tinny these days? You can thank your pregnancy hormones for giving everything you eat or drink that distinctly flinty flavour. This metallic taste is actually pretty common among newly minted mums-to-be. As with the morning sickness it often accompanies (doesn't misery love company?), metal mouth should taper off – or, if you're lucky, disappear altogether – in your second trimester, when those hormones begin to settle down. Until then, attack it with acid. Assertive acidic foods – such as citrus juices, lemonade, sour boiled sweets, and even pickles and other foods marinated in vinegar (often pregnant crowd-pleasers, anyway) – can dial down that metallic taste. Those acids will also step up saliva production, which will help wash that tinny taste away (hey, what's a little more saliva when your mouth's already flooded with the stuff?). Since the heavy metals in your antenatal vitamins, such as copper, zinc, chromium and iron, can (no surprise) leave a metallic aftertaste, ask your healthcare provider if changing to a more easily absorbed formula might help. Brushing your tongue (or using a tongue scraper) each time you brush your teeth can help minimise the metal, and rinsing with a bicarbonate of soda solution (¼ teaspoon bicarb to 250 ml water), which neutralises pH levels in your mouth, can also provide relief.

---

vomiting, some of the tips for dealing with morning sickness (beginning on page 106) can help with aversions as well. Here are a few other things to bear in mind if you've lost that loving feeling for foods you've always been fond of:

If the aversion is to something you're better off without . . . embrace your aversion. Consider yourself lucky if you suddenly can't stand coffee, or wine smells sour, or beer tastes bitter. It'll never be easier to give them up than when they're turning your stomach.

If the aversion is to something you feel you should eat, but just can't . . . just say no for now. Even if it's the healthiest food on the planet – or several of the healthiest foods on the planet, or seemingly all of the healthy foods on the planet – don't force yourself to eat it. Try, when possible, to find a substitute that's acceptable to your tender tummy and taste buds but approximates the nutrients in the food you can't handle (maybe it's peanut butter instead of chicken, or almond milk instead of cow's milk, or a mango smoothie instead of a salad). Are meat, fish, chicken, eggs and other animal proteins off your menu for now? Happily, protein comes in all kinds of packages, not just in the standard steak-house favourites. Instead of the meat or seafood counter, head to the dairy aisle, where you'll find cottage cheese (225 g easily subs for a 115-g chicken breast, protein-wise), yogurt (Greek or skyr are especially protein packed), as well as eggs.

Dairy's too close for comfort to cows, and eggs make you think too much of chickens? If the carb card is the only one you can easily play right now, play away. You can net that carby comfort plus a protein punch with a spin down the bread, cereal and pasta aisles – where high-protein grains, seeds, nuts and legumes (pulses) have found their way into a carb-lover's variety of meat-free products. Remember, too, that a small hill of beans can stand in for a mound of meatballs (that is, if your tummy can handle the side effects of wind). And don't forget that peanut butter (and almond butter) can spread a little protein on your toast, your apple slices . . . or even your pickles, if that's where your cravings have been taking you.

Not ready to give up on meat? Consider that it might be the sight of that slab that offends, in which case you might try hiding the meat rather than headlining it. Beef mince that's lost in a sauce, or soup, or stew – instead of front and centre as a burger. Chicken that's minced up and camouflaged in a casserole instead of confronted on the bone (or as a boneless fillet). Diced prawns that are barely recognisable in that sea of pasta.

Can't look at anything green? Until this aversion passes (which will likely be by the end of your first trimester, or soon afterwards), take a break from the salad bar – or from any vegetables that turn you into a Kermit look-alike. Take a walk on the sweeter side of the produce aisle, where you'll find mellow yellow and orange veggies, such as carrots and sweet potatoes, that offer the same beta-carotene benefits without the bitter taste. Or trade in your vegetables entirely for now and turn to fruit that can fill your need for those nutrients

---

Beyond Eating Well

Non-diet-related tips for fighting all of the pregnancy symptoms discussed in this chapter can be found in *What to Expect When You're Expecting*.

---

such as cantaloupe, mango, papaya, nectarines, peaches and apricots.

Can't sublimate or substitute? Not to worry. Though occasionally an aversion to a healthy food (or foods) plays for keeps during pregnancy (or new ones keep popping up), it doesn't typically outlast the first trimester. Which means you'll probably be back on the egg (or spinach, or beef) express before you know it – and before your still-teeny baby could possibly miss the nutrients in the foods you're skipping. You may find, in fact, that nutrient-packed foods you can't look in the face (or wing, or drumstick, or fillet) now, become foods you can't get enough of later. For example: you couldn't eat meat in the first half of pregnancy, but by the time you reach week 20, you can't get enough of it – perhaps nature's way of reminding you that it's time to step up your iron intake.

Constipation

As if getting food down (or keeping food down) weren't challenging enough these days, maybe you've discovered that getting it out can also be a struggle when you're expecting. The real bottom line: constipation clogs up the works for at least half of all expectant mums.

As with so many pregnancy discomforts, constipation is a crappy symptom that's around for a good reason. Here's why it happens: during pregnancy,

The Poo Scoop

Assume you're constipated as you're not having a daily bowel movement? That's a popular assumption, but not an accurate one. Constipation is defined as the passage of small amounts of hard, dry bowel movements, usually fewer than three times a week, and often with difficulty and pain. It's usually accompanied by wind, bloating and a 'sluggish' feeling (cue the laxative commercial).

Not have a bowel movement daily but you're eliminating with ease – and without discomfort – when you do? Having infrequent bowel movements, by itself, isn't a sign of constipation – in fact, there is no 'right' number of daily or weekly bowel movements. Normal is what's normal for you – whether that's three times a day or three times a week.

progesterone (one of the hormones responsible for a healthy pregnancy) relaxes the muscles of the bowels and causes the digestive tract to move at a much slower pace. The positive result of this digestive relaxation: better absorption of nutrients earmarked for baby making. The not-so-positive result: stools that stick around too long becomes harder (often literally) to eliminate. As pregnancy progresses, mounting pressure on the bowels from a growing uterus often compounds constipation.

How do you combat constipation without interfering with intestinal best (for baby) intentions?

■ Focus on fibre. Of course you've heard that fibre helps fight constipation – but do you really know how? It's easy: foods high in fibre absorb water, softening stools and expediting and easing their passage, essentially preventing or clearing up clogs in your digestive pipes. Not a bran flake fan? Think pensioner when you think of prunes? There are plenty of other fibre foods to focus on: wholegrains of all kinds (grains that are 'whole' include the bran, so no need to go all-bran – you'll get plenty in a bowl of any wholegrain cereal, a

slice of wholemeal bread or a plate of wholewheat or lentil pasta). Vegetables (especially raw or lightly cooked). And fruit (fresh, dried or freeze-dried). You should aim for about 25 to 35 g of fibre a day, but there's no need to count. You'll know you're fitting in enough fibre when your stools are large and easy to pass, not hard or pellet-like (poo frequency is less important than its consistency). But also know when enough of a good thing becomes too much. An excess of fibre in your diet can loosen stools up too much, and pass them through the digestive process too quickly, leading to diarrhoea and a loss of needed nutrients.

■ Don't clog up the works. So now you know why getting plenty of fibre is the key to keeping your pipes clean and running smoothly. But just as important is knowing which foods can clog you up. Common constipators: white rice, white bread, cereal that's made from refined grains (such as cornflakes), bakes made with refined grains (especially if they're also packed with sugar), and white pasta. Bananas may be the only fruit that's constipating instead of regulating, but they still come with nutritional benefits and are soothing for many queasy mums. So while it's smart not to go bananas with bananas if you're super-constipated, there's no need to ban them from your diet either.

- Drink up. Fluids keep digestive by-products moving efficiently through your system, so keep your water bottle handy. Experts recommend aiming for about 2.4 litres of fluid a day – and you can reach your share with water and other drinks as well as with fluid-rich foods such as melon, citrus fruits, lettuce, cucumbers, smoothies and soups. Stepping up your fibre? You'll need to step up your fluids, too (the fibre needs to absorb water to soften stools – otherwise the fibre itself can constipate you). Another time-honoured way to get things moving: turn to warm liquids, including that spa staple, hot water and lemon. It'll help stimulate peristalsis, those intestinal contractions that help you go.

- Befriend bacteria. The good kind, that is. Probiotics (aka good bacteria) are pro-digestion – they'll stimulate the friendly bacteria that's already in your digestive tract to break down food more efficiently, keeping it moving more effectively. Enjoy probiotics in yogurt and yogurt drinks (such as kefir) that contain active cultures. You can also ask your healthcare provider to recommend a good probiotic supplement – in capsules, chewables or a powder form that can be added to smoothies.

- Make use of magnesium. It's a pregnancy nutrient touted for easing leg cramps. But did you know that an adequate intake of magnesium may also help kick constipation in the buttocks? It works by relaxing the muscles in your bowels and drawing

Fine Fuzzy Friend

Eating prunes is definitely one way to combat constipation, but if you like your fruit fresh – and not too sweet – look no further than the kiwi fruit to get things moving. Besides providing that prune-like laxative effect (with no stewing required), this diminutive fruit packs plenty of nutrition within its fuzzy skin. In fact, gram for gram, the juicy kiwi provides more vitamins C and E than any of its produce peers. Peel kiwis, then slice them into salads, into yogurt, on top of cottage cheese or into cereal (they pair well with strawberries) – or simply split one in half and scoop out that yumminess with a spoon.

water into the intestines, allowing smooth passage of poo. Definitely ask your healthcare provider before you consider popping supplementary magnesium (you'll probably get the go-ahead at a safe dosage), but there's no need to check before adding plenty of magnesium-rich foods to your diet. Many of them are also high in fibre, including beans, dried fruit, brown rice, bran cereal, nuts, peanut butter, spinach and other green leafies, and oats. One dietary source of magnesium that's almost sure to put a smile on your face: dark chocolate.

- Be supplement savvy. Sometimes, supplemental iron can contribute to constipation, as well as other tummy troubles. Talk to your healthcare provider about whether a switch in your antenatal supplement (or your iron supplement, if you've been prescribed one) may help relieve your constipation. And though they may be a mum's best friend when heartburn strikes, popping too many antacids may also be constipating – so limit those if you're feeling clogged up.

Looking for overnight relief? Consult your healthcare provider before using over-the-counter laxatives or herbal or home remedies.

Wind and Bloating

Wondering how that bump can be so big when your baby is still so small? Chances are that's wind, baby. Gassiness – and its uncomfortable buddy bloating – often appears early in pregnancy, keeping your trousers from buttoning even while baby's still pea-sized. For some expectant mums, it's happily short-lived. For others, it can linger through the entire nine months.

And, once again, you can blame your pregnancy-relaxed digestive system. As the system that processes your food slows down, wind production (resulting in flatulence) steps up. Constipation (and bowel distention) compounds the bloating problem by keeping both stools and wind trapped inside the digestive tract.

The production of wind isn't harmful to you or your baby, of course. But it can be endlessly annoying and, let's face it, potentially embarrassing. To diminish the discomfort and beat the bloat, try the following:

- Go slow. A slow digestive system calls for slower eating. Taking meals on the run (one hand filled with a breakfast wrap, the other with car keys as you dash out the door), tossing down snacks (trying to beat nausea to the punch by gobbling up an extra-large tray of watermelon chunks while you're racing through the market on the way home from work), or mixing business with food pleasure

(negotiating a crucial deal on a conference call while simultaneously negotiating a chicken baguette) can lead to air swallowing. The gulped air forms pockets in the intestines that cause pressure, fuelling more painful wind. Instead, make time for your meals and snacks (even if that means getting up 10 minutes earlier in the morning to build in breakfast or signing out for an actual lunch break) and take them sitting down. As hungry as you are, or as keen as you are to get a little something in your stomach, chew on this: chewing is the first part of digestion, and breaking food down thoroughly with your teeth gives your sluggish system a much-needed head start on the process. And then, to avoid extra air, swallow with care (instead of inhaling your food).

- Avoid overload. Stuffing yourself will – obviously – only make you feel fuller and more bloated while leaving your digestive system with too much to tackle at once. Again, even if you're feeling like a bottomless pregnant pit, try not to fill your stomach to capacity. Eat enough to sustain and satisfy yourself but not to bloat yourself – grazing on six small, closely spaced meals and snacks a day instead of two or three gut bombs.

- Keep it moving. The more trouble you have passing stools, the more wind you'll accumulate – and the more wind you'll pass. So take steps to combat constipation.

- **Phase in fibre.** Does your battle to beat constipation have you going crazy for kale and bananas for bran cereal (without the bananas you were afraid might clog you up)? Doing too much too soon in the fibre department can overtax your digestive system before it has a chance to adjust. Take your fibre intake down a notch or two and then, as your tummy acclimates, gradually step it up again.

- **Bypass the beans.** They're a great source of fibre, protein, vitamins and minerals – but they're also a notorious source of flatulence. So until wind eases, consider limiting the amount of beans you eat (or even banning beans altogether for now), along with other common wind producers, such as onions, broccoli, cabbage, Brussels sprouts, cauliflower, green pepper and greasy, fried foods.

- **Be less bubbly.** For now, favour still water if sparkling water (or other carbonated drinks) gets your tummy bubbling, too.

Heartburn

What do pregnancy and pepperoni pizza have in common? That's easy – they both deliver heartburn, and lots of it. In fact, no one does heartburn like a pregnant woman (except, of course, for a pepperoni-pizza-eating pregnant woman).

Despite its name, heartburn has nothing to do with your heart – though that's approximately the area where you'll feel that burning sensation when acid from the stomach leaks up into the oesophagus. Normally, the oesophagus acts as a one-way valve – allowing food to enter the stomach, but not letting anything back up. During pregnancy, however, the muscle at the top of the stomach that usually prevents digestive acids from splashing up relaxes (like all those other muscles in the digestive tract), causing heartburn and indigestion. Even if you order in a grilled chicken salad, instead of that pepperoni pizza.

More than 1 in 4 women experience heartburn at one time or another during pregnancy (or all the time), but it usually worsens in the third trimester. That's because as the baby grows, the uterus puts pressure on the stomach, crowding the digestive tract and making it even easier for those acids to back up where they don't belong.

Reflux Redux

If you have gastroesophageal reflux disease (GERD), heartburn's nothing new, but treating it during pregnancy might be. Many of the dietary tips for fighting heartburn can also help with your reflux, but be sure to ask your healthcare provider about whether the prescription medication you're used to taking is still okay. Some are not recommended for use during pregnancy, but most are safe.

Heartburn, like so many other pregnancy symptoms that bug you, will not bother your baby. And, as with so many other pregnancy symptoms, the best cure for heartburn is prevention. Taking these steps can help cool the burn:

- Take it slow. Eating quickly may save you time, but you'll pay in heartburn. So take a tip from your digestive system, and relax. Don't rush through your meals, and chew thoroughly (so that your stomach doesn't have to work so hard digesting food).

- Take it early. Try to eat dinner at least 2 hours before going to bed at night so your body has time to digest the meal. An easy-to-digest bedtime snack (as recommended for a better night's sleep, anyway) is fine, though.

- Take it easy. Though heartburn is technically caused by a relaxed digestive tract, it's often related to stress – especially if you're stress-eating or eating while stressed. To prevent the burn, try to chill out while you eat. Avoid checking messages or emails or news apps that are likely to aggravate you, and try not to talk or think about stressful topics. Make mealtimes as zen as you can, and don't eat on the run if you can manage to sit.

- Keep it small. Large meals will stuff up your stomach, making it more likely that some of the food (and accompanying stomach acid) will find its way back up the oesophagus. Yet another reason to eat small meals more frequently.

- Keep fluids separate. There's a place for fluids and a place for solids, but when you're suffering from pregnancy heartburn, there may not be a place for both at the same sitting. Drink before and after meals instead of with them, or just drink a little. Too much fluid mixed with too much food will distend the stomach, aggravating heartburn.

- Keep your head up. Sit in an upright position when you're eating, and avoid lying down, slumping, slouching or bending over immediately after meals.

- Keep your weight on track. The heavier a load you're carrying, the more pressure you place on your oesophageal sphincter, the gatekeeper of the stomach. So try to gain your pregnancy pounds at the recommended pace (see Chapter 6).

- Don't pull the heartburn triggers. It doesn't take long to figure out which foods fire up the worst burn – once you do, you can eliminate them (at least temporarily) from your diet. Though your offenders may vary, common culprits include tomato-based foods, highly seasoned, spicy foods (that pepperoni pizza comes to mind, as does a vindaloo), caffeinated drinks (because they also relax the oesophageal sphincter), mint (particularly peppermint) and citrus. A diet high in fat can also contribute to heartburn, so ease up on the greasy foods (another strike against the pizza and vindaloo). Some mums even find that cold water can lead to heartburn, and sadly that chocolate can get high heartburn marks.

- Chew it away. Chew some sugarless gum for a half hour after meals to increase saliva production. Naturally alkaline, saliva helps neutralise the acid in the oesophagus. If peppermint is a trigger for you, try switching to cinnamon or fruit-flavoured gum.

- Go on an almond offensive. These tasty nuts neutralise stomach juices, relieving or even preventing heartburn.

Grab a few almonds for an after-meal chaser, or soothe the burn with an icy glass of almond milk (you'll get a calcium bonus).

■ Search for other soothers. Some mums-to-be find sweet relief by eating fresh, dried or freeze-dried papaya (which scores vitamins A and C, too). Others find comfort in warm milk mixed with a tablespoon of honey (or even honey straight up) – especially taken just before bed, to prevent night-time heartburn. Some say milk or yogurt can soothe, but your results may vary (you may actually find that dairy gives you heartburn). Some mums-to-be swear by small amounts of bicarbonate of soda or cider vinegar in water, and others say fizzy soft drinks work for them. Experiment to see what spells relief for you (or at least, what doesn't make your heartburn worse).

■ If you can't prevent, try popping. An over-the-counter antacid that contains calcium (such as Rennie or Rolaids) is safe to take during pregnancy and may keep the burn at bay while boosting your intake of that important mineral. If your heartburn is severe, see your healthcare provider to ask for a prescription for a safe medication that might help.

Fatigue

Used to be, you could hit the gym before you hit the morning commute – now you're hitting the snooze button . . . over and over again. You could top off a client lunch with an afternoon of meetings before capping it off with a client dinner – now your shoulders are sagging, your feet are dragging, and your eyelids are drooping by 3 p.m. Your weekends were always packed with activities – now they're packed with naps. And like most pregnant women, especially in the first and last trimesters, you're wondering where your 'get-up-and-go' has gotten up and gone.

The answer is simple. The energy you used to take for granted is now being taken up with the monumental physical challenge of making a baby. Your body is currently working harder at rest (the rest you're always yearning for) than it used to work when you were on the run – yes, even during those 10-km runs you once had the energy for. In addition to nurturing and nourishing a baby, you're fuelling its factory. Your heart rate and metabolism are up. You're producing more blood. You're using up more water and nutrients. And if that's not enough to knock you down, higher levels of the hormone progesterone are circulating in your system, making you feel fatigued when your day's just starting, and sleepy hours before bedtime.

Looking to put more pep in your pregnancy step? Clearly, giving your body the sleep it needs and the rest it craves will help relieve some of your fatigue. But how you eat can also make a difference. To eat your way to more energy:

■ Cash in on those extra calories. Your baby-making factory will need extra fuel as it kicks into high gear, which means you'll need extra calories (about 300 extra calories each day during the second and third trimesters, fewer in the first trimester). Undercutting this

The Flip Side of Fatigue

Could this be another pregnant paradox? You're so tired all day, you can hardly keep your eyes open . . . and then you fall into bed and can't sleep? Here's how to eat well to ease expectant insomnia:

- Have your cup of coffee in the morning. It can take 8 hours for caffeine to leave your system – and that can leave you buzzing at bedtime if you don't time your intake wisely. The better-sleep takeaway: Avoid caffeine in any form (coffee, tea, caffeinated fizzy drinks) in the afternoon and evening so you're not all wound up when you're trying to wind down. Ditto for dark chocolate – have your fix earlier in the day.

- Snack before you snooze. Remember milk and biscuits? It's time to revisit your childhood bedtime snack routine, with maybe a few modifications. The right bedtime snack will not only help you fall asleep, but stay asleep. Milk (warmed for those fuzzy slipper feelings) plus a wholegrain muffin or digestive will provide the protein and complex carbs you need to keep your blood sugar on an even keel all night long. So will cheese and wholegrain crackers. Or a banana and a yogurt. And presto, you're getting sleepier . . . and sleepier . . .

- Limit fluids after 6 p.m. so you aren't kept awake by (even more) frequent toilet runs. Get your fluid fill, but get it early. (Of course, if you're thirsty, drink up no matter what time it is.)

- If your healthcare provider has prescribed a magnesium supplement for constipation, take it before bed. Magnesium has relaxing properties that can help you drift off (while warding off the leg cramps that can stand between you and a good night's sleep). Plus that laxative effect you may be seeking will kick in just when you need it to . . . in the morning.

amount will undercut your body's already overtaxed energy reserves.

- Pack in extra nutrition. It may sound obvious, but a healthy diet provides higher-grade fuel for your body as it tackles not only the demanding job of baby growing, but also the other demands of your busy life. Simply put: more nutrients equal more energy. Another reason to be faithful about taking your antenatal vitamin, too.

- Breakfast like a champion. After a foodless night, your body needs to refuel before you start your engine – so start your day with a healthy breakfast that would make your own parents proud.

Stay away from quick fixes that don't last (like sugar and caffeine), and stick to the dynamic duo of protein and complex carbs that will stick with you all morning long (or at least until your mid-morning snack), keeping your blood-sugar level up and your body revved: porridge with walnuts and raisins, almond butter and sliced banana on a wholegrain bagel, a cheese-and-tomato melt on wholemeal.

- Eat extra often – and extra sensibly. That's right: the early-and-often approach to pregnancy eating applies to fighting fatigue, too. You'll keep your energy up by keeping your blood sugar up – and you'll keep your blood sugar up by eating small amounts of healthy food throughout the day (aka the Six-Meal Solution). Eat too much at a time, on the other hand, and the energy your body needs to get through the day will be shifted to digestive duties – after all, it's hard work to process a meatball baguette. Also, try to eat for long-term energy as you graze through your day. You may think having a chocolate bar will give you an energy boost to get through those afternoon slumps, but there's little truth in that thought. You may get a quick lift from a Snickers bar, but it'll likely be followed by a blood-sugar crash that will leave you lagging. Caffeine will give you an energy rush, but it will do nothing to sustain your blood sugar. And because that jolt will trick your body into thinking it doesn't need rest when it really does, it may keep you from falling asleep and staying asleep, especially if you suck down that espresso drink late in the afternoon. For a lift that lasts, turn instead to snacks that combine protein and complex carbs: peanut butter on apple slices, a slice of cheese and wholegrain toast, a smoothie blended from Greek yogurt and fruit. Be sure, however, to get most of your calories during the day, instead of saving them up for a super-sized dinner. Your body needs the most energy (and so the most

food) when you're on the go, not when you're about to head to bed. Stocking up on food when you're most active will give your body energy when it most needs it. Plus, you'll sleep better if you're not stuffed. (Do make a bedtime snack part of your bedtime routine, however; see the box on the opposite page.)

■ Add extra fluids. Your body doesn't just need extra fuel when you're pregnant – it also needs extra fluids. Not getting your fill of those fluids can lead to fatigue.

■ Pump extra iron. Occasionally, extreme fatigue (as opposed to run-of-the-mill pregnancy fatigue) is related to iron-deficiency anaemia. Since iron reserves typically start dipping midway through pregnancy, your healthcare provider will do a routine check of your iron levels at week 28 (as well as earlier, at your booking appointment) to see if you're starting to run low – and may prescribe an iron supplement as needed. Don't take extra iron beyond what's in your antenatal without your healthcare provider's go-ahead (it could constipate you), but do try to include iron-rich foods (such as red meat, spinach and iron-fortified cereal) in your diet. Still inexplicably exhausted? See your healthcare provider.

Other Pregnancy Symptoms

Eating well isn't the answer to every pregnancy complaint (if only!), but it can have a positive effect on a surprising number of aches, pains and more pains. Here's a sampling of additional pregnancy symptoms that you may

encounter during your nine months and how diet can help:

Tooth and gum problems. Besides the obvious (see your dentist, brush your teeth at least twice a day and floss regularly), making sure you get enough calcium and vitamin C foods will strengthen your own teeth and gums, and ultimately your baby's as well. When you're nowhere near a brush, munching on some cheese or nuts, or chewing on some sugarless gum, can do a good stand-in clean-up. Crisp fruits and raw vegetables, such as apples, carrots and celery, can also help clean plaque from teeth.

Dizziness. Running on empty for long stretches (something you're more liable to do in the afternoon, when many dizzy spells strike) can cause your blood sugar to dip, leaving your knees weak and your head spinning. So can being dehydrated. Snacking and drinking regularly to boost your blood sugar and keep yourself hydrated can ward off those woozy moments – especially if pregnancy nausea and vomiting are making it hard to stay well hydrated.

Leg cramps. Nothing cramps a good night's sleep like leg cramps, which keep many mums-to-be tossing and turning in the second and third trimesters. Hormones play a role, but some say diet can contribute, too. One theory suggests that an excess of phosphorus and a shortage of calcium circulating in the blood trigger leg cramps. Another implicates a shortage of magnesium or potassium (usually due to dehydration). To get a leg up on leg cramps, be sure your diet includes adequate calcium, magnesium, potassium and fluids.

Swelling. Nobody thinks puffy ankles are swell, but a certain amount of swelling (also called oedema) is normal and healthy during pregnancy. And it's common, too: about three-quarters of all expectant mums experience some. But excess water retention, especially when your shoes don't fit by the end of each

day and you can barely stand on those swollen feet, can make pregnancy (especially the second half of pregnancy) a pain. Not surprisingly, excesses of salt (say, that whole jar of pickles) can increase water retention. But in a less intuitive twist, drinking extra water can keep you from retaining too much, by helping you flush out waste products. And, of course, saltier foods can make you thirstier, making you reach for more water (so maybe those pickles aren't such a bad idea after all).

Headaches. Pregnancy can sometimes be a headache . . . and for some expectant mums, headaches can strike more often during pregnancy. The number one culprit: those pregnancy hormones. But headaches (especially the migraine kinds of headaches) can also be triggered by diet. To keep headaches at bay as best you can, stay away from your headache triggers (caffeine or chocolate, for instance) and be sure to eat regularly. A grazing approach keeps your blood sugar level, so you'll avoid those headaches brought on by low blood sugar. Keep a supply of high-energy snacks (such as lentil crisps, fruit-and-nut bars, peanut butter and crackers) to hand (in your bag, at home, in your office) so those headaches never even get off the ground in the first place. Also, drink lots of water, since dehydration can lead to headaches. Since going cold turkey on coffee can also trigger headaches (these from caffeine withdrawal), it's smart to cut down on a hefty coffee habit gradually.

Mood swings. As with headaches, mood swings can be brought on by low blood-sugar levels – and that's yet another compelling reason to ditch your usual three-meals-a-day eating routine and switch to the Six-Meal Solution. Keep complex carbs and protein front and centre in your mini-meals so that your blood sugar – and mood – stay stable. And keep sugar and caffeine consumption to a minimum, since both can give your blood sugar a quick spike – followed soon after by a downward spiral that can take your mood down with it. Getting plenty of omega-3 fatty acids in your diet (from walnuts, fish and enriched eggs) may also help with mood moderating. And here's some news that's sure to keep you in a good mood: a daily dose of dark chocolate can help boost your mood.

Skin and hair troubles. So your complexion didn't get the glow memo? That's actually true for many mums-to-be. But no matter what's wrong with the pregnancy skin you're in, it's possible that a healthy diet can help make it right. Dry, flaky, itchy skin? Try upping your fluids and adding some healthy fats (such as walnuts and avocados). Skin discolouration? Some blotchiness comes with the pregnant territory, but too much may be linked to a folic-acid deficit – so make sure you're taking your antenatal supplement faithfully, as well as eating plenty of green vegetables and wholegrain breads and cereals.

Teenage-style breakouts, and bacne? Hormones are the culprit (as they were when you were 15), and a doctor-prescribed vitamin B_6 supplement – which seems to help treat hormonally induced skin problems – may be the answer. But since some research also links acne to inflammation (possibly triggered by a diet that's high in sugar and other simple carbs), cutting back on refined foods may get you in the clear. Skin and nail beds that are paler than usual? You may be low on iron. Ask your healthcare provider whether you might need a supplement, and make sure you're getting enough iron-rich foods.

Spider veins and varicose veins starting to spin their unsightly webs? Turn to sources of vitamin C, known to promote elasticity. Ditto for all-over skin blahs – see the vitamin C light, and you may actually see the glow you've been looking for in the mirror.

Flaky scalp issues? Some research suggests that getting enough B vitamins from your diet can help reduce dandruff. Dry scalp, like dry skin, may benefit from a healthy dose of healthy fat. If your flaking dandruff is caused by yeast overgrowth, eating a diet low in yeast-friendly foods (sugar, refined carbs and bread, dried fruit, vinegar, soy sauce, peanuts and mushrooms) may starve that funky fungus and feed a healthier scalp.

CHAPTER 8

Eating Well Whenever, Wherever, Whatever

Y ou count your Daily Dozen at night instead of sheep. You've become a nutritious-food foodie and a serious label reader. You're completely committed to eating well while you're expecting. And then real life gets in the way. Your budget is blown by your first visit to the organic produce section, before you even picked up that organic steak. You have to work through lunch, again, and push 'select' on the vending machine, again. You have to work late, again, and end up at the drive-through on your way home, again. Business dinners challenge your resolve – and your ability to simultaneously feed your clients and your baby what they're hungry for (client: sushi and sake . . . baby: roasted salmon and steamed broccoli). The airline you've chosen for a 3-hour flight tosses a packet of snack mix your way and calls it lunch. The destination you've chosen for a 'babymoon' is known less for its green leafy vegetables and more for its gravy. The holiday buffet tables are covered with red flags (from the raw oysters to smoked salmon to the possibly unpasteurised Brie and eggnog). Not to worry – you can eat well whenever, wherever, whatever pregnant life throws at you.

On the Job

Mixing business with baby growing is always challenging (what you really need is an afternoon nap but what you really have is an afternoon presentation), but never more so than at meal and snack times. You packed a well-balanced lunch box (good for you!), but left it at your front door. Your morning meeting puts you face-to-face with the pastry tray. Your stomach's been growling since 11 a.m., but you're not on break until 2 p.m. Here's how to make sure that your 9-to-5 job doesn't conflict with your 24/7 job of feeding baby.

Stock up on supplies. Fill your desk drawer, your locker, your briefcase and your handbag with a selection of healthy snacks and quick bites to ward off hunger pangs between meals. A convenient fridge makes snack-stashing easier but isn't a necessity. For great snack ideas, see page 138. Also good to stock up on: containers for lunches and snacks. Be the cool mum with the bento box lunch – or the layered salad in a jar (see the box on page 267). Grab a flask while you're at it for hot lunch options.

Pack it. Leaving your next meal up to chance is never a good idea when you're trying to eat well, but especially when you're trying to eat well on the job. So unless you know where your lunch will be coming from (and you're afraid it may end up coming from the vending machine), don't leave home empty-handed. Pack up a healthy lunch (and a healthy breakfast, too, if you don't have time to eat before you run; see the recipes starting on page 191). See the box on page 132 for some lunch suggestions. See the recipes starting on page 210 for sandwich ideas.

Serve it hot. Cold sandwiches for lunch every day starting to leave you cold? Think hot instead. Bring a flask of chilli or hearty soup. Use the office microwave to warm up a chicken breast and some pasta, brown rice and steamed vegetables, or a tuna melt on multigrain bread.

Keep it cold. Take advantage of the office refrigerator (if there is one) and put any perishable foods you've brought from home in it. Or pack your lunch in an insulated bag with an ice pack to keep it cold.

Think drink. You're not just eating for two – you're staying hydrated for two, too. Which can be extra challenging when you're on the job instead of within steps of your kitchen fridge. Stay hydrated by keeping a large glass or a water bottle at your desk and refilling it often (giving you a chance to stretch your legs and catch up on the water cooler gossip). And though it's hard not to think coffee when you're thinking drink on the job, it's smart to limit your caffeine consumption (see page 69 for the reasons why).

Stick to a schedule. Never find time for meals when you're at work? Start thinking of baby's next meal as a clock you

> **CHEW ON THIS.** In Chinese culture, a pregnant woman is expected and encouraged to continue working throughout her pregnancy because it's believed that pregnancy 'labour' eases delivery. And if you have to work anyway – wouldn't that be nice to believe?

What's for Lunch?

Here are some lunch-in-a-box suggestions:

- Any of the sandwiches starting on page 210

- A flask of hot or cold soup (see the recipes starting on page 222), a cheese stick, wholegrain tortilla chips

- Leftovers from last night's dinner

- Layered salad in a jar. A great way to bring your salad to go. See the box on page 267 for tips on creating a salad in a preserving jar.

- A bento box lunch – perfectly portioned meals separated into distinct compartments

- A baked potato stuffed with leftover steamed broccoli and cheese (heated up in the office microwave)

- Cottage cheese, cut-up fruit, wholegrain muffin

- Greek yogurt, nuts, a granola bar, a peach

- A hearty salad, wholegrain bun

- Fresh roasted turkey breast and cheese wrapped in a wholemeal tortilla

- Turkey, beef or vegetarian chilli topped with cheese and chopped tomato, side salad

---

must punch, a deadline you must meet, or an appointment you've got to keep. Plan for a lunch break at the same time each day, and follow through as though your job (of baby feeding) depended on it. If your work takes you out to late lunches or dinners, have a healthy snack at your regular lunch or dinner hour to tide you (and baby) over until you and the clients can stop talking turkey and start eating it.

Make it easy. Feeding baby on the job doesn't have to be complicated, stressful or time consuming. Whenever possible, take the easy way out. Cook dinners with leftover lunches in mind. Toss juice or milk boxes (the kind that don't need refrigeration) into your bag so you won't have to run to the nearest corner shop for a drink. Let someone else do the peeling and chopping, and visit a nearby salad bar for lunch.

On a Budget

Watching your wallet? A tight belt may not be the most comfortable accessory when you're expecting – especially when you're always being advised to reach for the pricier organic produce or spring for the organic lamb. Still, there are plenty of ways to squeeze in good nutrition when you're feeling the financial pinch:

Pack your lunch. Need another reason to bring your own lunch? It'll save you money. Instead of paying a premium for a takeaway lunch, lay out for less on a delicious layered salad (see the box on page 267), dinner leftovers (that extra grilled chicken breast and brown rice you wisely made), a flask of hearty soup and some lentil crisps, or any sandwich on wholemeal. Wrap or bag it (or better still, pack it in reusable containers), and you'll save a bundle by the time your baby bundle arrives. See the recipes starting on page 210 for savvy sandwich ideas.

Tap into savings. You can save money multiple times a day – each time you reach for a glass of water instead of a soft drink or fruit drink. It's not only free, but it's the healthiest drink in the house. And in most houses (and offices, and restaurants), it's safe to drink straight from the tap. So instead of pouring money down the drain by buying bottled water (brands may be sourced from the tap, not from a spring, anyway), invest in a refillable water jug (with a filter as needed) – it'll pay for itself in no time. Bring a refillable water bottle to work, too.

Be a planner. Impulse shopping can cost you plenty. Use a menu planning/ grocery shopping app to keep you on the straight and narrow shopping list.

Go generic. While the packaging on store-brand foods isn't usually as pretty to look at, it's what's inside that counts. And generally, what's inside is of comparable quality and nutritional value to pricier brand-name products. Happily, most packaged foods are available in generic form – and more and more often, there are organic options in that no-name space as well. And here's something the food-industry giants might not like you to know: In many instances, the store brand is actually a brand name with a store label.

Stay seasonal. Buying fruits and vegetables in season isn't healthier just for you and baby, it's also healthier for your bank account. For instance, peaches and strawberries may be available year-round, but they're most nutritious and cheapest in the summer months. When the season is over for a certain fruit or vegetable, head to the frozen foods aisle, where the price and the nutrition are right year-round.

Pick and choose organic. No need to shell out more money for all organic products – just the ones where it'll make a difference. See the box on page 66 for the details on when it pays to pay for organic produce.

Eat a hill of beans. Or bean pasta. Or quinoa. Or eggs. Or tinned salmon. Lean sources of baby-building protein don't always have to come in pricy packages such as steak or fresh fish. So explore lower-cost protein options. (Who says you can't have an omelette for dinner?)

Keep it simple. Sauces add extra price – and extra calories. So choose simpler preparations: steaming, roasting, grilling.

Consider whether convenience is worth the price. Time is money, sure. But are the couple of minutes you save when you buy your carrots already peeled and cut or your cheese already grated worth the extra money you'll pay for these convenience foods? Sometimes they will be, sometimes they won't.

Buy in bulk. Bigger is almost always better when it comes to budget food shopping. So buy economy sizes of nearly everything you can – from chicken breasts to oats. Stock up on sale items, too, if they're not perishable and you're sure you'll be able to use them. (That case of grapefruit might look like a good deal, until you realise you can't fit them

Planning Ahead

The best way to ensure that your next snack or meal will be a healthy one – and that you'll have it when you're hungry for it? Plan ahead. That way, you'll have healthy eating in the bag (and your fridge, and your car, and your desk) whenever you're in the market for something to eat. Another perk to planning ahead? You'll often save time (in the long run) and money. Here are some realistic plan-ahead strategies:

- Plan for between-meal hunger. If healthy snacks are always within arm's reach, you'll never have to make a trip to the vending machine (for a packet of cookies) or to the corner shop (for a bag of crisps) when hunger strikes. Bag some crunchy freeze-dried peaches and toasted almonds to toss in your work tote, stash some kale crisps in your desk drawer and some fruit-and-nut bars in your car, and keep the fridge filled with ready-to-munch hard-cooked eggs, cheese sticks or individual wedges, cut-up raw vegetables, and fresh fruit. Prepping ahead will help: boil a big batch of eggs in advance (they'll stay fresh in their shells for a

week). Cut up those fruits and veggies twice a week, and keep them stashed in plastic containers. Or buy them pre-cut.

- Plan for shopping. Don't just stop and shop with some vague idea of what you'll be eating. Take a few minutes to make a weekly (or daily, if you shop that often) menu and arm yourself with a shopping list (on paper or an app) that covers it all. If that's too much prep work for the spontaneous you, at least make sure your cupboards, fridge and freezer are filled with healthy choices you can build meals from. If grocery delivery's your deal, place those carefully planned orders ahead.

- Plan for real life. Don't plan for meals you don't have time to make. The Beef Stew with Wild Mushrooms (45 minutes prep time; 1½ hours to braise) may have looked fabulous on your favourite food blog, but if you're likely to get home from work at 7 p.m. to an empty pot and an empty stomach, it wasn't the wisest choice for dinner (unless, of course, you're a slow cooker; keep reading).

all in your fridge – or eat them before they've gone soft.)

Get loyal. Download or sign up for supermarket loyalty programmes, where you may get weekly items at lower prices and be eligible for special discounts to bring the cost of your trip to the shops down.

Shop online and with apps. Online supermarkets and consolidators have

sales on every type of food – from cereal to bananas, wholegrain bread to oranges, healthy soup to nuts. Take advantage when you see online sales, and then multiply your savings by using discount sites and/or apps.

Grow your own. Whether it's fresh herbs on your windowsill, a small crop of tomatoes on your balcony, or a full-on garden of seasonal produce, cultivating green fingers can save you money.

- Plan on taking it slow (cooker). A small investment of time in the morning can pay delicious dividends in the evening when you come home to a ready-to-eat meal, thanks to your slow cooker. Sure, you can go all traditional with slow-cooked soups and stews, but you don't have to limit yourself to just those dishes. The slow cooker is plenty versatile, allowing you to whip up chilli, pulled beef, sweet-and-spicy chicken, lasagne, meatballs, sweet potato casserole and even puddings with minimal prep and little kitchen mess.

- Plan for leftovers. There's no rule that says you have to cook from scratch every single day. But when you do cook, consider doubling the recipe and freezing the extra portion for a different day. Or make just enough extra one night so that the leftovers can do double duty for a delicious meal the next day. The leftovers from your grilled chicken and broccoli dinner can turn into a leafy green salad with chicken strips and broccoli the next day, for instance. Baked salmon can be eaten hot and fresh from the oven one night, with the extra saved to be shredded and turned into salmon-and-quinoa patties for later in the week.

- Plan for tomorrow, tonight. If mornings are rushed for you, there's a good chance you'll dash out the door without breakfast. And as for packing a lunch box when you're already running late? Forget about it – it'll never happen. So instead of leaving tomorrow's meals up to chance – and up to the twists, turns and snooze buttons of real life – spend a few minutes before you turn in at night doing some advance work. Combine the yogurt and fruit and refrigerate it in the blender jar, so you can crush your morning smoothie, or pile some fresh spinach and cheese on a wholegrain tortilla and roll it up, ready for the morning microwave. When you're done prepping tomorrow's breakfast, pack both tomorrow's snacks and lunch – and hey (why not?), fill up tomorrow's slow cooker dinner so all you have to do in the morning is set it and forget it. (And don't forget to make an extra batch of that stew to freeze – one less thing to plan for next week.)

When Time Is Tight

Feel like you barely have time to eat, never mind eat well? Not to worry. Even if time isn't on your side, good nutrition can be. Following these time-saving tips will help:

Stock up. No time to stop at the supermarket after work? No problem – as long as your kitchen's well stocked. Keep your cupboards, fridge and freezer filled with all the ingredients you'll need to make quick, healthy meals all week long.

Shop once. With a good shopping plan and list to hand (or on your phone), do a week's worth of shopping for staples at once, supplemented, if necessary,

Microwave Smarts

I t cooks, reheats, defrosts – and saves time. That is, if you know how to use it. Armed with the following tips, you might really be able to turn your microwave into the little appliance that could:

- Start with microwave-safe containers. Use only cookware that is specifically manufactured for use in the microwave (look for a microwave-safe BPA-free container), and don't let cling film touch foods during microwaving. Better still, use kitchen paper or a paper plate to cover your food before you zap it.

- To maximise the retention of nutrients when cooking vegetables in the microwave, add only a few drops of water. Too much water, and the nutrients will be washed away. Even better, keep your vegetables on top of the water (with a microwave-safe rack) so you're steaming, rather than boiling. Be sure, too, to keep your microwaving time to a minimum, so that your broccoli ends up crisp and green, not soggy and grey. To cook to crisp-tender, 3 minutes (for 175 g) should be the ticket. Easiest of all: omit the water entirely (and the washing and cutting up) by choosing microwave-in-the-bag vegetables. (Those steam-in-the-bags don't contain BPA or other chemicals and are safe to use in the microwave as directed by the instructions.)

- Use your microwave for all it's worth. Sure, it's great for reheating those leftovers from last night. But there are plenty of other ways to work microwave magic. Here are a few:

  ◆ Before squeezing an orange, lemon or lime for its juice, microwave the fruit on high for 20 seconds. You'll get more juice flowing.

  ◆ Toast nuts in a flash by spreading them out on a plate and heating them on high for 2 to 3 minutes, stirring every minute.

  ◆ Make your own breadcrumbs by cutting a slice of bread into cubes and microwaving on high for 1–2 minutes, stirring once. Then crumb in a blender and toast like nuts.

  ◆ Poach an egg: crack it into a microwaveable mug, cover it with water (add a dash of vinegar if you wish), then cover with a plate. Microwave on high for 1 minute, then at 10-second intervals until cooked.

  ◆ For tear-free onions, slice off the ends off a whole onion and heat on high for 30 seconds.

---

by quick trips to the fish market for fresh fillets. Or forget trips to the shops altogether. Do all your shopping online and get your groceries delivered.

Equip yourself. So you got home from work at 7 p.m., have a class at 8 p.m. – and somehow have to cook and eat dinner in between? The right kitchen equipment can shave many valuable minutes off your food-preparation time:

- A microwave. Use it to defrost frozen foods fast, reheat leftovers in no time and even cook a whole dinner. A microwave cookbook or online microwave-specific recipes can show you how to make zap magic happen. See the box on this page.

- A slow cooker. Despite its name, a slow cooker can save more time than practically any appliance in your home. Chances are you got at least one as a present or on a whim at some point – dust it off and get busy. Just toss some dried beans and meat or chicken, some vegetables and flavourful stock, and a few herbs into the slow cooker before leaving the house in the morning, and a delicious stew will be ready and waiting when you walk in the door. Instant dinner! And yes, some slow cookers are Bluetooth enabled.

- An instant pot. This multitasking appliance is more than a pot – and depending on the brand you get, it could be a pressure cooker (which cooks food quickly – up to 70 per cent faster than traditional cooking methods), a slow cooker (see above), a rice maker, a steamer, a sauté pan, an egg boiler, plus more . . . potentially making mealtime magic happen in one pot, in no time. It also allows prepped meals to go directly from freezer to piping hot to satisfied tummy without pausing for defrosting. An added bonus: instant pots are extra smart – thanks to sensors, they won't overcook your food. Not smart enough? Pick one that's Bluetooth enabled.

- An air fryer. Sure, it's another appliance, but with no need to preheat and a faster cooking time, vegetables come out perfectly crisp and proteins perfectly cooked – in less time than it would take in the oven. (An added perk: you get your foods crisped perfectly without all that extra oil.)

- A wok (or large frying pan). The secret of really speedy – and healthy – cooking is stir-frying. Throw some chunks of chicken, broccoli, carrots and water chestnuts into the wok – and in a matter of minutes, a delicious dinner is served.

- A blender. You can enjoy a breakfast smoothie in just 30 seconds.

- A food processor. Who has time to chop? Who would bother when there's a food processor to do the work for you? These handy appliances can dice, slice, mince and purée onions, vegetables, potatoes, fruit or just about anything else that would otherwise take time and elbow grease.

- A really good knife. Don't have the budget or the space on your kitchen worktop for a food processor? Invest in the next best thing: a good-quality knife. A really sharp blade will chop hours off your food-preparation time.

Cook fast foods. Instead of going out for fast food, choose foods that cook up fast. A fresh fillet of fish or a boneless chicken breast can be grilled, poached or air-fried in minutes. Thinly sliced strips of lean beef or chicken can be stir-fried in moments. Vegetables can be air-fried or steamed to just-tender more quickly than they can be boiled, and you'll have saved not only time, but also the vitamins and minerals from going down the drain with the cooking water. Dinners prepared in instant pots are ready in a flash. Many recipes in this book can be prepared in 20 minutes or less.

Or don't cook at all. Serve vegetables raw. Eat leftover grilled chicken cold on a bed of salad leaves. Enjoy some chunks of cheese and a pear straight from the refrigerator. Open a bag of baby carrots, snack on dry cereal or freeze-dried fruit, or peel a banana and slice it into a single-serving container of cottage cheese or yogurt. All nutritious – all in no time at all.

Concentrate on convenience. When feeding yourself and your baby is going to take more than just reaching into the refrigerator and chewing, look for ways to make cooking and preparing meals easier and faster. Instead of buying heads of lettuce that need to be torn,

Launch a Snack Attack

Poking around the fridge, the freezer or your local market for some good healthy snacks to round out your day and your Daily Dozen? Give these a try:

- Hard-boiled egg (keep a supply in your refrigerator for a quick protein fix)

- Avocado toast with sliced egg (add sriracha for a kick)

- Drinkable yogurt or kefir

- Low-fat yogurt with granola, nuts and/or berries sprinkled on top

- Freeze-dried cheese

- Parmesan crisps (see box, page 252)

- A mozzarella stick and frozen grapes

- Mango, lime, chilli powder, pasteurised feta

- Babybel cheese and an apple

- Sliced tomato topped with pasteurised feta (or mozzarella) and olive oil (add some basil for a caprese salad)

- Wholegrain savoury biscuits or crackers with a cheese wedge

- Wholegrain tortilla, rolled up with grated cheese and tomato

- Wholegrain waffle

- Wholewheat pitta chips – ready-prepared or homemade (add your own salty, sweet or spicy flavourings)

- A healthy protein bar

- Carrot muffin (page 206)

- Ants on a log (peanut butter on a celery stick, studded with raisins or chocolate chips)

---

washed and spun dry and vegetables that need to be peeled and chopped, open a bag of pre-cut, pre-washed salad leaves, a bag of pre-grated carrots or cabbage, and a packet of ripe cherry tomatoes, toss them all into a bowl and top with oil, vinegar, dried oregano and some pre-grated Romano cheese. Presto – you've just made a fresh salad (and that took how long?). Scan supermarket shelves for other time-saving ingredients: grated low-fat cheese, pasta-ready tomato sauces, pre-peeled baby carrots, pre-grated cabbage for coleslaw, bags of microwave-ready vegetables, chopped, sliced or diced fruits and veggies, chopped garlic. Though these might cost more at the shops, you'll likely find they're worth the price when time is at a premium. Look also in the freezer section for frozen vegetables and fruit, as well as for healthy frozen mains. And don't forget the ready-prepared aisle, where you can pick up a roast chicken to go (a healthy choice once you've removed the skin and added that 10-second salad, a microwave-baked sweet potato or pre-cooked brown rice, and quick-to-cook frozen vegetables).

Cook for an army. If you cook enough for two or more meals at once (which takes only a few moments longer) and tuck the extras, in meal-size portions, in the freezer for future use, you'll save loads of time. (Mark the meals, so you won't be left with unidentified frozen objects.) Make a big batch of wholemeal pancakes or waffles on Saturday and freeze, and reheat for quick weekday breakfasts. Do the same when you're simmering up a batch of chilli. Bake or grill a multipack

- Almond butter spread on wholegrain crackers

- Peanut butter and dark chocolate between 2 apple slices

- A handful of almonds or walnuts mixed with raisins or freeze-dried blueberries or strawberries

- Dark chocolate chips with nuts or coconut flakes

- Fruit smoothie (see the recipes starting on page 345)

- Dried or freeze-dried fruit

- Frozen blueberries

- Frozen banana, spread with nut butter, sprinkled with dark chocolate chips

- Sliced banana topped with fat-free Greek yogurt and chopped walnuts

- Watermelon cubes, lime, a sprinkle of salt, a sprinkle of pistachios

- Carrot and celery sticks with hummus or guacamole

- Cucumber hollowed out and filled with hummus

- Baby cucumbers and tzatziki

- Toasted seaweed

- Broccoli crisps (homemade or ready-prepared)

- Bean chips, lentil crisps, veggie crisps, soya crisps, wholegrain tortilla crisps, kale crisps, root vegetable crisps

- Crunchy freeze-dried green peas or snap pea crisps

- Air-popped popcorn, sprinkled with Parmesan cheese and chilli powder

- A cup of soup sprinkled with cheese

- Crunchy roasted chickpeas (see page 252)

of boneless, skinless chicken breasts and freeze them individually so you'll always have some to top a salad, fill a sandwich, or add to a veggie stir-fry or pasta dish. Cook a huge batch of brown rice or other grains, and freeze flattened in portioned-out sizes. Just remember to date your freezer stash, so you'll know which items to use first. Have an instant pot? You can use it to heat up your stash without needing to defrost first.

Prep for an army. Cut up fruits and vegetables twice a week, and keep them stashed for easy snacking in airtight plastic containers. Boil up a big batch of eggs so you'll have them at the ready for snacking, slicing on top of salads or on toast or chopping into egg salad. They'll stay fresh in their shells for up to a week in the fridge.

Give leftovers a new lease on life. Roast a large turkey breast (or large chicken) on Sunday, have warm turkey leftovers on Monday (along with leftover sweet potato mash), turkey salad for lunch on Tuesday, turkey stir-fry with brown rice for dinner Tuesday night and (as you'll probably be sick of turkey by Wednesday) freeze the rest for turkey cacciatore (just add a jar of tomato sauce and some pasta) whenever the turkey mood strikes again. Or freeze the leftover turkey in slices, ready for workday sandwiches. Make a double batch of steamed broccoli, have it hot the first night and cold with a vinaigrette or warmed up in a pasta dish or casserole on the second.

Put time on your side with planning. See the box on page 134 for tips on planning ahead.

Ordering Up Labour

Are you over being pregnant (or even overdue)? Looking for a miracle meal to bring on those contractions sooner or help them get the job done faster? A last pregnant supper? Choose from this menu of supposedly cervix-friendly foods, some of which have become labour legends in the mum community, others of which have some medical evidence to back them up:

Dates. Thinking dates will be the last thing on your mind when you're pushing nine months of pregnancy? You might want to think again – and stock up on dates. Not the kind with your sweetie (though you might as well stock up on those dates, too, while you still have the chance), but the kind you can eat – also sweet. Not because they'll bring on labour sooner, but because research shows that eating dates in the last month of pregnancy can lead to a shorter, easier labour. Date-munching mums appear less likely to have premature rupture of the membranes and appear more likely to go into labour spontaneously (avoiding labour induction), have a shorter first phase of labour and have greater cervical dilation upon admission to the hospital or birthing centre. What's in a date that makes it so labour-friendly? Besides all the nutrients that are packed into those tiny sweets (including potassium, magnesium, vitamin K and folate), dates have an oxytocin-like effect on the body, helping to stimulate uterine contractions. Their laxative effects (rivalling those of their dried-fruit friend the prune) also stimulate uterine contractions. How many dates will you need to pop to expedite becoming a mum? The researchers had expectant mothers eat six dates daily beginning at week 36 of pregnancy. Just remember that dates are very high in fruit sugar, so if you've been instructed to mind your sweets (for instance, if you have gestational diabetes), ask your healthcare provider before you start dating that much.

Liquorice. Real black liquorice contains glycyrrhizin, an ingredient that, eaten in very large quantities (repeat: very large quantities), may speed up the onset of labour. The theory: glycyrrhizin interacts with cortisol levels and/or increases prostaglandins, bringing on contractions. But beware: that same compound can also cause potassium levels to drop, and in some people, possibly lead to heart arrhythmias. And while liquorice is safe in pregnancy, the root isn't. For mums with gestational diabetes, there's also a downside to all the sugar that liquorice sweets contain.

When Eating Out

Whether you're grabbing a lunch-break bite from a takeaway van, lingering over a leisurely brunch with friends or stopping for a quick dinner on the way home from work because you don't have the strength to lift a wooden spoon, chances are you'll be eating at least some of your pregnancy meals out. Maybe most of them. But how do you make sure eating well is on the menu, even when cooking isn't? And how do you keep the pounds from

Spicy foods. In the category of no harm and no proof: spicy foods. While there isn't any evidence that wolfing down some spicy chicken wings or anything doused in sriracha will bring on contractions, plenty of mums swear they've gone straight from a spicy meal to the labour and delivery floor. Of course, if your tummy (and your heartburn) can't take the heat, you probably won't want to turn it up – especially not in the last, extra-uncomfortable weeks of pregnancy.

Pineapple. Prefer a sweeter option? Pineapple or pineapple juice contains the enzyme bromelain, which (when consumed in large quantities), some believe, can contribute to cervical ripening and uterine contractions. There is no scientific proof confirming this theory, but if you're pining for labour, it's worth giving pineapple a try.

Italian food. Some mums credit the balsamic vinegar in popular 'labour salads'. Others point to those tasty Mediterranean herbs, such as oregano and basil, used in Italian cooking. Still others swear it's the aubergine that edged them closer to delivery. But scientists aren't buying it (though they may be eating it).

Castor oil. Hoping to sip your way into labour with a castor oil cocktail? Women have been passing down this yucky-tasting tradition for generations on the theory that the powerful laxative will stimulate a mum's bowels, which in turn will stimulate her uterus into contracting. The caveat for this one: castor oil (even mixed with a more appetising drink) affects your bowels more than it affects your uterus – causing diarrhoea, severe cramping and vomiting. Before you gulp it down, talk to your healthcare provider – and make sure you're ready to begin labour that way. A less aggressive way to get your bowels (if not your uterus) in an uproar: have a bowl of all-bran cereal.

Herbal teas and remedies. Raspberry leaf tea, black cohosh and evening primrose may be just what your ancestors (and Instagram buddies) ordered for the overdue, and some studies show that these herbal remedies may actually help trigger or speed up contractions. However, since there's no proof of their safety or effectiveness, it's best to ask your helathcare provider about whether (and how much of them) you should take and how. And turn to them only once you've reached full term.

For more DIY labour-induction tricks that may (but probably won't) do the trick, see *What to Expect When You're Expecting.*

---

piling on too fast when eating out comes with your job or your lifestyle? Easy – just keep these tips in mind:

- Choose a baby-friendly restaurant. It won't be high chairs you'll be scouting for when you're taking your baby out to dinner (at least not yet) – it'll be healthy eating options. Realistically, you won't always get to pick the restaurant, but when you do, be picky. Before you ask for a table, ask for a menu. Better still, scope it out online ahead of time, and scan it for nutritious items (most restaurants have at least some).

- Have your order in mind. Again, you can't always plan ahead or run the dinner show. But when you can, try to have at least a general idea of what you'll order before you sit down. One, because you'll be able to order it faster, which means you'll be tucking into your meal faster (especially important if you're running on empty). Two, because it will leave less room for impulse orders (if you've mentally prepared for grilled chicken and a salad, you're less likely to end up wandering to the fried side of the menu).

■ Take the hunger edge off. Whether it's a handful of almonds or a wedge of cheese, have a light snack before you head out to eat, so you won't be starving by the time your food arrives.

■ Ask . . . and you will probably receive. Rare is the server (and kitchen) who won't accommodate a pregnant woman's special requests. So make them.

■ Be on portion patrol. Many restaurants dish out portions that well exceed suggested serving sizes for most foods – whether it's a huge steak or a dish piled high with pasta. Too much food (which you may feel obligated to eat, since you're paying for it) can lead to too many calories . . . and/or too much heartburn. Especially if you eat out often, consider sharing a main course or bringing home half (and there's tomorrow's lunch, ready to roll). Or skip the main course and go appetiser-happy: order two of them – one for your starter, one as your main course.

■ Look before you leap into the bread basket. Check the contents for wholegrain options. If none turn up there, ask your server if there are any available from the kitchen. If you're still out of luck, try to go easy on the white stuff, saving your appetite for more wholesome foods still to come. And mind the butter and olive oil, since that fat can add up fast – and your meal's just getting started. Dip and spread with a light hand.

■ Go for green. Select a salad as a first course or a side, so you're sure to score your green leafy vegetables. Ask for the dressing on the side so you can choose how much you want to spoon on or dip in. Not feeling like a salad? Start with grilled vegetables instead.

■ Seek soup. In many restaurants, some of the most nutritious dishes come in bowls (or cups). Look to lentil, bean or vegetable soups (from minestrone to tomato, sweet potato to butternut squash), and don't forget to consider cold ones, too (gazpacho, for instance, is a veritable salad-in-a-soup-bowl). Clamouring for a clam chowder? Choose one that isn't cream-based – in fact, avoid all cream-based soups, which are typically heavy on the fat.

■ Keep it simple. Stick to lean meat, poultry, fish or seafood, and order them simply grilled, roasted, baked, steamed or poached – 'fried' and 'sautéed' are often keywords for 'full of fat'. Ask for sauces and gravies to be served separately on the side, so you can drizzle as desired.

■ Be side savvy. The company your meat (or fish) keeps is important, too. Since restaurants usually offer a choice (or will allow substitutions), choose wisely: opt for a side salad, steamed or grilled vegetables, beans, a baked potato, sweet potato or, if it's offered, brown or wild rice or another wholegrain. Since vegetable servings are often skimpy (are those orange slivers the carrots you ordered?), you might consider asking for an extra portion.

■ Treat yourself with care. Is the dessert menu sweet-talking you? Try talking yourself into fresh berries, or maybe a scoop of ice cream or fruit sorbet, instead of the dulce de leche cheesecake (or other desserts that come with a hefty calorie tab). Cravings are calling? Give in while still being sweets-smart: Consider sharing with the table, instead of attacking it all by yourself.

While Travelling

Never again will it be so easy to travel with baby on board. (No nappies! No car seats! No childproofing hotel rooms!) Still, whether you're flying from Edinburgh to India, driving from Cardiff to Sheffield, or on the road for business, pleasure or a little mix of both, being a pregnant traveller poses certain challenges – especially when it comes time to feed your hungry load. After all, it's easy for your eating habits to wander when you're roaming.

How do you schedule regular meals when you're on an irregular schedule (you just lost 3 hours to a time change, or 2 hours sitting on the runway)? How can you handle blood-sugar dips on take-off – or 2 hours from landing? A grumbling tummy between train stations or miles from the nearest motorway rest stop? And what do you do when you can't drink the water or eat the local produce?

You won't have to stick close to home to stick close to healthy pregnancy eating. What you will have to do is include baby's nutritional needs – and yours – in your travel plans:

On a Plane

■ Plan ahead. As you know if you've travelled before, meal service on some airline flights has just about disappeared in economy (you still should find it on long-haul flights). The best you can expect is a sandwich or snack for purchase, if that. Call ahead or check online to find out exactly what will be served and if meals are available for purchase (or for free on international flights). Sometimes a snack means nothing more than a beverage and a packet of pretzels. Take-off delays can result in mealtime delays, food service carts can move at a maddeningly slow rate down the aisles and special meals sometimes don't show up at all (plus, let's face it – they're not all that special).

■ Pack a snack (or a meal). Even if you'll be served a meal or have the option of buying one, chances are that what you'll find on your tray table won't fill your stomach. Not by a long shot. Plus, you have no control over when it will arrive or whether they'll run out of the only healthy choice by the time it's your turn to choose. So don't leave meal service up to chance. Always pack a healthy meal or a substantial snack, as well as a few light snacks, in your carry-on bag. Consider a cold sandwich or salad, a cheese stick and crackers, fresh or freeze-dried fruit, a fruit-and-nut bar, a bag of trail mix, lentil chips or vegetable crisps. Check your airline to find out what you can bring along from home and what you'll have to purchase once you've passed through security (like drinks and yogurt).

- Keep the fluids flowing. Flying can be dehydrating because of the low humidity in aircraft cabins, so be sure to drink a lot before and during the flight. Besides keeping yourself from becoming dehydrated, increasing your fluids will send you to the toilet often – a great way to stretch your legs and prevent circulation problems. But plan on picking up or filling up your own bottle of water before you board. That's because beverage service can take forever on a jumbo jet, and those tiny plastic cups may not satisfy your thirst. Never drink the tap water on an airplane.

In a Car

- Plan ahead. If you have many miles ahead of you, check travel apps or road maps to see if there are frequent rest stops on the motorway and what kinds of restaurants are available on the road you'll be travelling. (Bear in mind the eating-out tips on page 140 when making those pit stops.)

- Pack a bag. Wherever you're headed, don't leave home without a snack bag. Options to include: beverages, non-perishable snacks (those nuts, that freeze-dried fruit and cheese), a flask of soup for easy sipping and (if you're

carrying a cooler) a selection of cheese sticks or wedges, hummus and cut-up vegetables, and sandwiches (pittas and wraps make for neater eating). If you're in it for the long haul, you can always pull off the motorway and restock your snack supply at a local supermarket.

On a Train

- Check to be sure there's a dining car with a full menu. If not, pack enough meals and snacks for the ride. The snack bar, most likely, won't cut it.

- If you're travelling to the continent, check to see if there will be stops between transfers for a quick trip to restaurants or shops in the station.

On a Ship

- Assuming you're allowed on a cruise ship (your trip will have to be completed before week 24), it's practically impossible to go hungry on an all-you-can-eat cruise. But it is pretty easy to eat more than you're hungry for – and far more calories than you actually need. Fortunately, most cruise kitchens offer healthy options, and many will honour special requests. There will be plenty of temptations for sure, but try to shop the buffet and the menus with an overall healthy big picture (and your Daily Dozen) in mind.

- Be aware of bugs on board. Outbreaks of norovirus and other gastrointestinal illnesses are not uncommon on cruise ships and may be especially dangerous when you're expecting. Check a ship's safety record before you book, and follow the safe eating tips on the pages that follow when you're cruising with a baby aboard you.

Fill 'Er Up

Stopping to fill up your car with petrol doesn't mean you'll have to fill yourself up with junk food. Many petrol station shops will carry frozen fruit bars, bananas, yogurt, nuts, cheese, wholegrain crackers, healthy crisps and healthy snack bars, and some have fresh fruits.

At Your Destination

■ Build meals into your itinerary. Whether you'll be sightseeing or meeting, shopping or swimming, schedule in breakfast, lunch, dinner and snacks. Keep as close to the rhythm of your daily eating routine as you can, but when you can't (you slept through breakfast after a late hotel check-in, or the local restaurants don't open for dinner until 8 p.m. and your tummy can't wait), have a snack to tide you over until mealtime.

■ Pack snacks (again). Because you never know when those hunger pangs may strike (and in case they hit when you're far from a restaurant or shop – or before the dining room opens or after it has stopped serving), carrying easy-to-munch, energy-boosting snacks is a roaming-mum must.

■ Request a mini-fridge. Don't be held captive to the high-priced contents of the hotel minibar (if there is one). Most hotels will provide guests with a small, empty refrigerator upon request (sometimes for a fee) or allow you to empty the stocked minibar. Ask about fridge access ahead of your arrival if you can, and stock your mini to the max with milk, juice, cheese, yogurt, fruit pots, veggie trays, and other drinks and nibbles that need refrigeration. You'll be glad you did when midnight snack attacks strike. Want to avoid the sticker shock of hotel-provided bottled water? Stock up on your own supply and keep it chilled in your mini-fridge.

■ Play it even safer. Eating carefully – avoiding raw fish and shellfish, under-cooked meats and eggs, unpasteurised soft cheeses – is even more important on the road, especially if the road has taken you to a foreign country. If it's a foreign country with poor sanitation, you'll have to avoid even more. Any food that hasn't been cooked could be contaminated, so stay away from salads and raw fruits and vegetables that haven't been peeled by you (unless you've checked with the hotel to be sure sanitation protocol has been strictly followed – for instance, the kitchen washes all produce with purified water before prepping). Stay away also from milk and milk products (like cheese) that you're not positive have been pasteurised. Thoroughly cooked foods that are still hot are generally safe to eat, though you shouldn't eat any food (hot or otherwise) that appears to have been prepared or stored under unsanitary conditions. If food that is served to you seems questionable, send it back and order something safer. Lovingly rubbing your bump translates in any language: 'I'm not trying to be difficult – I'm just watching out for my baby.'

■ Hydrate with care. Getting your pregnancy quota of fluids when travelling is important, particularly if your flights were long or your destination is hot. But before you quench your thirst with a glass of cold local water, make sure it is safe to drink. (Visit www.travelhealth pro.org.uk/countries before you visit your destination.) If you're not sure whether the tap water is safe, avoid ice cubes and reconstituted juice or milk unless they are made with bottled, boiled or purified water. They will be in most good hotels, but always ask. Drink bottled water instead, preferably sparkling. (If the water is still carbonated, you can be sure the bottle hasn't been refilled from a tap and resealed.)

■ Don't ask for tummy troubles. A case of traveller's tummy can take the fun out of any trip. But when you're pregnant, cramps, vomiting and diarrhoea can be much more than a miserable inconvenience – and if they lead to dehydration, they can become dangerous. (Besides, who needs another reason to be nauseous when you're pregnant?) To make sure you don't pick up anything but souvenirs at your destination, follow food-safety rules like a mummy maniac – especially if you're travelling in a developing country. If Montezuma does claim revenge, be wary of self-treating. Many over-the-counter diarrhoea medications are not recommended for pregnant women, though electrolyte drinks and rehydration fluids are okay. Put in a call, email or text to your doctor or midwife back home for advice.

At Parties

So maybe you're not the party animal you used to be. (Those cocktail parties aren't quite as much fun without the cocktail, your eyelids can't stay open past 10 p.m. and your dancing feet are too swollen to fit into your dancing shoes.) That doesn't have to make you a pregnant party pooper. You can still kick up your heels (maybe just not those 5-inch stiletto ones) and enjoy a few rounds (just not the alcoholic kind) on the social circuit – much as you did when your little black dress was actually little. You just have to party . . . like you're pregnant. Bear these tips in mind:

Have one for the road. Because you never know what'll be on the menu when you're not the one planning it, eat a healthy snack before you leave home to take the edge off your appetite – just in case food isn't served promptly (or at all – as in, the cocktail party is cocktails only). Or the party buffet is just desserts – or simply sushi. And for the same reason, make sure you cram a snack into your evening bag, too.

Don't pass the bar. Sure, your party (or holiday) spirit will have to come from within – not from alcohol – when you're expecting. But that doesn't mean you'll need to work the room without a cocktail in your hand. Many cocktails can easily become mocktails – from a virgin Bloody Mary to a no-tequila sunrise or a rumless piña colada. Or keep it simple: an orange juice and fizzy water with a twist, or icy cold grapefruit-and-cranberry (stirred or shaken). Unspiked house punch or hot mulled apple juice won't be the same – but still fun and festive.

Survey the buffet. There may be plenty of can-do canapés: make a beeline to the veggie and fruit trays. Nibble on nuts; olives; cheese cubes, sticks or crisps; cocktail prawns or other cooked seafood; devilled eggs; grilled skewers (just make sure any meat you eat isn't rare); meatballs; vegetable or cooked-fish sushi; grilled vegetables. Pass on the smoked fish; raw, seared or otherwise rare meat or fish (as tempting as you might find that tuna tartare); raw seafood (those oysters and clams); sandwich meat (unless you're sure it's freshly roasted and carved); soft cheese (unless you're sure it's pasteurised or steamed to bubbly – see pages 82–83). Clearly, some buffet dishes will be worth

Healthy Holidays

'Tis the season to be jolly? No problem – and no need to get thrown off course, even with all those extra courses of food at family feasts. Eating well all year round is easy peasy, if you just remember these tips:

- Make room for tradition. No need to diss traditions – just dish up more of the right ones. Pile on the turkey and Brussels sprouts. Load up on the sweet potatoes. Find the medium-well cooked end of the roast and get busy. Go on the easy side when it comes to holiday trimmings that don't exactly fit the Daily Dozen profile – enough can be a feast. Your family's traditions don't include vegetables, wholegrains, or salad or fruit in any form? Start a new tradition, and bring along a tray of roasted carrots, a quinoa salad or a festive fruit medley.

- Feast but don't fast. Don't take a holiday from regular meals and snacks – even if you want to save up for a big Christmas dinner, you and your baby still need breakfast and lunch. Just make them a little lighter than usual.

- Don't be a Scrooge. Eating during pregnancy isn't about denying yourself – especially during the holidays.

Instead, make moderation your motto when it comes to the treats and sweets of the season. Where there's no wiggle room because of safety concerns – the eggnog is homemade with eggs missing a British Lion stamp (and rum), as is the holiday hollandaise, there's cold smoked salmon on the canapés, and the Brie from the local farm isn't baked – just take a pregnant pass (see Chapter 5 for other foods to table).

- Don't invite trouble. Enjoy the holidays, but bear in mind sensible eating tips as you do. Watch your overall consumption of calories (so you don't end up with a 10-pound gain during a two-week holiday season), try not to stuff yourself silly (so you don't pay the price in heartburn or painful wind), and while you're making merry, try to make as many healthy choices as you can.

- Look forward to next year (and years to come). If you feel a little deprived this season, bear in mind that you have more non-pregnant holidays ahead of you than pregnant ones. So take this year's holiday cheer with moderation, and look forward to being just a little jollier when next season rolls around.

digging into (those chicken breasts, that pork loin, those grilled prawns, that wild rice pilau) . . . others, not so much (that super-creamy Alfredo, those fried potatoes, that greasy sausage or those unidentified fritters). And of course, don't forget to leave room on your plate for salad and steamed or grilled veggies.

Be selective with sweets. If you really want it, you deserve it – so have it, in moderation. That's what celebrations are for. But try not to bust your calorie bank with sweets that are just so-so – and maybe don't take the all-you-can-eat sundae bar literally. Also be wary of desserts, such as mousse, that might have raw egg in them from home-reared chickens. Is there fruit on the dessert table? Go to town.

CHAPTER 9

Eating Well When Eating Is Complicated

I t's not always easy to eat well when you're expecting, even when you can (at least in theory) eat almost anything. But it's definitely more difficult to follow a healthy pregnancy eating plan when what you can eat – or should eat – is restricted by a chronic condition (such as coeliac disease) or a pregnancy complication (such as gestational diabetes). Or if eating – or gaining enough weight – is doubly (or triply) challenging because you're expecting multiples. Or if you're in bed with a bad cold – or on bed rest – and eating's just too much like hard work. Luckily, with a little nutritional know-how, there's a way around just about any obstacle to healthy eating.

If You Can't Handle Dairy

M ilk and dairy products are nature's finest sources of the calcium your body and your baby need when you're expecting. But if milk leaves you with more than a moustache (think wind, lots of it), you may think twice before reaching for a glass. Or before pouring milk on your cereal. Or dipping into frozen yogurt. Or cheesing up your sandwich.

What's causing all your tummy troubles? It could be that you can't tolerate the lactose or that you're sensitive to one of the naturally occurring proteins in milk. But which is it, and how can you tell those conditions apart?

Lactose intolerance results from a lack of (or inadequate supply of) lactase, the enzyme needed to digest the milk sugar lactose. Those who are lactose intolerant experience a range of symptoms, including wind, bloating, indigestion, cramping that can range from mild to severely uncomfortable and diarrhoea. Wondering if you're among the seeming legions of lactose intolerant? There actually may be fewer of them around than you might think. Studies show that many people who believe they are lactose intolerant actually aren't. Bear in mind, too, that there are degrees of intolerance. While some people can take up to a glass of milk without hearing rumbles from their stomachs, a few may be so lactose deficient that even a sip of milk triggers tummy turbulence.

To tell if you're lactose intolerance is legit, take this simple test: when your stomach is empty (2 to 3 hours after a meal or first thing in the morning), drink two glasses of milk. If you experience the symptoms associated with lactose intolerance, it's likely you are unable to digest lactose. Need even more confirmation (just to make sure pregnancy symptoms aren't confusing the picture)? Stay away from dairy products for 2 weeks. If all symptoms disappear, you have a pretty definite diagnosis. If you find your tummy's still acting up, you'll have to blame something else for your gastrointestinal unrest.

Want a more definitive diagnosis? Ask your GP about a breath test that measures the amount of hydrogen your body produces in the digestive tract after drinking a lactose-containing drink. The presence of hydrogen in your breath indicates improper digestion of lactose in your colon.

Fortunately, there's no need to torture your tummy – not even during pregnancy, when you need to increase your calcium intake. If you're lactose intolerant, there are plenty of ways to get the calcium you need without the stomach upset you certainly don't want:

- Take it slow. Try drinking only 120 ml of milk at a time, eating a small dish of cottage cheese or a thin slice of cheese. In general, small quantities of the offending dairy products spread out during the day may cause less digestive disruption than a couple of large doses.

- Go lactose-free. Shop for lactose-free milk, cheese, butter, frozen yogurt and other dairy products. All the calcium gain, without the painful wind. Most supermarkets now stock them.

- Take it with food. Lactose is easier to digest when mixed with other foods (particularly wholegrains). So pour your milk into your bran flakes, or melt your cheese on wholemeal.

- Take two. Take lactase in tablet form (it comes in chewables or tablets) with your first bite or sip. Or add lactase drops to your next dose of milk.

- Say cheese. Since milk itself is usually the major culprit, the closer a dairy product is to milk, the more likely it is to offend. Aged cheeses (such as Cheddar, Swiss and Parmesan) may be easier on your stomach because more than half the lactose is removed during processing.

- Get active. Active cultures, that is – the kind found in yogurt, yogurt drinks and kefir. These active bacterial cultures (usually acidophilus) may help break down lactose. And though there's no hard evidence that shows taking a probiotic supplement will ease lactose intolerance, it could help with other tummy troubles (and there's no harm in trying one).

Don't have a problem with lactose but still end up with tummy troubles after drinking milk? You may have difficulty digesting one of the proteins in cow's milk (the A1 protein). Drinking A2 milk (available online), which comes from cows that naturally produce only the A2 protein and not the A1 protein, could be the answer you're looking for – allowing you to drink milk without the accompanying bloating, wind and discomfort. Not sure if your tummy turbulence is a reaction to the lactose in milk or the A1 protein? Try each type of milk for a week or two and see if your troubles subside on one or the other.

Still can't handle dairy? There's no need to force the issue, or force down that glass of milk or pot of yogurt and face the gastrointestinal music (and pain). But you will need to make up the nutritional shortfall if you're not doing dairy at all. Here's how:

- Look elsewhere. There are plenty of other sources of calcium, including tofu, calcium-enriched nut, soya and other plant-based milks, tinned salmon and sardines (bones included, but you'll never notice if you mash them up) and green leafy vegetables.

- Don't be D-ficient. Calcium is regulated in the body by vitamin D. Most people get enough vitamin from being outdoors in direct sunlight between April and October if they aren't wearing sunscreen or covered up. Taking an antenatal supplement that contains vitamin D (which you're probably already doing), eating enriched cereals, breads, eggs and mushrooms or drinking vitamin D-enriched milk alternatives can help fill the gap.

- Supplement. Ask your healthcare provider about prescribing a calcium supplement if you're not getting enough through your diet. If your pregnant tummy gives you plenty of trouble with or without dairy, you might want to consider taking the supplement in the form of a calcium-containing antacid, such as Rennie or Rolaids.

If You Have Coeliac Disease (or Gluten Sensitivity)

If you have coeliac disease, you already know that a strict gluten-free diet is a must. You also likely already know why: when someone with coeliac disease ingests gluten (a protein found in wheat and certain other grains), the body triggers an immune response that causes damage to the small intestines, resulting in the malabsorption of nutrients and other problems from diarrhoea to bloating. Something else that's not news to you: even though staying on a gluten-free diet is difficult, it's definitely worth the effort.

And that goes doubly when you're expecting. Untreated coeliac disease can cause pregnancy problems from miscarriage to premature birth and low birthweight. But staying completely gluten-free before, during and after those nine months can prevent all of those increased risks. Here's how to eat well for two without gluten:

- Ask for your gastroenterologist to be part of your pregnancy care team. Adding a registered dietitian with expertise in both pregnancy and coeliac disease can help, too, as you formulate your pregnancy eating plan.

- Stay gluten-free, of course. You know the drill. Strictly avoid wheat and wheat varieties (such as khorasan/kamut, spelt, farro, couscous and bulgar wheat), rye, barley and triticale and all foods with even trace amounts of those grains. Seeking baby-nourishing wholegrains that are free of gluten? There are plenty to pick from, including brown, black and wild rice, corn (just check to be sure no other grains have been added to the corn products you choose), quinoa, millet, teff, buckwheat and amaranth. Oats are iffy; see below.

- Consider oats carefully. Pure oats are gluten-free, but while most people with coeliac disease can eat them safely, a small percentage may experience a gluten-like reaction to them. If you're not sure whether you're in that percentage and you've always avoided oats, check with your healthcare provider before adding them to your pregnancy diet. If you do reach for oats, reach only for those that are certified gluten-free. Oats and oat products are more likely than most grains to have contact with gluten-containing grains before making it to store shelves.

- Be a label reader. According to the Food Standards Agency (FSA), by law food manufacturers must list in bold lettering any of 14 allergens – including cereals such as wheat – on labels of pre-packed foods that contain them. But (and again, this likely isn't news to you) don't assume that wheat-free means gluten-free. Other grains besides wheat contain gluten and plenty of gluten-containing ingredients that might not be obvious ('natural flavouring' or added 'seasonings' may contain gluten). Screening ingredients lists carefully is a good start – if you really know your gluten and all the forms it can come in – but it doesn't protect against the possibility of cross-contact during processing or manufacturing. That's why your safest bet is to look for foods that are labelled 'gluten-free'. That indicates that a product has undergone a stringent review process and contains fewer than 20 ppm (parts per million) of gluten. A number of manufacturers include the crossed-grain logo as a quick way of identifying gluten-free products.

- Look for hidden gluten. Another reason to reach for products that are labelled 'gluten-free'? Gluten lurks in products you might never associate with it (unless you've been gluten-free for years): soy sauce, salad dressings, sauces – even chocolate or potato crisps. Nuts, seeds and peanuts are naturally gluten-free, but always reach for ones carrying the 'gluten-free' label, since some may have been processed near gluten-containing ingredients. Check the labels of supplements, too.

- Keep an eye on your kitchen. Cross-contact (between gluten-containing and gluten-free foods) can happen anywhere there are gluten eaters. You probably know what to look for, but look anyway: double dipping in the peanut butter jar (the knife leaves errant crumbs of wheat bread), or dipping a wheat-containing tortilla chip into the salsa. Dishing out the gluten-free salad dressing with a spoon that has touched the regular salad dressing. Reusing the pot that cooked the regular pasta to cook the gluten-free one. Experts suggest it's safest to use separate chopping boards, toasters, strainers and other utensils when possible (unless everyone who lives with you goes completely gluten-free, too).

- Be a wary diner. Something else you almost certainly already know: According to the FSA, restaurants and other food businesses must label menu items with allergens, adhering to the same strict standards as manufacturers of food products. Will the kitchen in a restaurant always be that careful? That's hard to know for sure. So always ask the waiter to ask the chef about the gluten status of menu items. Ask not only about the ingredients used, but the preparation and cooking standards. (Do they use separate pots, pans, fryers, prep spaces and kitchen utensils for gluten-free menu items?) If you have coeliac disease (as opposed to a sensitivity), be clear that your health depends on staying gluten-free. It might be easier to say that you have a 'severe allergy to gluten' – the kitchen may be more likely to take your request seriously.

- Omit the gluten without missing out the nutrients. Since many processed gluten-free products are made from nutritionally meaningless starches (white rice flour, tapioca starch, cornflour, potato starch), they may be nutritionally poor performers, lacking in (or low in) iron, B vitamins and fibre. Select healthier gluten-free products by looking for those that are enriched and contain nutritious gluten-free wholegrains and seeds.

- Keep out the gluten, keep up the vitamins and minerals. Straying from a completely gluten-free diet can result not only in intestinal damage, but also in vitamin and mineral deficiencies caused by malabsorption of nutrients (especially zinc, selenium, iron, vitamin D and folic acid). With pregnancy's increased nutritional need for these and other vitamins and minerals, that's a doubly significant risk. Besides staying on a strict gluten-free diet when you're expecting (which can be a rich supply of vitamins and minerals that come from naturally gluten-free foods such as fruits and vegetables), it's especially important to take your daily antenatal vitamin and any additional supplemental vitamins and minerals as directed by your healthcare provider (just make sure that all your supplements are labelled 'gluten-free').

Don't have coeliac disease, but do have a suspected or diagnosed case of non-coeliac gluten sensitivity – one that triggers significant tummy troubles when you eat gluten, if not serious health risks? Ask your healthcare provider to discuss a pregnancy diet protocol – and make sure that if you're avoiding gluten entirely, you're getting your fair share of nutrients from the foods you do eat.

If You Have Irritable Bowel Syndrome

Whether it's constipation, wind, bloating, nausea, vomiting or all (or a combination) of the above, most mums-to-be can expect their tummies to take a hit during pregnancy. Add irritable bowel syndrome (IBS) to the mix, and the normal digestive pains of pregnancy can multiply. (A few mums with chronic IBS find their symptoms ease during pregnancy, but they're the lucky exception.) Since a diet that's free of foods that trigger IBS symptoms can also be low on nutrients that are important during pregnancy, eating well while still feeling well can be extra challenging. Here are some tips to keep your symptoms in check while ticking off your Daily Dozen of nutrients:

- Stick to the old tricks. A lot of the strategies you probably already use to keep your IBS symptoms under control are actually smart strategies for every pregnant woman: eat small, more frequent meals, stay well hydrated, avoid excess stress and, of course, stay away from foods or drinks that make your IBS symptoms (and likely your pregnancy symptoms) worse, like anything fried or that produces extra wind.

- Slowly step up your fibre intake. If you're used to avoiding fruits, veggies and wholegrains to avoid diarrhoea, increase your fibre intake gradually. Too much too soon can tax your tummy as it adjusts.

- Enlist a professional. Following a low-FODMAP diet to manage your IBS? This diet eliminates foods containing short-chain carbohydrates that, if poorly digested, ferment in the lower part of your large intestine. The problem is it can also eliminate a lot of healthy foods that can normally do a pregnant body (and a baby) good such as dairy, certain fruits and vegetables, nuts and some grains. To make sure you manage your IBS and your nutritional needs during pregnancy, ask that your gastroenterologist and dietitian work with your pregancy care team to help create an eating plan that does both.

- Get cultured. Adding some probiotics to your diet (in the form of yogurt or yogurt drinks, if you can handle them, or in the form of a supplement) can be surprisingly effective in regulating bowel function, and they're safe during pregnancy. Ask your healthcare provider for a recommendation.

If You Have Food Allergies

Whether you developed a food allergy early in life or later in the eating game, you probably already know how to avoid the triggers in your diet, and depending on how serious the allergy is, you may already be used to playing food detective – and being extra assertive about giving strict orders with your restaurant orders. Pregnancy is definitely not a time to play around with serious food allergies, but it's also not a time to shortchange yourself on nutrients. Here's how to work around both challenges:

- Always remember to read food labels extra carefully, and always alert restaurants to your allergy before ordering.

- Find substitutes where you can, to fill in the missing nutrient gaps.

- Keep your healthcare provider in the loop. He or she can determine if additional supplements beyond an antenatal vitamin are necessary.

- It goes without saying, but: if your allergy is severe, make sure to carry an EpiPen with you at all times in case of emergencies.

Wondering if your history of food allergies (or your family's, or your partner's) should keep you from eating foods that are considered highly allergenic (such as wheat, soy, milk, fish, shellfish, peanuts, tree nuts and eggs) during pregnancy and breastfeeding, to avoid exposing your baby and increasing his or her risk for developing food allergies? Actually, research has confirmed that the reverse is true: not only is there no reason to avoid allergenic foods during pregnancy and breastfeeding (assuming you're not allergic to them yourself), but eating them may reduce your baby's future risk of food allergies. Ask your healthcare provider about specifics in your case.

If You Have Gestational Diabetes

If you've been given a diagnosis of gestational diabetes (GD), you have plenty of company – and it's growing. It's estimated that up to 5 per cent, or one in 20, mums-to-be develop this pregnancy-related condition, which occurs when the body becomes more resistant to insulin (the hormone that lets the body turn blood sugar into energy) and isn't able to produce enough insulin to keep blood sugar under control. Unlike other types of diabetes, GD is temporary – blood-sugar levels usually return to normal after delivery (though mums with gestational diabetes are at much greater risk for type 2 diabetes later in life). But for a pregnant woman who is suddenly faced with major restrictions to her diet, it can seem to stretch on and on. That's the bad news. The good news is that gestational diabetes can usually be controlled by those dietary restrictions (as tough as it may seem to follow them, at least at first). Other measures can help manage gestational diabetes (such as getting regular exercise; see *What to Expect When You're Expecting* for much more), but eating well when you have GD will mean:

Diet changes. There's really no way around it: managing gestational diabetes usually takes plenty of diet changes – changes you may not be super happy about, especially if you have a sweet tooth or you're a carb-craver. Your healthcare provider will tell you to follow a special diet, which probably won't be all that different from the Pregnancy Diet. Working with a dietitian who has experience with GD (ask your GP for a referral) will make working out the best eating plan – and sticking to it – a little easier. There's no one-size-fits-all food plan for every mum-to-be with GD because everybody tolerates carbs differently, but in general it's recommended that women with GD do the following:

- Be carb conscious. You'll likely be told to limit the amount of refined carbs you eat (white rice, white potatoes, white bread, white pasta) because they turn quickly to sugar when digested, raising blood-glucose levels. Focus, instead, on high-fibre complex carbs that have a low glycaemic load, such as wholegrains, beans, peas, lentils and vegetables. So-called low glycaemic index foods release sugar into the blood more slowly, helping to keep blood-sugar levels stable and within normal range.

You'll find that they offer more long-lasting energy boosts, too. Chances are that fruit (another complex carb) may be limited but won't be off the menu (fruit juice may be; keep reading). Some women are told to count and curb even complex carbs, or at least to limit the amount taken at one sitting – but again, take your dietary marching orders from your doctor.

- Unfriend fruit juice. Even fruit sugar can raise your blood sugar, which means that naturally sweet 100 per cent fruit juices will have to be restricted, too. Your GP or dietitian may (or may not) give you the green light on occasional small amounts of juice (up to 120 ml, taken with meals). Mixing the juice with sparkling water will dilute the fruit sugar while making your treat last longer.

- Be choosy with fruit. Can you still be best friends with fruit? Unlike juice, fruit contains fibre, which slows the absorption of sugar into the blood. Still, don't get too friendly with fruit. Depending on how your body processes carbs and sugars, you might be told to eat fresh or fresh-frozen fruit in moderation, limit it to 75–150 g at a time, or (less likely) strictly avoid fruit altogether. Some fruits contain more sugar than others – you might be told to avoid only those that do such as grapes, cherries, pineapple, mango and banana. Dried fruit contains more sugar than fresh, so it's more likely to be restricted.

- Stay low-fat. Fat is an essential nutrient – especially during pregnancy. But fat lingers in your bloodstream, causing sugars to stay elevated and insulin to be less efficient, which means your body will need more insulin to keep blood-sugar levels within normal range. Choose lean sources of protein

and calcium, and stick to healthy fats such as those in nuts, seeds and avocado.

- Pass on sugar. Chances are your sweet tooth won't get much wiggle room. To keep your blood-sugar levels from rising to unsafe levels, you'll need to stay away from foods that increase them. Not surprisingly, foods (and drinks) that contain added sugar in any form and by any name (white sugar, muscovado sugar, raw sugar, turbinado sugar, fructose-glucose syrup, high-fructose corn syrup, honey, maple syrup, molasses, agave, coconut sugar and so on) top that list. You may be allowed to eat small amounts of sugar-sweetened foods and drinks in moderation (or they may be officially off-limits), but try to stay away from high-sugar standards such as cakes, tarts, biscuits, ice cream, chocolate bars and soft drinks. See page 74 for a list of sugar substitutes. Watch out, too, for added sugar in places you might not expect to see it such as ketchup and other condiments.

Meal control. The grazing approach to eating works best for most pregnant women, but is especially important for those trying to regulate their blood sugar. Aim for three meals and two to four snacks each day – spaced as evenly as possible (so that you're eating a small amount every 2–3 hours). Another rule that applies to all pregnant women but must be more strictly stuck to by those with GD: no skipping your meals. Regularly skipping meals (or snacks) can result in hypoglycaemia (low blood sugar), which can make you feel miserable – irritable, shaky, headachy.

In general, try to combine a protein with a carb at each meal and snack – especially at breakfast, when blood sugar tends to be higher. A bedtime snack will be superimportant, too, since it will help ward off the lower-than-normal blood-sugar levels that are common during the night in pregnant women with gestational diabetes. Before turning in, eat a snack that contains protein (such as low-fat cheese) and complex carbohydrates (such as wholemeal bread). The carbohydrates will stabilise your blood-sugar level early in the night, while the protein acts as a long-acting stabiliser.

Weight control. Since too many pounds can send blood-sugar levels soaring, you'll have to pay even more attention to your weight gain than other mums-to-be. You'll also need to pay extra attention to the rate of gain. Gaining too much weight too quickly (2 lb/900 g or more per week) results in extra body fat, which, in turn, can produce an insulin-resistant effect. See Chapter 6 for ways to help you gain the right number of pounds at the right rate during pregnancy.

If You're Carrying Multiples

Expecting twins (or more)? Then you'll need to pay at least twice as much attention to your diet as a mum with only one baby on board. As it turns out, good nutrition during a multiple pregnancy has an even greater impact on baby birthweight than it does during a singleton pregnancy. And quality alone won't do it – you'll also need to add some quantity. For each extra baby you have on board, you'll have extra requirements above and beyond those of an expectant mum-of-one. Fortunately for you (and your bump, which will be stretched to capacity anyway during your multiple pregnancy), that doesn't mean you'll have to consume twice as many calories or vitamins for twins, or three times as much protein for triplets. Just bear in mind the extras you'll need when you're eating for three or more:

Extra weight. Not surprisingly, toting an extra baby means you'll have to tote around extra weight. Also not surprisingly, the healthier your weight gain (and your diet), the healthier your babies' weight gain is likely to be. Most experts say that women of normal pre-pregnancy weight who are pregnant with twins should gain 37–54 lb (17–24.5 kg) – roughly 50 per cent more than the recommended weight gain for a single pregnancy (for triplets, 50–60 lb/22.7–27 kg). And because you can expect your babies to arrive somewhat earlier than single babies (full term for twins is usually considered 37 to 38 weeks), you'll need to pack in that weight gain (and all those extra nutritional needs) in a shorter period of time. Challenging? You bet, especially because you're also likely to experience more nausea and vomiting in your first trimester and beyond than a mum expecting a single baby. But, with a little extra efficiency, it can be done.

Extra calories. So how do you gain all that extra weight? The usual way, by piling on extra calories. There are no UK guidelines, but US experts recommend 150–300 extra per foetus per day. If you're carrying twins, that's an extra 300–600 calories, and if you're carrying triplets, that's an extra 450–900 calories per day (ask your healthcare provider to determine your magic number). A food dream come true? Depending on what your food dreams are made of, maybe (peanut butter on everything!), maybe not (fries with everything!). Most of those extra calories should come from nutrient-dense foods that best nourish your babies and your pregnancy. Studies show that a high-calorie diet that's also high in nutrients significantly improves your chances of having healthy, full-term babies.

So get ready to eat more – but to eat well. Use the Pregnancy Diet in Chapter 3 as your guide to adding more nutrient-dense food, keeping an eye on the scales to ensure your weight gain is on target (no calorie counting necessary). With your bigger goals in mind, efficiency will be extra important. Instead of trying to squeeze the extra calories and nutrients into only three meals, try eating five or six small meals and several light snacks throughout the day. Another reason to eat more often: research has suggested that women who eat at least five meals plus snacks a day are more likely to carry to term. Plus, you'll likely be less bothered by indigestion and heartburn – just a couple of the tummy troubles that are often doubled in twin pregnancies. (See page 107 for mini-meal tips.)

Extra iron. Being pregnant means your body's in the blood-making business big-time, since blood volume must increase significantly to nourish a developing foetus. Naturally, the more foetuses that blood volume must support, the more it must increase. Enter extra iron – the mineral that helps manufacture red blood cells. Most women end up needing more iron than their diets can provide at some point in their pregnancy – you'll need lots more, lots sooner. To fill that need, your healthcare provider will probably prescribe an iron

supplement early in your pregnancy. Be sure to supplement that supplement by eating iron-rich foods such as red meat and dried fruit. Take iron sources with a vitamin C–rich food to aid absorption, but avoid taking calcium supplements or eating calcium-rich foods along with iron, since that can block absorption.

Extra vitamins. More babies means a greater need for baby-building vitamins of every variety. Your one-a-day antenatal supplement will cover the basics, but you and your babies will benefit when you increase your vitamin intake the old-fashioned way – by eating vitamin-rich foods.

Extra minerals. Your antenatal vitamin is a good place to start, but it won't give you with all the extra minerals you'll need when building an extra baby. Some doctors recommend, for instance, that women carrying twins supplement with magnesium and calcium – and for good reason. Magnesium may reduce the risk of preterm labour – something most multiple pregnancies are at risk of. Calcium, of course, builds strong bones and teeth, and with at least two sets of each growing inside you, you'll need plenty of help from that essential mineral.

Extra fluid. Being dehydrated can also lead to preterm labour, so step up the fluids – drinking at least ten glasses daily. Drinking between meals (rather than attempting to sip with them) will keep the fluids from competing with the solids for coveted room in the closer and closer quarters of your stomach. Even better: try to eat plenty of fluid-rich fruits and veggies such as watermelon and lettuce.

Extra help eating well. Your GP may refer you to a dietitian who can help you work out how to fit all those nutrition extras in.

When You're Sick

It doesn't seem quite fair, and yet it's true. As a mum-to-be – probably already saddled with a variety of uncomfortable pregnancy symptoms, from nausea and vomiting to heartburn and indigestion – you're actually more likely to become sick than members of the non-pregnant population. That's because your immune system is slightly lowered during pregnancy – nature's way of ensuring that your baby (who is a foreigner to your system) won't be rejected by your body. This immune suppression, as well intended as it is, leaves you particularly susceptible to infections, coughs, colds, gastrointestinal bugs and the flu. And it's not just the glow that goes when a pregnant woman gets sick. It's often her appetite and her ability to eat a regular diet as well.

Should you find yourself sick in bed with more than just the usual pregnancy symptom suspects, be sure to ask your healthcare provider for a diagnosis and a treatment plan. But also plan to eat well while you're feeling unwell. These tips should help:

When you have a cold. It's never a good idea to starve a cold, especially when you're expecting. (The same goes for the flu, but a case of flu – or suspected flu – also requires prompt medical attention during pregnancy.) Since your body needs energy (from food) to heal, you'll get better faster if you eat. Of course, that's easy to say, but not so easy to do when your nose is stuffy, your head achy, your throat sore and scratchy, and your mouth busy coughing. Still, try to push:

■ Soft, soothing foods. Porridge, scrambled eggs, apple purée, smoothies – really, whatever is easiest for you to swallow. And don't forget to sip on some soup – any soup, but especially chicken soup, which research shows isn't good just for the soul, but also for relieving congestion.

■ Fluids. You'll need your usual quota of fluids when you're laid up with a bug, plus extra fluids to replace those lost through a runny nose and to promote a quicker recovery. Staying hydrated loosens the mucus in your nose and sinuses, helping to reduce congestion. So keep a bottle or flask next to your bed (or at your desk if you've brought your cold to work) and sip whatever you can, as often as you can. Water, ginger tea and diluted juice are all good choices, and warming up the fluid (yes, even the water) will make it more soothing to sip. Soup counts, too, as do juicy fruits. And although milk has long been rumoured to increase nasal congestion, there is no scientific evidence to back up that theory. So unless you find that it makes you stuffier, there's no need to miss out on milk while a cold has you down. Warm milk might be extra soothing, especially mixed with a teaspoon of honey.

■ Vitamins. Getting your share of vitamins and minerals may help keep you from coming down with a cold in the first place – or, if it's too late for that, help you beat it back. So take your antenatal supplement as usual (but no extra doses of vitamins without your healthcare provider's go-ahead), and focus on concentrated sources of vitamin C such as citrus and melon.

Stomach bug. You finished weathering morning sickness, and thought your tummy had nothing but smooth sailing ahead. Then those all-too-familiar rumblings began anew – this time, courtesy of a stomach virus or a mild case of food poisoning. While morning sickness can last for months (as probably nobody needs to tell a pregnant woman), symptoms of a stomach bug are usually brief, if intense – lasting no more than 24 or 48 hours. But because diarrhoea and vomiting can rob your baby of vital nutrients and fluids – even in a short time – you'll need to pay as much attention as possible to your diet while you're waiting for the misery to pass. Push yourself on:

- Fluids. You've likely heard it before, but it's worth repeating: in the short term, fluids are more important than solids. Even when you can't keep as much as a crust of bread down, you'll need to prevent dehydration by getting enough fluids. Try plain water, sparkling water or ginger tea. If you're vomiting, taking small sips every 15 minutes may give the fluids a fighting chance of staying down. If you can't stomach sipping, suck on ice chips or ice lollies. If symptoms are severe or you can't manage to get enough fluids into you (or both), your healthcare provider may recommend a rehydration fluid (or frozen rehydration lollies) as a precaution. Coconut water may be helpful, too. Once clear liquids (diluted fruit juices – particularly white grape, which is easier on the tummy – and clear broth) go down and stay down, you can add nutritious smoothies and fruits with high water concentration such as watermelon. Don't forget that ginger can also ease the quease when you're down with tummy troubles. Drink it in tea, ginger ale or other ginger drinks (you can also suck or chew on ginger sweets).

- Foods you can handle. If you can stomach solids, focus on whatever you can

Weighing In on That Ounce of Prevention

The best kind of medicine – especially during pregnancy – is the preventive kind. Giving your immunity a shot in the arm – by keeping yourself well rested and well nourished – can keep you from coming down with mild infections in the first place, or help you recover from them faster when they do strike. Some of nature's finest immunity boosters also happen to be Daily Dozen hall-of-famers, including yogurt (the probiotics naturally found in it are excellent fighters against bad bacteria) and foods rich in vitamin C and beta-carotene.

On the other hand, you should definitely not reach for alternative remedies sometimes used (though not scientifically proven) to prevent or help treat infection – say, extra doses of vitamin C or zinc or such purported immunity-boosters as echinacea to stop a cold in its tracks or minimise symptoms. None of these remedies are recommended for pregnancy use. It's smarter – and safer – to reach for an orange instead.

get down and keep in such as crackers, unbuttered toast, bananas, apple purée, porridge, brown rice or pasta. No need to restrict your diet if (or when) food is appealing, even if you have diarrhoea – though it makes sense to stay away from difficult-to-digest foods such as anything fried, greasy or spicy.

- Vitamins as usual. Try to take your daily pregnancy supplement at a time when it's least likely to come back up, and never on an empty stomach. But don't worry if you need to skip it for a day or two. Once the bug stops bugging you, you'll be able to make up those lost nutrients.

Urinary tract infection (UTI). UTIs are so common during pregnancy that an estimated 5 per cent of pregnant women can expect to develop at least one. They're also serious business during pregnancy. Untreated, a UTI is more likely to progress to a kidney infection in pregnant women. So don't try to self-diagnose or self-treat a UTI – call your healthcare provider if you suspect you have one.

Prevention is always the best strategy, especially when you're expecting. But these preventive tips, when used in conjunction with your healthcare provider's prescribed treatment, can also help you speed up recovery from an infection:

■ Drink plenty of fluids. Water can help flush out any bacteria that are hanging out in your bladder. Some say that cranberry juice, which changes the alkilinity of urine, may keep bacteria from sticking to urinary tract walls, making it an especially beneficial fluid.

■ Avoid coffee and tea (even decaffeinated) since they may increase irritation – the last thing your urinary tract needs right now.

■ Ask your healthcare provider about taking probiotics to help restore the balance of beneficial bacteria. Probiotics could be especially helpful if you're taking antibiotics.

When You're on Activity Restriction

Just about everyone dreams of being able to kick off her shoes, put up her feet, plump up the pillows and lounge the day (or even the afternoon!) away in bed or on the sofa – binge-watching her favourite TV shows and (hey, since it's a dream anyway) popping chocolates. But for mums with complications who end up being prescribed any amount of enforced rest – whether it's bed rest (at home or even in the hospital), restricted activity, shortened work days, limited standing or a combination of these, it can be less dream, more nightmare. And mealtimes? Not exactly the room service experience dreams are made of either – especially when no one's around to deliver it.

Fortunately, bed rest in any form is rarely recommended anymore, primarily because most of the evidence shows that it's not only ineffective in treating or preventing complications (such as preterm labour) but that it can do far more harm than good. Still, if you've been issued no-marching orders (or periodic marches to the sofa for some lying-down time), you may be wondering how it's possible to stay off your feet and on the Pregnancy Diet at the same time. Here are some strategies if you're on activity restriction or enforced rest:

Stay hydrated. Reducing your activity may also have you reaching for your water bottle less often – after all, you may feel less thirsty if you're moving around less. Getting enough fluids will help minimise swelling and constipation, both of which may be compounded when you're often parked on the sofa. Staying hydrated is especially important if you're trying to head off contractions.

Break for meals and snacks. All those rest breaks may put the brakes on your appetite (it may be hard to get hungry when you're not getting a move on) – or the time you have to break for meals and snacks. Keeping stocked up at the office and at home on healthy, easy eats and setting reminders to refuel on schedule may help. On the flip side, if you're pretty sure the couch potato in you will cry out for potato crisps – and you're prone to snacking when you're prone and bored – be extra mindful of mindful eating. And make sure your nibbles are carefully curated to include more carrots than biscuits. Either way, tap into healthy food delivery options to save yourself the time spent on your feet shopping and cooking.

Give yourself props. Not because enforced rest can be hard (it can). But because you'll feel the (heart)burn more when you're lying down. So prop yourself up with pillows as you rest, and especially if you're resting while eating.

Keep an eye on the scales. Limiting your activities will limit the calories you're burning – but it may also limit the number of calories you eat (if you never feel hungry). As always, the best strategy is to watch your weight gain, to be sure it's rising at the right rate. Also, ask your healthcare provider about exercises you can do while sitting (or even lying down), if only to boost your circulation, flexibility and muscle strength.

For more on activity restrictions during pregnancy, see *What to Expect When You're Expecting*.

CHAPTER 10

Eating Well Postnatal

....

Your baby-making days are officially over, at least for now – but your baby-care days (and nights) have only just begun. Especially if you're breastfeeding, the demands of new-mum life – and the demands of your hungry baby – will be at least as great as the demands of pregnancy were. At 3 a.m., maybe even more so.

Happily, the demands on your diet (and your eating habits) won't be nearly as heavy a lift. Postnatal eating – and drinking – allows for a lot more leeway than pregnancy eating does. Can't wait to dig into a fully runny egg (or an uncensored Caesar) from your own home-reared chickens? Your time has come! Love the way that wine with dinner winds you down after a hard day with baby? Uncork that bottle! Having sushi withdrawal? Whip out those chopsticks and get busy, and even pass the sake!

Still, there are plenty of perks to healthy postnatal eating – and to keeping some of those healthy eating habits you picked up during pregnancy. Eating well postnatal can help you recover from those long months of pregnancy and those long hours of labour and delivery. But it can also help you put your best new-mum foot forward (and keep you on your feet after two solid hours of rocking). It can boost your energy (what there is of it), lift your mood, ease that postnatal constipation and those haemorrhoids, help you sensibly shed those leftover pregnancy pounds and, if you're breastfeeding, help pump up your milk supply.

The Postnatal Diet

Now that you're on the other side of pregnancy, continuing to eat well can help your body bounce back. And just as the Pregnancy Diet wasn't all that different from the average healthy diet, the Postnatal Diet isn't either.

Nine Ways to Eat Healthy Postnatal – and Beyond

The nine basic principles that steered you through nine months of healthy eating can continue to be your guide during the postnatal period and beyond – whether you're breastfeeding or not:

Choose calories you can still count on. Looking to lose the pregnancy love handles you're not exactly loving? It will help to remember that all calories are not created equal. The calories eaten in the form of an iced pastry, for instance, are less likely to be burned as fuel and more likely to accumulate in those hard-to-trim areas than the calories consumed in almond butter spread on an apple. Try to take most of your calories through lean protein, fruits, vegetables, wholegrains and healthy sources of fat – you won't only have more energy to burn (something you'll need a lot of these days!), but you may also find those inches melting off faster.

Continue being an efficient eater. When you focus on foods that multitask in nutritional categories – a serving of Greek yogurt (protein and calcium) with half a mango (vitamin A and vitamin C) – you're eating efficiently. Selecting foods that pack the most nutrition for the calories is a winning strategy – for your overall health and for your waistline.

Feed yourself, feed your baby. Missing meals (who has time for breakfast when baby needs to be fed, burped, have a nappy changed, dressed – and repeat?) can leave you with less energy when you need it the most – and when baby most needs you to have it. And if you're breastfeeding, inadequate nutrition can, over time, compromise milk supply.

Be complex with carbs. Your postnatal body will still need the energy-sustaining vitamins and minerals that are naturally found in wholegrain breads and cereals, brown rice, beans and other legumes (also called pulses). Complex carbs also pack a natural punch of fibre – something that will do a postnatal (possibly constipated) body good.

Spare the sugar. Maybe you've heard (and would like to believe) that nothing beats a chocolate bar for giving you the energy boost you so sorely need these days (and nights). But the truth is, sugary treats will lift you only briefly before sending you into an energy crash-and-burn. And while having the occasional sugary treat won't throw your postnatal eating plan into a tailspin, making them your most frequented food group will. Not to mention make it harder to (gradually) drop those pregnancy pounds.

Feature fruits and vegetables. Looking for a tasty, low-cal and low-fat food to help keep weight loss on track? Something that's a powerhouse in vitamins, minerals and phytochemicals? Something high in fibre to help keep constipation at bay? And something that will give you energy when baby's pulling an all-nighter? Look no further than the produce aisle, where you can load up on fruits and vegetables that provide vitamins, minerals, fibre, phyto-chemicals and energy-producing carbs in each delicious bite.

Choose foods that remember their roots. Foods that are highly processed have not only lost a lot of their natural nutrition and (more than likely) gained a lot of unhealthy saturated fat, salt and sugar in the processing plant, but may also contain chemical additives that could find their way into your milk supply (and your baby) if you're breastfeeding. Best, as always, to stick to foods that haven't ventured far from their natural roots.

Cave to the crave. Deprivation usually doesn't work when you're trying to eat well or when you're trying to lose weight – and you're trying to do both postnatal. So have your cake in moderation, and eat it without guilt. Just know your limits and stick to them (especially if a sliver of cake will inevitably lead to a slab . . . or two).

Eat well family-style. There's never been a better time to join nutritional family forces for a healthier future. After all, there's a new mouth to feed in the house. How that mouth will be fed (and how it will eventually choose to eat) will depend a lot on what fills your plate, as well as what fills your store cupboard, fridge and freezer. A little one who's raised in a home where the protein is lean, the snack of choice is fruit, salad is friend not foe, sandwiches come on wholemeal, cereals aren't sweetened and fast food isn't a first choice is likely to grow up thinking that eating well is, well, natural.

The Postnatal Diet

What makes a healthy postnatal diet? The same Daily Dozen that covered your nutritional bases during pregnancy. With just a few tweaks in the number of servings – more if you're breastfeeding, fewer if you're not:

Calories. After months of putting on weight, you're probably keen to start taking it off. But drastically slashing calories isn't the smart way to rediscover your waist. Instead, you'll need to strike a balance: enough calories to keep you on the go, not so many that the numbers on the scales don't start gradually dropping. Operative word, 'gradually'. Remember, it took nine months to put those pregnancy pounds on, and it may take at least that many to take them off.

Breastfeeding actually requires more calories than pregnancy does (after all, you're still feeding baby – only baby is much bigger now). So, though you don't literally need to count them, you may need up to 500 more calories a day when you're breastfeeding than you would need to maintain your pre-pregnancy weight (double that if you're exclusively breastfeeding twins, triple if you're the sole food source for triplets). Many mums find that breastfeeding helps melt the pounds away, even with the extra calories – other mums find that baby feeding makes them so hungry that losing baby weight becomes a losing battle. Either way, be careful not to restrict your calories too much, or you may end up reducing your milk supply.

If you're not breastfeeding, your extra calorie allowance has expired – at least, if you'd like to start losing the pregnancy weight. Eating about the same number of calories as you did to maintain your pre-pregnancy weight will get you back there sooner or later – sooner if you're more active than you

Help for the Zombie Mum

Feeling more zombie than mummy? Finding the little things in life – putting one foot in front of the other (and the right shoe on the right foot), pouring the milk into your coffee (not into your orange juice), putting the dirty clothes into the washing machine (not the dryer) – harder and harder to achieve in your chronically sleep-deprived state? Of course you are – that's part of the new-mum package, especially when your package includes around-the-clock breastfeeding. Still, while sleep deprivation will probably be a given for months to come, utter exhaustion doesn't have to be. Just fight fatigue with food.

In general, the same tips that helped you (sort of) deal with pregnancy fatigue can help now, too (sort of). For instance, opt for eating small amounts of energy-sustaining food frequently throughout the day instead of three hearty meals (as if you had time to sit down for even one). Mini-meals won't give you more sleep, but they will help keep your blood sugar (and thus your stamina) up. And because they don't put as much demand on your digestive tract, they won't tap into those energy stores as much as a gut bomb would. (The bigger the meal, the more energy it takes to digest, so the more tired it makes you feel.) Try also to include a combination of carbohydrates and protein in each mini-meal so that you get the energy-enhancing benefits of both nutrients.

Hold the simple sugars (like that doughnut you're contemplating), which pick you up only briefly before sending you crashing. Instead, snack on some of the following (you can also revisit the snack and mini-meal ideas on pages 138 and 107).

- Trail mix. You don't need to be planning a trek to munch on a combo of dried and/or freeze-dried fruit, nuts and seeds. It has a good balance of complex carbs and protein – plus it's high in iron, which helps combat the fatigue caused by postnatal anaemia. Toss in a few dark chocolate chips for extra energy (and extra happiness).

- Wholegrain cereal with milk. Chock-full of B vitamins that help break down food into fuel, wholegrain cereal is a great way to energise your day after an all-nighter. And don't save the cereal for breakfast. It makes a high-energy lunch or snack, too.

- A real-food protein bar and a banana. Or a cheese stick and an apple.

- Half a wholemeal bagel, topped with melted Emmental cheese. A tasty way to combine carbs and protein, plus an energy boost that comes with a calcium bonus.

- Half a peanut butter and banana sandwich on wholemeal, or apple slices and almond butter.

- Hummus in a wholemeal pitta – protein plus carbs, it doesn't get easier.

- Fruit and yogurt sprinkled with chopped walnuts or sliced almonds. Complex carbohydrates in the form of fruit provide sugar the way nature intended, supplying longer-lasting energy for your body. The nuts deliver protein and healthy, brain-boosting fats, and the yogurt adds protein (even more if you go Greek) and calcium.

Time to Shake the Salt?

No need for an all-out assault on salt – everyone needs some sodium, a component of salt, in their diet. Still, if you picked up a pickle habit while you were expecting, it's probably wise to cut back now. After all, most people in the UK consume too much salt, which is linked to a higher risk of heart disease and stroke. And too much salt in your diet certainly isn't helpful when you're trying to lose pregnancy water weight. So as a sensible rule, limit those super-salty foods (like the ones you'll run into at fast-food chains) and salt lightly at the table. Your baby will get the salt (and sodium) he or she needs through breast milk or infant formula: less than 1 g of salt (0.4 g of sodium) up to 12 months. But get into the practice of not adding salt when cooking, so when you start introducing solids baby won't get more than the recommended 2 g of salt (0.8 g of sodium) for one- to three-year-olds.

used to be, later if you're less active. But don't cut calories too drastically until you've completely recovered from pregnancy and childbirth (at least six weeks after giving birth) – even if you're keen to expedite weight loss. Once you've got your healthcare provider's go-ahead, you can go ahead and reduce your number of calories by 200–500 per day. Even then, slow is the better way to go when it comes to weight loss.

Protein: three servings daily if you're breastfeeding; two if you're not. See the list of protein choices on page 34, bearing in mind (as always) that many also double as a calcium serving. If you're breastfeeding twins or triplets, get ready to eat hearty: you'll need an extra serving of protein for each additional baby.

Calcium: At least four servings daily if you're breastfeeding; three if you're not. Whether you're making milk or not, you should still be drinking it (or taking the equivalent in other calcium sources) to strengthen your bones. Remember that many of the calcium choices on page 40 also serve up a good amount of protein, so take full advantage of this nutritional overlap. If you're breastfeeding twins or triplets, you'll need an extra calcium serving for each additional baby. An important note for breastfeeders: while your baby won't suffer if you don't meet your calcium requirement, your bones might. To keep your milk calcium rich, your body will draw this essential mineral from your bones for milk production, possibly setting you up for osteoporosis later on if you don't take in enough calcium from your diet. If you find it's hard to reach your calcium quota through your diet, fill in the gaps with a calcium supplement. Choosing calcium-fortified dairy-free products will also help boost your intake.

Vitamin C: two or more servings daily whether you're breastfeeding or not. See page 40 for vitamin C choices – and remember that many vitamin C foods also fill the vitamin A bucket.

Vitamin A: three to four servings daily whether you're breastfeeding or not. See page 41 for good food sources, bearing in mind that many of these also fill the requirement for vitamin C.

Other fruits and vegetables: one or more servings daily whether you're breastfeeding or not. See page 45 for good choices.

Wholegrains and legumes: three or more servings daily whether you're breastfeeding or not. See page 47 for good choices.

Iron-rich foods: some daily whether you're breastfeeding or not. You'll need iron to replenish your blood stores after delivery and to prevent fatigue caused by anaemia (you'll be plenty tired without it). See page 48 for good choices. If you're low on iron stores, your healthcare provider may tell you to continue (or begin) taking an iron supplement.

Fat and high-fat foods: small amounts daily. Even though a breastfeeding mum needs fat (half the calories of breast milk come from fat), you don't need as much as you did when you were pregnant. If you're gaining weight (or not losing any), cut back on the amount of fat you're taking in. If you're losing too quickly, add more fat servings into your diet. See page 50 for a list of fat servings.

Omega-3 fatty acids: some daily. In your quest to drop those postnatal pounds, remember that fat isn't the enemy and some fats are still your friends – namely, those DHA-supplying ones. DHA is just as important while you're breastfeeding as it was during pregnancy, and here's why. The DHA content of your baby's brain triples during the first three months of life, and getting enough of this vital nutrient through your milk (which already contains DHA) will help fuel that growth. It's recommended that breastfeeding mums – like pregnant mums – eat at least two portions of low-mercury fish (see page 72) per week to meet their omega-3 requirement, so definitely go fish when you're breastfeeding. Your antenatal vitamin, which likely includes omega-3s, will also help you fill your quota. For other good sources of DHA see page 51.

Back on the Postnatal Menu

With your pregnancy days behind you, it's time to enjoy what is back on the menu (and hopefully some favourites). Whether you're breastfeeding or not, you can go back to eating raw or rare fish and seafood (but restrictions on high-mercury fish still apply if you're breastfeeding or planning to become pregnant again – see page 74), and you can enjoy other foods that had been shelved (see pages 81–84), whether in the UK or when overseas, such as rare meat, raw dairy, unpasteurised cheese or juice, runny eggs, cold meat, smoked fish, raw bean sprouts and fermented foods. (See page 173 for breastfeeding caveats on alcohol and caffeine.)

Fluids: at least twelve 240-ml daily if you're breastfeeding; approximately ten 120-ml glasses daily if you're not. Here's one requirement you might expect to increase when you're in the milk production business – and it does, somewhat. The best way to tell if you're getting enough fluids is to keep an eye on your urine. If you're not getting enough, it will be darker and more scant. If you're getting enough, your urine will be clear and plentiful. Since you'll be nursing eight to 12 times a day, one of the simplest strategies for keeping up with your fluid intake is to drink when baby drinks – keeping a bottle or glass of water close during breastfeeding sessions. As always, remember that other fluids work towards your quota (including milk, stock and juice), as do juicy fruits and veggies. Think more of a good thing is even better? Actually, drinking too many fluids can decrease your milk supply.

Not breastfeeding? You don't need fluids for milk production, but you do need them to help recover from childbirth and flush out extra fluids retained during pregnancy. Dehydration can also contribute to fatigue, headaches and other postnatal symptoms you definitely don't need.

Vitamin supplements. Continue to take your antenatal vitamin or a breastfeeding supplement daily if you're breastfeeding. Though it's likely you'd make good-quality milk without it (just by eating well), taking one provides a dose of insurance, providing you with the extra vitamins and minerals you need during breastfeeding, including vitamin A, vitamin C, vitamin E, biotin, calcium, choline, chromium and copper iodine. Ask your healthcare provider for supplement advice if you're a breastfeeding vegan – you may need additional supplements, such as vitamin D and B_{12}. If you're not breastfeeding, continue taking your antenatal for at least the first six weeks postnatal, and then talk to your healthcare provider about whether you should stick with it or switch over to a standard multiple vitamin and mineral supplement (a formula with enough folic acid to keep you covered throughout your reproductive years, just in case).

Eating Well When You're Breastfeeding

All new mums (and new dads, for that matter) can benefit from eating well, especially during those early endless days and nights after a baby's arrival, particularly during the first three months postnatal (dubbed the fourth trimester, since this period is an integral part of the reproductive cycle). Sleep deprivation plus recovery from pregnancy and delivery can drain energy and put a strain on nutritional status. But mums who are also taking on the (literally) draining job of breastfeeding have an extra reason to eat well. Here's what you need to know.

What to Eat

Wondering if feeding your baby well on the outside will take as much effort as feeding him or her well on the inside did? Actually, because the basic composition of breast milk isn't directly dependent on what you eat, breastfeeding makes minimal demands on your diet. Quantity isn't affected either, unless a mum's diet and nutritional reserves are severely deficient (as they might be if she were living under famine conditions). That's because Mother Nature puts a breastfeeding baby's needs first. Skimp on the calories, fall short on the protein or come up behind on minerals, and your body will tap into its own stores of nutrients to make milk – at least until reserves run out. In other words, your milk isn't likely to become deficient in nutrients, but you could. Eating a well-balanced and well-varied diet will help keep you healthy while your milk helps keep your baby healthy. And because there are fewer restrictions on your postnatal diet, eating well won't be nearly as challenging as when you were pregnant (though finding the time to eat at all – well, that's a different story).

There's yet another reason to eat a variety of healthy foods when you're breastfeeding – and believe it or not, it's got nothing to do with nutrition. Because what you eat affects the taste and smell of your breast milk, your breastfed baby is exposed to different flavours before he or she is ready for that first bite of solids. In fact, studies have shown that babies fed breast milk are more accepting of new foods when they start on solids than babies who are formula-fed – probably because they've already got a taste for them. Enjoy a lot of highly flavoured foods while breast-feeding, and your baby's more likely to grow into an adventurous eater. (Forget the chicken nuggets, mum – pass the pad thai!) Eat your vegetables now, and your baby may be more likely to eat his or her vegetables later.

You already know the Daily Dozen drill: lean meat and poultry, low-mercury fish (experts recommend at least two portions per week when you're breastfeeding to ensure enough omega-3s in your system and in your breast milk), plenty of fruits and vegetables, wholegrains and legumes (pulses), and iron-rich foods. Just adjust your servings for breastfeeding. To find out what's back on the menu now that you're no longer pregnant, see the box on page 167. To find out what's off-limits or still restricted, see page 173.

What about lactation foods and supplements you've heard increase your milk supply? Should you be dunking lactation cookies in coconut water, or chasing a bowl of porridge down with a blue electrolyte drink? Taking mother's milk tea for two, along with fenugreek capsules and a big spoonful of brewer's yeast? Here's a breakdown of some of the foods, drinks and supplements that are touted as milk-making miracles but don't necessarily stand up to the science.

■ Fenugreek (and other herbs). The most popular ingredient in the vast

Colour Your (Breast Milk) World

You don't have to be Irish to celebrate St Patrick's Day with green breast milk – all you have to do is eat a plateful of asparagus. What you eat can change the colour of your milk (though it doesn't always, and you may not notice the change unless you're pumping), and from there, even the colour of your baby's urine. And it's easier being green than you might think. Kelp, green jelly, sea-weed (in tablet form) and some other natural supplements can be linked with green breast milk. Green not your colour? Going carrot crazy can lend a slight orange hue. Eat beetroot (or red jelly), and you may see pink, or slightly red. Unless a colour change comes with tummy troubles for your baby, there's no need to worry, or to take a pass on asparagus.

Bear in mind that breast milk naturally comes in slightly different colours. Foremilk (the milk at the beginning of a feed) usually runs a little blue, or somewhat watery look-ing. Hindmilk (the milk your breasts release later in a feed) is creamier looking, white or yellowish. Blood (usually from cracked nipples) can turn breast milk pink or rusty red – even brown if the blood is residual. Medication you take can also change the colour of your breast milk (make sure that any medicine or supplement you're taking is cleared by baby's healthcare provider). If there's a mys-tery in your milk or your baby's urine colour that can't be easily solved, or if an unusual colour continues, talk to your healthcare provider. See your baby's doctor straight away if baby's urine is darker and more concen-trated than usual or if it is scant, since this can be a sign of dehydration.

CHEW ON THIS. Old wives are fond of passing down this less-than-wise tale: eating onions and garlic will help with weaning. Obviously, this tale is rooted in another tale – that babies don't like the taste of garlic, onions or other strong flavours in their breast milk. But studies have shown that this is likely to be the case only when mum's been a bland eater throughout her pregnant and lactating days. In fact, lots of babies especially enjoy breast milk when it's spiked with flavours such as garlic – possibly because they picked up a taste for garlic-infused amniotic fluid while dining at Cafe Uterus. If you're a fan of Aubergine with Garlic Sauce, it's likely your baby will be, too.

majority of lactation products, fenugreek also comes alone in capsule, powder, tincture or tea form (alone or in mother's milk tea blends). Fenugreek has been recommended for centuries by midwives, and more recently by some lactation consultants and mummy bloggers, as a milk-supply booster. While fenugreek is considered safe for most breastfeeding mums when used in moderation (it's smart to ask your doctor first), studies of its effectiveness have been mixed at best. So have real-life results as reported by mums. Some mums challenged by milk-supply issues find it works for them, increasing supply within a day to weeks of starting fenugreek, but others find that it doesn't help a bit. Coming to a scientific conclusion on fenugreek's effectiveness (or lack of it) is complicated by the fact that most women trying fenugreek (and other purported milk makers) are trying something else to boost their supply at the same time

– say, pumping more often or nursing more frequently. Was it the pumping, or the extra feeds, or the fenugreek that did the trick – or was it actually a psychological benefit (placebo effect)? That's hard to identify. Plus there are side effects to fenugreek and products containing it. Some side effects are more or less harmless (like your urine, sweat and milk – and possibly baby's – smelling like maple syrup). Other side effects are more uncomfortable (for mum, these can include loose stool, tummy troubles and nausea; for baby, green, watery stools and fussiness). And still others are potentially dangerous (severe allergies, hypoglycaemia or worsening asthma symptoms).

What about other herbs, herbal tea blends (including mother's milk tea, which blends fenugreek, fennel, anise, coriander, blessed thistle and more), herb-containing lactation products (such as chews and bars) and supplements (such as garlic and basil)? There are many on the market targeting mums looking to boost their milk supply (or their let-down), but there's little scientific evidence that they actually get the job done. Some carry a risk of side effects in high doses. Another case for: ask you or your baby's healthcare provider before brewing or dropping them into your diet.

■ Oats. Can a bowl full of porridge help you make two breasts full of milk? Maybe. Certainly, traditional wisdom passed down from mum to mum (and lactation specialist to lactation specialist) indicates that eating oats can boost milk supply. How, exactly? There are several theories. One: by pumping up iron levels – after all, oats are a good source of iron, and low iron levels have been linked to lower supply. Two: with its cholesterol-reducing

Pass the Broccoli . . . and the Wind?

Of course you know that wind can't really be passed through breast milk. It's produced in the intestines, and babies normally produce a whole lot of it, due to their age-appropriately immature digestive systems. Still, it's easy to blame baby's tummy troubles, fussiness or even colic on something you've eaten. Many mums claim that eating wind-producing foods (such as cabbage, onions, broccoli, Brussels sprouts or beans) produces bouts of wind in their babies. Or that downing dairy causes colic. Or that coffee triggers the fussies (in baby, not mum).

It's just not usually the case. Passing wind and crying are two things that babies do a lot of, usually unrelated to what mum had for breakfast (if she ever got around to eating it) or dinner (ditto). Some babies seem to excel in producing wind, or spitting up, or crying – but every baby does some of all three. And some days will be windier or fussier than others (and that goes for breastfed and formula-fed babies). The reality is that few babies are actually sensitive to something in their mum's diet, and that wind (or crying bouts, or both) is usually just newborn-baby business as usual. At least that's what the research shows, for the most part.

Still, scientific studies don't amount too much when it's your baby who's windy and uncomfortable after you've wolfed down a burrito. Or is crying overtime after that extra-large latte. And once in a while, a breastfed baby does show sensitivity and a consistent reaction (that wind, that fussiness, that crying) to something in a mum's diet. A super-sensitive baby might even have an allergic reaction (such as a rash, hives, wheezing, diarrhoea or bloody stool) to something in a mum's diet, but that's even less common.

Thinking that something you're regularly eating or drinking is rubbing your baby up the wrong way, or worse? Ask your baby's healthcare provider – especially if you think your baby might be allergic to something in your diet. You'll be able to screen for a sensitivity (or allergy) simply by eliminating suspect foods (whether it's those vegetables or that dairy) from your diet one at a time (in the case of dairy, it would mean eliminating the entire dairy category). Eliminate more than one at a time and you'll never know what, if anything, was causing the reaction. If baby's symptoms improve dramatically after two to three weeks of eliminating that food (though in most babies the symptoms will begin to improve within a week), chances are you've found your culprit. Give that food or drink a break, and then consider reintroducing it at a later date, or just wait until after you wean.

effects, which may (in theory) nudge up milk supply. Three: by offering a nourishing, sustaining dose of comfort food – comfort that can make a mum feel (potentially) more relaxed, which can, in turn, make her produce more milk and let it down more effectively. Plus, oats are a good source of B vitamins, often touted for breast milk boosting (and energy boosting). There's no scientific proof that oat-eating mums produce more milk, but many mums claim success. And with only nutritional upside, there's no reason not to start your day (or your night shift with baby) with a bowl of oats. You can also shake them into a smoothie.

Nursing Twins (or More)

Double (or triple) the mouths to feed? If you're nursing twins or triplets, you'll need extra rest and, yes, extra food – more calories, in fact, than when you were pregnant. Be sure to follow the Postnatal Diet for breastfeeding – increasing your calorie requirement by 500–600 calories and adding an extra serving of calcium and protein for each additional baby.

■ Lactation cookies, bars and shakes. You may be able to buy them, and you can make them at home – and there's no harm in eating (or drinking) them, as long as they don't include herbs you haven't cleared with your or baby's healthcare provider. But do lactation cookies, bars and shakes work? Not surprisingly, there's only anecdotal evidence that they do – and there's a chance that much of the reported success may, in fact, be caused by a placebo effect (a mum believes that eating lactation cookies helps her make milk, she relaxes while eating them . . . and the milk magic happens). Most contain oats, often as the first ingredient. Other healthy (if not proven milk-producing) ingredients in many of these lactation treats include linseeds (flaxseeds), peanut butter, nuts and seeds. Most also contain brewer's yeast (another purported milk booster that isn't backed by evidence but can lend a bitter taste to some recipes). And some contain significant amounts of sugar (that's the cookie talking), which brings up the only real downside to eating lots of them: they can add up in the calorie department.

■ Electrolyte drinks. From sports drinks (including Lucozade Sport and blue Gatorade) to coconut juice blends, you'll find plenty of mums who credit an 'electrolyte' beverage for boosting milk supply. But do they work? There's no scientific reason why they would, unless a mum were seriously dehydrated (say, from an extreme workout). Maybe it's the placebo effect at work again, but most experts feel confident that it's not the electrolytes (or the dye that turns Gatorade – and often breast milk – the requisite blue . . . or green). The downside, again, would be the sugar and empty calories in most drinks, along with any artificial flavours and colours. Coconut water is refreshing (look for one that doesn't include added sugar), even if it's not all it's cracked up to be in the milk production department.

■ Beer. You've waited nine months to have one, so go ahead – make your night. But don't count on beer (and make sure you do keep count; see the next page) to boost your milk supply. Again, mum tales (these from way back) may claim otherwise, but there's no evidence that the beer makes milk, as happy as it may make you. In fact, alcohol of any kind is known to decrease supply. The theory is probably rooted in the barley many (but far from all) beers are made from. Some say that barley can increase levels of prolactin (that's the breastfeeding hormone), which in turn bumps up milk supply. Without a doubt, barley's a good wholegrain to add to your diet – it's packed with fibre and B vitamins every new mum needs – but it definitely doesn't have to come in the form of a beer, and if it does, it should come only occasionally, in limited amounts.

▪ Chicken soup, papaya, dates, root vegetables – you name it. There are plenty of other foods said (but not conclusively proven) to help with milk production and let-down.

So should you give these foods, drinks and supplements a go? You could – and when it comes to healthy foods, such as oats and root vegetables, you definitely should. But consider, before you spring for big-ticket lactation products or commit to gagging down something you can't stand, that most women who think they have supply issues actually don't. And if you do, the best step you can take (besides taking the many milk-supply-boosting steps listed in *What to Expect: The First Year*) is to see a lactation professional who can diagnose the problem and help you find a remedy that's really tried and true, as well as medically sound.

What Not to Eat (or to Limit)

Maybe you barely noticed pregnancy's diet limitations – you weren't a raw fish fan to begin with, you didn't have a soft spot for raw soft cheese or cold meats, you always took a pass on cocktails or raw oysters. Or maybe aversions or morning sickness had you turned off to all – or some – of the above, making giving them up a piece of cake (especially because you could still have cake). Still, chances are you're looking forward to putting at least one of pregnancy's off-the-menu items back on the table. And for the most part, you can, even while you're breastfeeding. You can tap into beer and pop that champagne. Eat your cold meats cold and your salmon barely seared. Order your beef burger rare and your steak practically mooing. Embrace the Brie

and blue cheese when you're overseas without giving a thought to whether it's pasteurised. And pour the coffee you crave (though you could have poured it while you were expecting, too – at least, in moderate amounts).

But a few restrictions are still standing – some items to keep avoiding, others that can be added back in, but in moderation, and others (like that coffee) that you'll still be limited on. Here's a list of foods and drinks you'll have to watch for when breastfeeding:

Too much alcohol. The pub has reopened now that you've delivered – just in time to celebrate your baby's arrival. But remember to keep the bar low: no more than one drink at a time and preferably no more than two servings per week. Have a beer or a glass of wine, but to avoid sharing the alcohol with your baby (it will end up in your breast milk), drink it right after a feeding or pumping. Wait a few hours (two or three is usually enough) before you feed or pump again, since that will allow enough time for the alcohol to be metabolised. Pumping and dumping won't help speed up that process. Not sure whether you've exceeded your alcohol limit or if your body has finished metabolising it? Don't be

---

CHEW ON THIS. Here's one more for the old wives' hall of fiction: according to folklore, if you get frightened, your breast milk will go sour. While it's true that stress hormones (produced when you're scared, for instance) may temporarily suppress the let-down reflex, your milk won't taste any different to baby. So go ahead and push 'play' on that horror flick. Then take a deep breath, relax and don't get yourself worked up over soured milk.

Losing the Baby Weight

Here's something you might not have expected when you were expecting: still looking pregnant months after you've delivered. While you'll lose far more weight the day you give birth than you could ever hope to lose in many weeks of dieting (about 12 lb/5.5 kg, give or take), you'll likely have plenty of pounds to shed before you return to your pre-pregnancy weight. Some will be lost quickly after delivery, thanks to fluid loss. Most will linger a lot longer – and that's what you should expect. Remember, the body lays down extra pounds, beyond what it needs for baby building, to fuel breastfeeding after baby arrives – and that's a good thing.

Yet, if you're keen to wear trousers that zip up again, it can also be a frustrating thing. Try not to sweat the pounds (you'll be doing plenty of sweating anyway postnatal, nature's way of draining some of those accumulated fluids). Instead, remember that you've earned those inches in the service of a healthy pregnancy – and if you're breastfeeding, in the service of feeding your baby. Wear them with honour for now while looking ahead to reaching a healthy weight sensibly, bearing in mind these tips.

If you're not breastfeeding:

- Take a break. Sure, you're in a hurry to see your waist again. But it's not smart to embark on a weight-loss programme until your body has a chance to recuperate from childbirth. So wait until at least six weeks postnatal (three months is considered more reasonable) before starting any weight-loss campaign.

- Give yourself time. You didn't put on those pounds overnight, so you can't expect to lose them that quickly either. For most women, it takes six months to a year for pregnancy weight to come off.

- Add in exercise. The best way to lose weight postnatal is by combining exercise and diet. Once your healthcare provider has given the green light, resume or begin an exercise programme (preferably one that includes cardio and strength training) to help you shed the pounds.

If you are breastfeeding:

In addition to the tips for new mums above, also:

- Take a longer break. If you're breastfeeding, you should wait at least three months before starting any weight-loss plan. Ask your healthcare provider for specific guidelines for you.

- Go slow. Much of the weight you put on during pregnancy was set aside as fat stores earmarked for lactation. Lose those fat stores too quickly and your milk supply could suffer. Slow and steady will win this race (though it's definitely not a race). Once you start on your weight-loss programme, aim to lose no more than half a pound (225 g) a week (1–2 lb/450–900 g per month).

- Don't depend on breastfeeding. Although breastfeeding burns about 500 calories a day (the same as a daily 5-mile/8-km run, and all without even breaking a sweat), nursing alone won't guarantee weight loss. Though plenty of mums find the pounds melt away when they're breastfeeding, others have trouble losing weight, and some can't manage to lose an ounce until after baby is weaned. As long as the healthy foods in your diet outweigh the unhealthy and you've incorporated a consistent exercise routine into your day, it'll come off eventually.

tempted to test it with a DIY kit sold online that uses test strips to detect the volume of alcohol in your breast milk. If you strayed from limiting yourself to one drink, it's best to play safe. When it's time for a feeding, feed baby from your stash of pre-pumped and stored breast milk instead. If you need to relieve engorgement, you can pump a little, but you'll have to dump it.

Avoid heavy drinking when you're breastfeeding. Not only can large doses of alcohol make baby sleepy, sluggish, unresponsive and unable to suck well, but too many drinks can also impair your own functioning (whether you're nursing or not), making you more susceptible to depression, fatigue and lapses in judgement. And even moderate amounts of alcohol can reduce your milk supply.

Too much caffeine. During those early, sleep-deprived postnatal weeks, a little jolt from your local coffee bar may be just the pick-me-up you need. So go ahead and give it a shot – just not too many shots at a time. Sticking to the same 200 mg of coffee (or the equivalent in other caffeinated foods and drinks) per day as you did while you were expecting won't affect your baby, and may actually allow you to stay vertical when you'd really rather be horizontal. But exceeding that limit can make junior jittery and keep you both from getting any sleep – and no amount of caffeine is going to help you then.

Questionable herbs. Watch out for herbs, even some seemingly innocuous herbal teas. Stick to regular (black) tea that comes flavoured, or choose other teas that are considered safe during lactation, including white tea, chamomile and rosehip (you can ask your health-care provider for a list of safe teas). Read labels carefully to make sure other

---

Eating Well for the Next Baby

Is there a baby in your near future? If you're planning an encore, there's a lot more to the preparations than working out where yet another new nursery will go. You'll also have to prepare your next baby's very first source of bed and board: you. And one of the best ways to get yourself into tip-top baby-making shape during the pre-conception months is by getting your diet into shape (or getting it back into shape). Even before you start eating for two, you can start eating well for your future baby's health. For all the information you'll need on eating well before you're expecting, see *What to Expect Before You're Expecting.*

---

herbs haven't been added to the brew, and drink them only in moderation.

Some herbal preparations touted for their milk-producing properties can have unpleasant side effects, including nausea, and other herbs, such as chasteberry, jasmine and sage, can actually reduce milk supply. In general, because not all herbal remedies are regulated in the UK and little is known about how herbs affect a nursing baby, play it safe and consult your doctor before taking any herbal remedy.

Certain sugar substitutes. Most sweeteners are considered safe during lactation in sensible moderation. The one sweetener that's not sweet when you're breastfeeding: Sweet'N Low (aka saccharine). And, of course, avoid aspartame entirely if you have phenylketonuria (PKU) or your baby does.

Fish high in mercury. Though it's safe to reel in the sushi again, continue to avoid high-mercury fish, such as shark, swordfish and marlin, while breast-feeding. And if you travel to the USA, add tilefish from the Gulf of Mexico, king mackerel, bigeye tuna steaks and orange roughy to the list. You should also limit seafood that may contain moderate amounts of that heavy metal. But because guidelines recommend that breastfeeding mums eat at least two portions per week of low-mercury fish, be sure to cast your net widely to benefit from the brain-boosting nutrients found in safe fish (see page 72 for a list).

CHAPTER 11

Safe Cooking and Prepping When You're Expecting

M aybe you're already hyper when it comes to hygiene around your house, especially in your kitchen. Maybe you're a little laxer about kitchen conditions. Maybe bacteria is always on your mind when you're prepping, cooking, storing and serving food – or maybe it's on the back burner (literally, because you haven't cleaned the back burner since that soup you were simmering boiled over 4 days ago). Maybe you regularly take your food's temperature before you eat it, check use-by dates religiously and toss questionable foods without question. Or maybe you've been known to eat straight out of the takeaway container that sat out for 3 hours last night before you remembered to stick it in the fridge. Wherever your sanitary standards stand – whether you're sure you'd ace an inspection from your local health department or pretty certain you'd fail – everyone has something to learn about food safety, especially when they're trying to eat safely for two. That's because pregnant women, in general, are more susceptible to foodborne illness – and more likely to get sicker from it.

Consider this chapter your Food Safety 101 – the bacteria basics. A little on the boring side, yes. A lot of extra precautions, true. But following at least some of the advice here, at least some of the time, can sure beat getting hit with a bad bug (especially when you're already bugged by pregnancy symptoms). For information on foods you should avoid entirely because of the risk of bacterial infection they may carry, see Chapter 5.

Keeping Your Kitchen Safe

Think that you have months before you'll have to worry about making your kitchen safe for baby? While it's true that you can hold off on installing childproof latches on the cupboards and knob covers on the cooker, there are many other precautions you should be taking around your kitchen right now to protect your growing baby – not from pinched fingers or accidental burns, but from food-borne bacteria that can make both of you sick. So, before stepping up to the kitchen worktop:

Wash your hands. Mum (and the health experts) does know best when it comes to this first rule of safe cooking and eating. Washing your hands in hot soapy water before preparing food is your best line of defence against the spread

of bacteria in the kitchen. Break out the soap, too, after you've handled raw meat, poultry, fish or eggs – all of which can harbour dangerous bacteria. Stating the obvious but not always observed: also wash your hands after blowing your nose, going to the toilet, changing a nappy or attending to another germ-charged activity.

Wash your towels and sponges. That tea towel you just dried your hands with looks pretty clean, doesn't it? Take a closer look (like under a microscope) and you might change your mind – as well as your towel. Do the same with your sponge (a sponge for bacteria) and you'd do the same. Sponges and tea towels provide a perfect breeding ground for bacteria, which thrive in moist environments. To avoid drying your hands, wiping your worktop and cleaning your dishes with a veritable petri dish of microorganisms, wash dishcloths and towels often in hot soapy water or in the washing machine. Replace sponges at least once a month, and wash them thoroughly with soap and water or in the dishwasher at the end of the day (it turns out microwaving them won't kill all the bacteria). To avoid spreading germs around your kitchen, use kitchen paper for kitchen clean-up.

Wash (and watch) your surfaces. Bacteria multiply far faster than rabbits, especially when left to their own devices on kitchen surfaces. To keep those bugs from breeding in your kitchen, clean worktops and sinks often with soapy water or cleansers. Take precautions in the fridge, too. Don't put a package of raw chicken or meat or fish directly on the shelf for defrosting (even if it's

---

Home Is Where the Health Is . . . or Is It?

Myth: Food prepared at home is much safer than restaurant food. Most food-borne illnesses are contracted from food at restaurants.

Fact: Actually, you're more likely to pick up a bug dining at home than at your local cafe. That's because most (though certainly not all) professional food handlers have been trained in hygiene and food safety protocol and are more likely to be careful about following those standards. Plus, they know their restaurant can be shut down if those standards aren't met. Think about this, too: most home kitchens probably wouldn't pass inspection by the health department.

wrapped, it's likely to leak, so put it on a plate). Wash chopping boards in the dishwasher after each use – or if they're too large to fit, with hot soapy water. When boards get scarred from too much use, discard them. (Bacteria like to hide – and multiply – in pitted surfaces.)

Cut out cross contamination. One knife that gets around – from the raw chicken breasts to the cheese to the tomatoes – can spread a whole lot of bacteria around your kitchen. If you're using one knife for several food-prep steps, wash between uses with hot soapy water. Better still, keep different knives for different purposes (one for raw meat and poultry, another for produce). Something else to keep separate: chopping boards: use one for produce, another for fish, meat and poultry.

Keeping Your Foods Safe

You've shopped for the most nutritious ingredients, and you're ready to test your cooking chops (and your dicing, sautéing and saucing skills). Or maybe your plan is a little less ambitious – you're going to slice a peach and a banana, toss in some yogurt and nuts, and call it dinner . . . and a night. Or dive into that box of leftover pizza with a side salad. Either way, one thing you'll want to incorporate into your dinner (or breakfast, or lunch) plans is safety. So bear in mind these safe-food strategies when storing, preparing and serving:

■ Don't wait to refrigerate. Make sure anything that must be kept refrigerated (that meat, fish, poultry, cut raw or cooked produce, eggs, cheese, yogurt, milk) finds its way into your fridge as soon as possible after purchase, but definitely within 2 hours (less in warm weather). If you can't get to a fridge that quickly, bring along insulated bags and ice packs to store your cold purchases in until you return home. Clearly, if you've ordered perishables via an app for delivery, make sure you're home to receive them – or that you will be

> **CHEW ON THIS.** Not surprisingly, old wives have spent a lot of time in the kitchen over the ages – and have stirred up more than a few tales there. Among them – you shouldn't put hot food in the refrigerator because it will spoil. In fact, the old wives are way off base on this one. The longer a food (hot or cold) sits out at room temperature, the greater the chances bacteria will multiply – and the faster it will spoil. A good mantra to remember when cooking foods that won't be eaten straight away: cool slightly – then don't hesitate, refrigerate.

soon – so they're not sitting on a hot doorstep (unless they're packaged in an insulated box).

■ Give perishables priority placement. Store highly perishable foods (milk, fish) in the back of the refrigerator. The storage areas on the door are fine for condiments, but they don't stay as cold. Make sure your fridge is set to 5°C or below and your freezer at -18°C or below.

The Dating Game

How can you tell if a food you're about to purchase or that's been sitting in your fridge for a while is too old to eat? Play the dating game by checking the label.

- Products that aren't perishable, such as flour and grains, bakes, crisps, cereals and tinned goods, have labels with a 'best before' or 'best before end' (or 'BBE') date. Think of this date as being about the quality of the flavour and texture. These foods won't be dangerous to dig into after the date given, but they'll probably start to taste stale. Some, such as passata or oat milk, may need to be stored in the fridge after opening and consumed within the number of days specified on the packaging.

- Perishable products that require refrigeration and have a shorter shelf life (such as cheese, juice or ready-to-eat salads) will have a 'use by' date. This date is about safety: the food should not be consumed after that date passes, even if it smells okay.

- Fresh meat, poultry and fish should be refrigerated and used by the 'use by' date. Freeze them if you won't be using them within that time frame. How long they'll last in the freezer depends on how well they are wrapped and how cold your freezer is.

- Frozen foods (the kind you get from the freezer section of the supermarket, not the leftovers you've frozen) will last for 6 to 12 months in the freezer. The 'best before' date lets you know when they won't taste as good as intended. That's because flavour and texture break down over time.

- Eggs come with two dates: a 'display until' date that tells the grocer how long they can have it on their shelves for sale. The second date is the 'best before' date, the last date by which they should be eaten. Though eggs are not chilled in the shops, you should refrigerate them at home – they should be stored below 20°C.

Another trick? To choose foods with the latest dates possible, check the back of the shelf. It's common shop practice to put the older items up front (to get rid of them before they expire).

- Cook or freeze promptly. Didn't have time to cook that salmon or those chicken breasts, as planned? If you haven't got around to cooking fresh poultry, fish or meat mince within 2 days of purchase, wrap it up and stick it in the freezer. Don't keep other cuts of meat in the fridge for longer than 3–5 days – freeze or cook before they've reached that window.

- Heat it like you mean it. That stew that you turned off after simmering for hours, because your dinner guests were running late? Bring it back up to a rolling boil before you dig in. Ditto gravies and soups. Reheat leftovers thoroughly until hot and steaming.

- Don't let your buffet overstay. Here's a buffet table downer: Food shouldn't be left at room temperature for more than 2 hours (1 hour outside on a hot day or in a hot room – so beware the summer BBQ spread or the picnic in the park on a hot day). Love lingering with your guests when the party's over? Make sure you refrigerate those leftovers first.

- Refuse to refreeze. Don't refreeze foods that have been thawed at room temperature, or have been brought to room temperature after thawing, or have been kept for more than a day or two after thawing, even in the refrigerator.

- Go by 'sell by' and 'use by' dates (see the box on the opposite page). When in doubt, throw it out – even if there are no obvious signs of spoilage. Definitely throw out any food that has an off colour or odour.

- Don't double dip (dip a carrot into salsa, take a bite, and then dip the same carrot again) or eat straight from a container unless you're planning to finish off the contents. Bacteria from your mouth (transferred via the spoon, vegetable, cracker, crisp or chip you're snacking from) can contaminate the food – even if it's refrigerated afterwards.

- Wash the lids of tinned foods before opening to keep dirt and bacteria from getting into the food. Also, clean the blade of the can opener or drop it into the dishwasher after each use.

Safe Produce

Nothing is more wholesome than fresh fruits and vegetables, right? For the most part, yes. That is, unless that fresh peach or carrot or apple you're eyeing is covered in bacteria – courtesy of a picker, a shop worker or even a customer who didn't wash his or her hands before handling the produce you're about to plop into your trolley. Or bacteria that comes from the trolley itself, or the conveyer belt at the till, if you haven't bagged your produce in clean reusable or plastic bags.

According to health experts, nearly half of all food-borne illness has its roots in fruits and vegetables. Luckily, the overall risks are low, and they're lower still if you take steps to make sure the produce that's supposed to keep you healthy won't make you sick:

- Cook your produce. One of the best ways to bid bacteria bye-bye is to cook your fruits and veggies – sauté that kale, steam those carrots, bake that apple (yes, even grill that watermelon, those romaine hearts). But clearly, not every member of the produce family can take the heat (say, cantaloupe) – and just as clearly, there will be many times when you'll want your carrots raw, your salad crisp and your apple crunchy. So read on for how to safely eat them raw.

- Give all produce that isn't pre-washed a good wash. Thoroughly rinse the surfaces of all fruits and vegetables with water and then pat them dry with a clean towel or kitchen paper – not only to keep them fresher and crunchier, but to rub off even more surface germs. Do this just before serving, preparing or cooking – not when you bring the produce home (unless you're planning to cut up and stash that watermelon for easy munching right from the fridge). If necessary, use a scrub brush or glove designed for scrubbing produce to remove visible dirt (use a softer brush for mushrooms, a stiffer brush for potatoes), and wash the brush after use with hot soapy water or in the dishwasher. Don't skip that rinse because you're planning to peel your fruit or veg before serving anyway – otherwise the knife or peeler you're using can pick up surface germs and transmit them to the part you'll be eating. So rinse that avocado, that lemon, that cantaloupe before slicing into it, that carrot before peeling. Stick to rinsing rules, too, even if you just picked a basket of organic (or locally grown) strawberries at the local farmers market – those berries are just as likely to be sprinkled with bacteria as those from the supermarket, and either can make you sick if you're not careful. Will rinsing remove all bacteria? No, but it's an important precaution to take.

■ Double-check before you don't wash. Some packs of spinach or ready-to-eat salad leaves are already washed but read the fine print before serving. You may not need to rewash ready-to-eat produce, but do wash herbs, heads of lettuce and other salad leaves that haven't been washed – and do so right before cooking or serving them.

■ Screen pre-cut fruit and veggies. They're the ultimate convenience (those neat cubes of honeydew, those berry medleys just begging to be popped into your mouth, those sliced carrots and cucumbers). But even if you're happy to pay the price of conveniently pre-cut produce, make sure you don't inadvertently pay another price, in the form of a tummy ache or worse. Be sure to check use-by dates and select only ready-to-eat produce that's been kept refrigerated while on display. That goes for half watermelons and coconuts. Refrigerate at 5°C or less as soon as possible after purchase.

■ Buy local, when you can. For one thing, local produce is usually fresher than imports, which means it's likely to retain more nutrients (same goes for seasonal produce). For another, while any produce can wear bacteria home from the market or stand, locally grown may be less likely to be contaminated than imported, since regulations on sanitation are more lax in some foreign countries.

■ Go organic, when you can. Whenever it's available and affordable and looks good, opt for organic. It isn't less likely to contain bacteria, but at least it won't be covered with pesticides. Check out page 66 to see when an upgrade to organic is worth the extra cost and when it probably isn't.

■ Be picky when picking fruits and veggies, even when you're picking them from your fridge. That 2-for-1 deal on raspberries sounded like a great deal – but try to buy only what you can eat before it spoils. Check for soft spots, little bits of fuzzy mould, a funny smell, a damp look or brown

---

Recall Alert

A great way to stay on top of food safety is by staying on top of food recalls. The Food Standards Agency (FSA) will, from time to time, issue recalls on foods that are found to carry unsafe bacteria, from E. coli in beef lasagne to salmonella in pre-cut cantaloupe, or that are unsafe for other reasons. For the latest recalls, keep an eye on notices in supermarkets and visit www.food.gov. uk/news-alerts, where you can also sign up for automatic alerts to let you know when there's a food recall.

edges on all produce before buying, and then again before eating. Bruised isn't a biggie, though.

■ Date your produce. Always check 'best before' dates on bagged or boxed produce when buying and before eating.

■ Keep up to date on produce recalls and safety warnings (see the box on the opposite page).

Safe Meat, Poultry and Fish

Building a baby? There's no more efficient source of baby-building protein than lean meat, poultry and fish. To cash in on the protein without tapping into any bacteria that may have come along for the ride – and might make you sick – try to bear in mind these tips:

■ When freezing pre-packed fresh meat, poultry or fish, remove the plastic or paper wrapping it came in and seal in cling film and then heavy-duty aluminium foil or specially designed freezer bags to prevent freezer burn.

Alternatively, using foil or cling film, wrap around the original wrapping. Don't forget to label your packets so you won't be left with unidentified frozen objects – and to date them, so you don't let them overstay their welcome in the freezer.

■ Defrost appropriately wrapped meats, poultry or fish in the refrigerator on a plate, in cold water (changing the water every 30 minutes) or in a microwave oven on 'defrost', rather than at room temperature. Food defrosted

Now You Tell Me (Part Two)?

Already ordered your beef burger rare before finding out you shouldn't have it your way when you're expecting (unless your way is medium-well)? Poked around in the poke department before you discovered that well marinated isn't the same as well cooked when it comes to fish? Didn't know you should be running from runny eggs without the British Lion stamp? Gobbled those strawberries right out of the farmers market basket without washing them first? Not to worry. First, because foodborne illness are relatively uncommon in the UK. And second, because in the case of most of the bacteria (or parasites)

that can cause these illnesses, the only risk is getting really sick (and if you didn't get really sick pretty fast, that risk has already passed). The exceptions are Listeria and toxoplasmosis, which can be more dangerous during pregnancy (see page 82 for the lowdown on Listeria).

The bottom line on bacteria when you're expecting: it's best to avoid those that can make you sick. Worrying yourself sick about what you've eaten – or what you might eat inadvertently – isn't best. Take what precautions you can (and know about), and then sit back at the dinner table and relax.

Is It Done Yet?

How do you make sure that your dinner isn't half baked (or half grilled or half roasted) – and still potentially harbouring germs that could make you sick? By taking its temperature. Reaching the right temperature means your meat, fish or poultry won't be serving you a side of bacteria. Don't rely on the pop-up thermometers that come with some poultry – invest in a good-quality instant-read or leave-in meat thermometer, and use it faithfully (wash it after each use with hot soapy water). Of course, you'll also need to know where to stick it – as well as what temperature to look for once you have. Here's a guide:

For roasts, steaks or chops made from beef, veal, pork or lamb: Insert the thermometer in the centre or the thickest part of the meat, away from any bone, fat or gristle.

For meat or poultry mince or escalopes, fish and casseroles: Insert the thermometer in the thickest part of the food. For burgers, insert sideways.

For chicken, turkey, duck or goose: Insert the thermometer in the inner thigh area, where the leg meets the body of the bird (but be sure the thermometer isn't touching the bone).

The following foods can be considered safely cooked when they reach these temperatures:

- Beef, veal, lamb, pork roasts, chops or steaks: 62.8°C

- Beef, veal, lamb, pork mince: 71°C

- Precooked ham: 60°C

- Whole chicken or turkey, chicken or turkey mince: 73.9°C

- Chicken breasts: 73.9°C

- Stuffing (cooked in bird or alone): 73.9°C

- Fish: 62.8°C

- Egg dishes: 71°C

in the microwave should be cooked immediately.

- Marinate meat, poultry or fish in the refrigerator, not at room temperature. Don't reuse marinade that has touched raw meat or poultry. Set some marinade aside before pouring it all on the raw meat, poultry or fish if you'd like to use it for basting (change the utensil between bastings so you don't double dip) or for sauce.

- Keep hot meats hot and cold meats cold. If you're bringing chicken salad to a picnic, be sure it's transported and served on ice. Don't let cooked hot meats stay out at room temperature for more than 2 hours (1 hour on a hot day or in a very warm room).

- Don't stuff meat or poultry until it is ready to go into the oven. Stuff lightly (about 12 oz/350 g of stuffing per 1 lb/450 g of turkey), keep it moist, and cook until the centre of the stuffing reaches at least 73.9°C on a meat thermometer. After cooking, store the stuffing and meat separately. Safer still, don't stuff at all. Bake the stuffing in a separate tray, basting occasionally with broth. A bonus: the stuffing will develop a crusty top. If you prefer soft stuffing, bake it covered with foil.

- Cook meat to medium. Yes, it's true what you've heard (and you may not be pleased about it): rare meat is off the menu when you're expecting. But when cooking, don't rely on colour, which can vary too much. Use a meat thermometer to get a better reading of meat safety (see the box on the opposite page for information on what temperature to cook foods to). Order beef, pork, lamb and other meat 'medium' or 'well' in restaurants, just to be on the safe side. With a thick fillet, that might mean asking for it to be butterflied or spatchcocked before cooking.

- Cook chicken and other poultry through. The easiest way to see if poultry is safely cooked is to take its temperature – in the centre, not near the bone (see the box on the opposite page). Juices should run clear, too. You can't tell bone-in chicken by its colour near the bone (traces of pink may remain even after it's well cooked, because of leaching from the bone). Unfortunately for rare-duck-breast lovers (there aren't many rare-chicken lovers), these rules apply to any form of poultry. Order duck 'well' in restaurants, too.

- Don't eat it raw. Any raw meat, from tartare to carpaccio (even if it's seared) to traditional raw meats served in certain cuisines, is considered unsafe during pregnancy. Meat can harbour microorganisms when it isn't cooked through – you can't see them, you can't taste them, but they can make you sick. See page 83 for more.

- Don't eat it raw, fish edition. In case you haven't had the pregnancy briefing yet from your GP or midwife: raw or rare fish or seafood is also off the menu when you're expecting. Rolls containing only cooked fish or seafood (not seared)

Mould and Mums-to-Be

You had good intentions of filling your fridge (and your tummy) with nutritious goodies when you bought that extra container of cottage cheese and punnet of strawberries. But somehow you never got around to eating them, and when you finally dig them out for a healthy breakfast, blue fuzz has started multiplying across the top of the cottage cheese, and a green one is sprouting on the strawberries. Do you scrape and eat them, or dump them? Here are some guidelines about mould for the mum-to-be:

- If small fruits (grapes, berries, strawberries) become mouldy, throw them out. If a few berries at the top of a box are mouldy, it's okay to eat the rest as long as you've checked them carefully.

- If a hard fruit or vegetable (apple, potato, broccoli, onion, for instance) or hard cheese has a small area of mould, it's safe to cut the mould away (plus a ½ in/1 cm margin of safety) and eat the rest. Mouldy soft fruits (peaches, plums, melons, tomatoes) should be tossed in their entirety.

- Soft dairy products (cottage cheese, yogurt, soured cream, butter) that are sprouting mould should be discarded – even if the mould is only on top. Ditto mouldy meat and leftovers.

- Mouldy bread, grains, peanut butter, nuts, sauces and jams should be thrown away (even if the mould is only visible in one spot).

And always remember – when in doubt, throw it out. Especially when you're expecting.

are a safe pick from the sushi bar, while cooked shrimp or crab can be selected from the raw bar (as long as they're handled separately and stored separately from raw options). All fish (including salmon, often prepared 'medium rare', because it's inarguably yummy that way) and seafood should be cooked through (see the box on page 184). See page 72 for a list of fish that's safe to eat, and page 81 for information about the safety of smoked seafood.

- Heat ready-to-eat sausages, sausage rolls and cold meats as well as meat or poultry leftovers until steaming hot all the way through.

For more on meat and poultry safety, visit www.nhs.uk/live-well/eat-well/how -to-store-food-and-leftovers.

A Meat Myth That's All Wet

Myth: Raw meat, poultry and fish should always be rinsed before cooking to wash away the bacteria on the surface.

Fact: Cooking meats, poultry and fish to the right internal temperature (see the box on page 184) will almost always kill all the bacteria lurking on the surface – and inside. Rinsing doesn't wash enough bacteria away – however, it does splash germs and bacteria into the sink (and, if you're not careful, on to worktops). So, both pointless and counter-productive.

Safe Dairy

There's no quicker way to fill your calcium requirement (and to pick up a good bonus of protein) than to stop at your supermarket's dairy counter. And most dairy products are as safe as they are nutritious. To ensure safe dairy eating:

- Stay away from raw (unpasteurised) milk or cheeses. See page 81 for more.

- Store all dairy products in the refrigerator (even pasteurised products can become contaminated), and don't use them after the 'use by' date (see page 180) or if they smell or look off.

Safe Eggs

Keen to crack open a great source of pregnancy protein (and in the case of certain eggs, of omega-3 fatty acids)? Though the cholesterol in eggs isn't considered a problem in pregnancy, contamination with salmonella used to

be. So before cracking open that box of eggs, consider these rules of egg safety:

- Eggs should always be stored below 20°C. European farmers are prohibited from washing their eggs, which

CHEW ON THIS. Expectant mums in Mexico are often told that eating eggs during pregnancy can make their babies smell bad after birth. Take it from the egg-sperts: all babies smell amazing, no matter how many eggs their mums eat.

have a protective cuticle on the outer shell that makes them safe to store at room temperature if below 20°C. Supermarkets are generally kept below that temperature, so they don't need to refrigerate the eggs they sell. However, once you get them home, the advice is to always store eggs in the fridge until you are ready to use them. This is because the temperature in domestic homes fluctuates and won't necessarily be below 20°C. Health regulations in Europe also discourage the refrigeration of eggs in supermarkets, because when chilled eggs are brought back to room temperature, they can 'sweat', cracking the door to mildew growth and possible bacterial contamination. This is why, before refrigerating the eggs at home, it's best to not wash them, even if they're dirty – though you can wipe off any visible dirt on them. Only rinse with water to remove visible dirt immediately before you use them. You should also ensure that you use the eggs by their 'best before' date.

- Refrigerate cooked eggs. Even hard-boiled eggs can become contaminated, so don't leave them at room temperature for longer than 2 hours (and don't eat hard-boiled eggs from an unrefrigerated buffet table or salad bar if you're not sure how long they've been out there). Eat refrigerated unpeeled hard-boiled eggs within a week. Peeled hard-boiled eggs are best eaten right away and not longer than 4 or so days after peeling.

- Don't crack open an egg that's already cracked. Whether it was cracked when you bought it or cracked on the way home, toss it. Disease-causing organisms can get in through cracks too easily.

- Order your eggs pregnancy-style. If you don't know if the eggs have a British Lion stamp – which means the chickens were vaccinated against salmonella (the dangerous bacteria that sometimes spreads in chicken coops) – it's safest to cook or order them cooked until whites are set and the yolks have begun to thicken. Scrambles and omelettes should be cooked through. Poached or soft-boiled eggs should not be runny. And raw eggs shouldn't be eaten during pregnancy at all (see page 82).

- Go free-range when you can. The more room chickens have to roam around, the better. That's because cramped coops are breeding grounds for infectious bacteria that can end up in your eggs. See page 62 for more about what cage-free and free-range means when it comes to eggs.

PART 2

Cooking Well

E ating well for pregnancy isn't all that different from eating well at
any other time in your life – and the same goes for cooking well.
Most nutrition-forward, health-conscious, lean-leaning, whole
food-focused recipes are pregnancy-appropriate, even pregnancy-perfect,
sometimes with just a few tweaks for safety's sake (say, cooking the salmon
all the way through instead of searing it rare, making sure those goats cheese
crumbs are pasteurised before they top your salad) or with a nod to aversions
or super-sensitive sniffers or troubled tummies.

So by all means, tap into recipes you've collected that fit the Pregnancy Diet profile (you know, concentrating on those Daily Dozen heavy hitters: veggies, fruits, grains, lean protein and dairy, and healthy fats) and pore over those health-foodie blogs and cooking sites for more. Tweak as needed for safety or your own personal eating quirks, beef up the nutrients when you can (add red pepper to that sauce, carrots to that stew, swap romaine for the iceberg) and enjoy.

But also turn to the pages that follow, where you'll find recipes that are made for the pregnant you in mind. Most of them are quick to prepare, so you'll be eating in a hurry and with a minimum of muss, fuss and standing on the feet you'd so much rather put up. Many of them are quease-easing, or may be easily adjusted to stay away from tastes you're finding offensive. All of them pack plenty of nutrients – and of course, all of them are delicious.

From soothing smoothies to soups that eat like a meal, from breakfast muffins to one-pan dinners, pancakes to pasta, from sweet to spicy to a little bit of both, Asian to Italian to Mexican to typical British dishes, from healthy twists on classic comfort foods (mac and cheese!) to tasty but enlightened takes on guilty pleasures (Alfredo!) – you'll find something to satisfy your every craving and every nutritional requirement, usually in the same bite.

Happy cooking well – and eating well!

Breakfast

M um said it first and best (and most often, probably repeating it every time you tried to sneak out to school without your cereal, toast and orange juice): nothing starts the day off like a good breakfast. And that's especially true now that you're on your way to being a mum yourself (or adding another baby love muffin to your family). A healthy breakfast will provide the fuel both you and baby need to start the day off right. Plus, it can mean the difference between a day filled with nausea, heartburn and fatigue and a day filled with . . . well, less nausea, heartburn and fatigue. Still sneaking out the door without breakfast these days? Whether you're breakfast phobic or time challenged, the recipes in this chapter are tempting and quick enough to lure you back to the table (though you can take many of these breakfast champions on the morning commute or to the office, too). From easy Cafe Eggs and a sumptuous Tomato and Roasted Red Pepper Frittata to portable Breakfast Burritos and Stuffed Eggy Toast, you'll have no problem braking for breakfast.

Cafe Eggs
SERVES 1

Fried potatoes and eggs rolled into one, minus the greasy-spoon heartburn – plus, you get an added healthy dose of vitamin A from the red pepper.

1½ teaspoons olive oil
2 small red potatoes with their skins on, cooked and diced (about 40 g)
½ small onion, chopped

¼ teaspoon dried oregano or thyme
Salt and black pepper
2 medium eggs
½ medium-sized red pepper, diced
30 g Cheddar or Monterey jack cheese, finely grated

From the Test Kitchen

Looking to score another yellow vegetable serving with your Cafe Eggs? Substitute sweet potatoes for the red potatoes. Want something more adventurous to toss into your morning frying pan? Try any of the following (depending, of course, on your tastes and your morning nausea status): diced apple, chopped avocado, diced tomatoes, steamed broccoli florets, sliced mushrooms or jalapeño peppers.

1. Heat the olive oil in a 20-cm non-stick frying pan over a medium heat. Add the potatoes, onion and herbs, and cook, stirring occasionally, for about 4 minutes until a golden colour. Season with salt and pepper to taste.

2. Meanwhile, place the eggs in a small bowl and whisk. When the potatoes and onion are nicely coloured, add the red pepper and cook for about 1 minute until it is slightly softened. Pour the eggs into the pan but do not stir them. Lower the heat to low and cook for about 3 minutes until the eggs are cooked through, lifting the edge to let the uncooked egg run underneath.

3. Scatter the cheese over the eggs and serve.

NUTRITION INFO: 1 portion provides:

Protein: 1 serving

Calcium: 1 serving

Vitamin C: 2½ servings

Vitamin A: 1 serving

Other fruits and vegetables: ½ serving

Fat: ½ serving

Omegas: some, if using omega-3 eggs

It's No Yolk

Cholesterol's not a worry for most pregnant women. But if you're in the market for a particularly low-calorie omelette, or you're feeding someone who's watching his or her cholesterol, just leave out the yolks. To make a basic egg white omelette, whisk 4 egg whites with 2 teaspoons water. Cook them as you would a regular omelette and add your choice of fillings. You can also find compromise in a 1 whole egg, 2 egg white omelette.

Mushroom and Spinach Omelette

SERVES 1

This veggie-stuffed omelette makes for one easy, hearty breakfast, or a filling brunch or dinner when paired with a simple side salad.

1½ teaspoon olive oil
40 g very finely chopped shallots (optional)
1 clove garlic, very finely chopped
17.5 g button mushrooms, sliced
1 sprig fresh thyme (¼ teaspoon dried)
85 g fresh baby spinach
Pinch of salt
Pinch of pepper
2 medium eggs
2 teaspoons butter
2 slices provolone cheese (about 45 g total) or Edam cheese if unavailable

1. Heat the olive oil in a 20-cm non-stick frying pan over a medium heat. Add the oil. Add the shallots, if using, garlic, mushrooms and thyme, and fry for 7 minutes, or until the mushrooms are coloured. Add the spinach and fry for 4 minutes, or until the liquid has almost completely evaporated. Remove the vegetable mixture from the pan; discard the thyme sprig. Wipe the pan clean.

2. Place the salt, pepper and eggs in a small bowl and whisk to mix.

3. Melt the butter in the pan over a medium heat. Pour the egg mixture into the pan and cook for 1 minute until the eggs start to set on the bottom. Lift the edge of the omelette with a rubber turner to let the uncooked egg run underneath. Cook for 1 minute more, or until the centre of the omelette just begins to set. Place the provolone on top and spoon the vegetable mixture over the cheese. Run the turner around the edge and under the omelette to loosen it from the pan, fold it in half and slide it onto a plate. Serve.

NUTRITION INFO: 1 portion provides:

Protein: 1 serving

Calcium: 1½ servings

Vitamin C: 4 servings

Vitamin A: 4 servings

Other fruits and vegetables: 2 servings

Iron: some

Fat: 1 serving

Omegas: some, if using omega-3 eggs

Egg Bites

SERVES 4

Order up an easy breakfast or snack with these tasty egg bites – easier still if you've made them ahead for speedy reheating. Add a salad and a wholegrain bun for a light lunch or dinner.

Cooking oil spray
1 tablespoon olive oil or butter
265 g broccoli florets, chopped into small
    pieces
2 teaspoons chopped fresh thyme
85 g mature Cheddar cheese, grated
125 ml full-fat milk
4 medium eggs
1 teaspoon salt
¼ teaspoon pepper
1 tablespoon chopped fresh chives,
    for serving (optional)

1. Preheat the oven to 190°C/gas mark 5. Spray 8 holes of a 12-hole muffin tin with cooking oil spray.

2. Heat the oil or melt the butter in a large non-stick frying pan over a medium heat. Add the broccoli and cook, stirring occasionally, for about 6 minutes until softened but not coloured. Add the thyme and cook for 1 minute more until fragrant and the broccoli is tender. Remove from heat. Leave to cool slightly, then distribute the broccoli evenly among the prepared muffin holes.

3. Whisk together the cheese, milk, eggs, salt and pepper in a medium bowl. Pour about 4 tablespoons of the egg mixture over the broccoli in each muffin cup. Bake for about 13 minutes until set and a knife inserted into the centre comes out clean.

4. Leave to cool for 3 minutes before removing from the muffin tins. To

From the Test Kitchen

Fill these bites with whatever you like. Change the cheese (Gouda, Emmental, double Gloucester). Or swap any of the following for the broccoli, or do a mix and match depending on what you're hungry for and what you have to hand.

- Sautéed baby spinach
- Sautéed mushrooms
- Cooked turkey sausage, crumbled or diced

remove, run a knife around the edges, and then gently lift each egg bite out of the muffin tin. Sprinkle with chives and serve immediately.

The egg bites can be stored in the refrigerator in an airtight container for up to 3 days. To reheat, wrap in aluminium foil and heat in a preheated 190°C/gas mark 5 oven for 8–10 minutes until warmed through. If using a microwave, loosely wrap in kitchen paper and cook on high for 1–2 minutes.

NUTRITION INFO: 1 portion (2 bites) provides:

Protein: ½ serving

Calcium: 1 serving

Vitamin C: 1 serving

Vitamin A: 1 serving

Tomato and Roasted Red Pepper Frittata

SERVES 2

A brunch-worthy dish that cooks up in minutes – especially if you use leftover or bottled roasted red peppers. Add a salad and some wholegrain bread, and call it dinner, too.

4 medium eggs
4 teaspoons milk
40 g Parmesan cheese, grated
1 clove garlic, very finely chopped
Salt and black pepper
2 small tomatoes, deseeded and chopped
1 tablespoon chopped fresh basil or
    1 teaspoon dried basil
1 tablespoon olive oil
85 g roasted red pepper, roughly chopped
    (about 1 large pepper; leftover or from
    a jar)
1 tablespoon chopped fresh flat-leaf
    parsley or 1 teaspoon dried parsley
    (optional)

1. Place the eggs, milk, cheese and garlic in a medium-sized bowl. Add a pinch each of salt and black pepper and whisk to mix. Add the tomatoes and basil and stir gently to combine.

2. Heat the olive oil in a medium-sized frying pan over a medium-low heat. Pour the egg mixture into the pan and cook for 5–8 minutes until nearly set, lifting the edge to let the uncooked egg run underneath.

From the Test Kitchen

Have some leftover steamed broccoli from last night's dinner? Toss it in the frying pan along with the eggs and buy yourself an extra serving of green leafies and vitamin C.

3. Sprinkle the roasted red pepper on top of the frittata and cook 1–2 minutes longer until completely set.

4. Slide the frittata onto a plate and scatter the parsley on top, if desired, before serving.

NUTRITION INFO: 1 portion provides:

Protein: 1 serving

Calcium: 1 serving

Vitamin C: 2½ servings

Vitamin A: 1½ servings

Fat: ½ serving

Omegas: some, if using omega-3 eggs

Breakfast Burritos

SERVES 1

The ultimate in portable breakfasts, a Breakfast Burrito brimming with avocado, tomato, black beans, eggs and salsa can find its way to your mouth almost as quickly as the fast-food variety (more quickly if there's a wait at the drive-thru) but contains much less fat and is much more nutritious.

Olive oil cooking spray
40 g drained tinned black beans,
    rinsed and drained
2 tablespoons ready-made tomato-based
    salsa
1 spring onion (white and light green
    parts), trimmed and thinly sliced
1 tablespoon chopped fresh coriander
2 medium eggs, lightly beaten
1 wholemeal tortilla or wrap
    (30 cm in diameter)
¼ medium-sized avocado (preferably
    Hass), chopped (optional)
½ plum tomato, seeded and chopped
45 g Cheddar or Monterey jack cheese,
    grated

1. Coat a medium-sized frying pan with olive oil cooking spray and heat over a medium heat. Add the black beans, salsa, spring onion and coriander and cook for about 2 minutes until heated through. Add the eggs and cook, stirring gently, for about 3 minutes until completely set. Remove from the heat.

2. Place the tortilla on a microwave-safe plate or sheet of kitchen paper and heat for 15 seconds in the microwave.

3. Place the tortilla on a work surface or on a plate. Spoon the egg and black bean mixture in the centre. Scatter the avocado, if using, tomato and cheese on top.

From the Test Kitchen

Beans aren't exactly what the doctor (or the guy who sits next to you at work) ordered? If tummy troubles have you avoiding wind makers, skip the beans and toss in 185 g of cooked edamame (soybeans); you'll be getting some additional protein in the bargain. For that matter, you can roll up just about any steamed or sautéed veggie (think last night's leftovers) in a Breakfast Burrito.

4. Fold the top and bottom of the tortilla into the centre. Starting at one side, roll up the tortilla to enclose the filling.

NUTRITION INFO: 1 portion provides:

Protein: 1 serving

Calcium: 1 serving

Vitamin C: 1 serving

Other fruits and vegetables: 1 serving

Wholegrains and legumes: 2½ servings

Iron: some

Omegas: some, if using omega-3 eggs

Baby's Big Bite

SERVES 1

Egg on a muffin without the McFat, but with plenty of grains and calcium. Pack one of these quick and convenient babies to go tomorrow morning.

**1 wholegrain muffin, split, or
  2 slices wholegrain bread**
1 tomato, sliced
1 slice Emmental or Cheddar cheese
1 medium egg
1 tablespoon milk
1½ teaspoons oil or butter

1. Toast the muffin.

2. Place the muffin halves split side up on a microwave-safe plate and arrange half of the tomato slices on each. Top each half with a slice of cheese. Microwave on high power for about 30 seconds until the cheese is slightly melted.

3. Place the egg and milk in a small bowl and whisk until well combined. Heat the olive oil in a small frying pan over a medium-high heat. Add the egg mixture and cook, stirring gently, for about 1 minute until completely set.

4. Spoon the scrambled egg on a muffin half and top with the other half.

From the Test Kitchen

Extra hungry this morning? Heat diced turkey breast or cooked crumbled turkey, chicken or vegetarian sausage, then add them to the egg while it cooks.

NUTRITION INFO: 1 portion provides:

Protein: 1 serving

Calcium: 1 serving

Vitamin C: ½ serving

Wholegrains and legumes: 2 servings

Fat: ½ serving

Omegas: some, if using omega-3 eggs

Stuffed Eggy Toast

SERVES 1

Want a sandwich that eats like breakfast – only neater? Slices of wholegrain bread stuffed with fresh peaches or banana and fruit preserve hit the spot when you're craving something sweet.

1 tablespoon peanut or almond butter
2 slices wholegrain bread
2 teaspoons all-fruit preserve or jam
    (any flavour)
½ fresh or frozen peach or banana,
    very thinly sliced
1 medium egg
4 tablespoons milk
½ teaspoon vanilla extract
½ teaspoon ground cinnamon
1½ teaspoons rapeseed oil or butter

1. Spread 1½ teaspoons of the almond butter on one side of each slice of bread. Spread the preserve over one coated slice of bread. Arrange the peach slices over the preserve, then top with the other slice of bread to make a sandwich.

2. Place the egg, milk, vanilla and cinnamon in a shallow bowl and whisk to mix.

3. Place the sandwich in the egg mixture and let it soak for 1 minute on each side.

4. Heat the oil in a small frying pan over a medium-high heat. Cook the sandwich for 2–3 minutes per side until well coloured.

5. Cut the sandwich in half and serve warm.

From the Test Kitchen

Not in the mood for sweet? Make a savoury Stuffed Eggy Toast instead: substitute cooked turkey sausage (protein) and Emmental cheese (calcium), or Emmental and thinly sliced tomato, for the almond butter and fruit.

NUTRITION INFO: 1 portion provides:

Protein: ½ serving

Vitamin A: ½ serving if made with peach

Other fruits and vegetables: ½ serving if made with banana

Wholegrains and legumes: 2 servings

Fat: 1½ servings

Any Day Breakfast Parfait

SERVES 1

Getting your Daily Dozen doesn't get any easier than this. Or any cooler. This parfait teams fresh fruit, yogurt and granola for a refreshing breakfast at home or on the go.

**1 ripe yellow peach or nectarine or
½ mango, roughly chopped
240 g fat-free vanilla Greek yogurt
60 g granola
75 g blueberries or sliced strawberries
Mint sprig (optional)**

Arrange the chopped peach, yogurt, granola and berries in alternating layers in a bowl or glass. Top with a mint sprig, if wished. Want to take the parfait with you? Layer the ingredients in a plastic container or cup, or a medium-sized preserving jar.

NUTRITION INFO: 1 portion provides:

Protein: ½ serving

Calcium: 1½ servings

Vitamin C: 1 serving if made with strawberries; 2 if made with strawberries and mango

Vitamin A: 1 serving

Other fruits and vegetables: 1 serving if made with blueberries

Wholegrains and legumes: 1 serving

From the Test Kitchen

Any fruit that suits your fancy – or fills your fridge – can be layered into a yogurt parfait. Try raspberries, blackberries, plums, cherries, pineapple or bananas, too. If winter leaves you with slim pickings in the produce department, opt for frozen fruit, but thaw and drain it first. And there's always room for some dried or crunchy freeze-dried fruit. Toasted nuts make a great topping, too.

Wholemeal Buttermilk Pancakes

MAKES ABOUT 12 PANCAKES

Pancakes made with only white flour just can't stack up to these. Plus, you won't have to give up fluffiness for nutrition – these pancakes have plenty of both.

150 g wholemeal flour
60 g plain white flour
3 tablespoons ground linseeds
    (flaxseeds, oat bran or wheatgerm)
1 teaspoon baking powder
1 teaspoon bicarbonate of soda
1 teaspoon ground cinnamon
Pinch of ground nutmeg
Pinch of salt
400 ml buttermilk
4 tablespoons milk
1 teaspoon sugar
2 medium eggs
1 teaspoon vanilla extract
2 tablespoons + 2 teaspoons rapseed oil

1. Place the wholemeal and white flours, linseeds, baking powder, bicarbonate of soda, cinnamon, nutmeg and salt in a medium-sized bowl and stir to combine.

2. Place the buttermilk, milk, honey, eggs, vanilla and 2 tablespoons of the oil in another bowl and whisk to mix. Pour the buttermilk mixture into the flour mixture and beat just until smooth. If possible, let the mixture rest for up to 30 minutes at room temperature before cooking the pancakes.

3. Heat the remaining 2 teaspoons oil in a 23-cm frying pan over a medium-high heat. Cook the pancakes two at a time, using 4 tablespoons of mixture per pancake, for about 3 minutes until it bubbles on top and the pancakes are firm on the bottom. Turn the pancakes over and continue cooking for about 3 minutes

until the second side is coloured. Repeat with the remaining mixture.

4. Serve the pancakes warm. They can be frozen for up to 2 weeks: cool completely, then wrap them in a single layer or individually in aluminium foil. To reheat, unwrap a pancake and microwave it on high power for 2 minutes, or heat it in a 180°C/gas mark 4 oven for 10 minutes.

NUTRITION INFO: 1 portion (about 4 pancakes) provides:

Protein: ½ serving

Calcium: ½ serving

Wholegrains and legumes: 2 servings

Iron: some

Fat: 1 serving

Pancake Add-Ins

Make basic wholemeal pancakes anything but basic by tossing in:

- Finely chopped apple or pear
- Chopped banana
- Blueberries – fresh, thawed frozen, dried or freeze-dried
- Dried cranberries or cherries
- Raisins
- Chopped dried apricots
- Chopped pineapple, peaches, cherries or mango
- Chopped pecans, almonds or walnuts

Ginger-Blueberry Wholemeal Pancakes

MAKES 10–12 PANCAKES

Feeling a little green this morning? Try some blues. These pancakes, infused with ginger and packed with blueberries and wholemeal, make a soothing and nutritious morning meal. What's better still is that these pancakes are surprisingly light – even with the wholemeal flour.

180 g wholemeal flour

1 teaspoon ground ginger

1 teaspoon ground cinnamon

Pinch of ground mixed spice

1 teaspoon bicarbonate of soda

250 ml milk

1 tablespoon butter, melted

2 small eggs

2 teaspoons granulated sugar

215 g fresh or unthawed frozen
    blueberries or 125 g freeze-dried

2 teaspoons rapeseed oil

1. Place the wholemeal flour, ginger, cinnamon, mixed spice and bicarbonate of soda in a large bowl and stir to combine. Set aside.

2. Place the milk, butter, eggs and sugar in a medium-sized bowl, and whisk to blend. Add the milk mixture to the flour mixture and whisk until blended. Add the blueberries and stir gently to combine.

3. Heat the rapeseed oil in a 23-cm frying pan over a medium-high heat. Cook the pancakes two at a time, using about 4 tablespoons mixture per pancake, for 2–3 minutes until a golden colour on the bottom. Turn the pancakes over and continue cooking for about 2 minutes until the second side is a golden colour. Repeat with remaining mixture.

4. Serve the pancakes warm with maple syrup or a Quick Fruit Syrup (see below). The pancakes can be frozen for up to 2 weeks: cool completely, then wrap them in a single layer or individually in aluminium foil. To reheat, unwrap a pancake and microwave it on high power for 2 minutes or heat it in a 180°C/gas mark 4 oven for 10 minutes.

NUTRITION INFO: 1 portion (about 4 pancakes) provides:

Other fruits and vegetables: ½ serving

Wholegrains and legumes: 2 servings

Quick Fruit Syrups

Feeling fruity? Warm some all-fruit preserve or jam in the microwave on medium-high power, then serve them syrup style over pancakes. If you like your syrup thinner, add some water after heating the preserve.

Power Breakfast Bars

MAKES ABOUT 20 BARS

These pack a lot more nutrition than the bars you buy. Pack them to go – with a side of yogurt or cheese, they make the perfect take-along breakfast, mini-meal or snack.

55 g packed soft brown sugar
80 g maple syrup or honey
65 g smooth peanut butter
2 medium eggs
4 tablespoons rapeseed oil
30 g butter, melted
1 teaspoon vanilla extract
225 g porridge oats
120 g wholemeal flour
½ teaspoon bicarbonate of soda
1 teaspoon ground cinnamon
2 tablespoons oat bran or ground
    linseeds (flaxseeds)
100 g walnuts or almonds, chopped
150 g raisins or mixed dried fruit such
    as chopped apricots, blueberries,
    cranberries and/or cherries, chopped

1. Preheat the oven to 190°C/gas mark 5.

2. Place the sugar, maple syrup, peanut butter, eggs, oil, butter and vanilla in a mixing bowl and beat until well mixed.

3. Place the oats, wholemeal flour, bicarbonate of soda, cinnamon, oat bran, walnuts and raisins in another mixing bowl and stir to mix. Add the oat mixture to the sugar and oil mixture and stir until thoroughly combined.

4. Line a baking tray with baking paper. Shape heaped tablespoons of the mixture into bars about 5 x 10 cm, arranging them about 2.5 cm apart. Bake the bars for about 15 minutes until the bases are brown and the tops are golden brown. For crisper bars, reduce the oven temperature to lowest setting and bake for 5–10 minutes longer.

5. Leave the bars to cool completely before sliding them off the baking sheet. Wrap individually in foil or cling film if you plan to transport them. The bars can be stored in an airtight container for 3 days at room temperature or frozen for up to 1 month.

NUTRITION INFO: 1 portion (2 bars) provides:

Protein: ½ serving

Vitamin C: ½ serving

Vitamin A: ½ serving if made with apricots

Other fruits and vegetables: ½ serving

Wholegrains and legumes: 1½ servings

Iron: some

Fat: 1 serving

Omegas: some

No-Bake Energy Bites

MAKES ABOUT 18 BALLS

These easy-to-make energy bites can pull triple duty as breakfast, snack or wholesome dessert. Store them in an airtight container in the fridge.

90 g rolled oats
130 g smooth peanut butter
30 g ground linseeds (flaxseeds)
85 g mini dark chocolate chips
85 g honey
50 g raisins or dried chopped cherries
1 teaspoon vanilla extract
½ teaspoon salt

1. Stir the oats, peanut butter, linseeds, chocolate chips, honey, raisins or cherries, vanilla and salt together in a medium-sized bowl until thoroughly mixed. Cover and chill in the refrigerator for about 30 minutes.

2. Lay out a sheet of greaseproof paper on a work surface. For each bite, scoop out a heaped tablespoon of the mixture, roll into a 2.5-cm ball and set it on the greaseproof paper. Store in the refrigerator in an airtight container, with the layers separated with greaseproof paper, for up to 1 week.

NUTRITION INFO: 1 portion (2–3 balls) provides:

Wholegrains and legumes: 1 serving

Iron: some

Omegas: some

Muffins

M ad about muffins but wondering whether there's a place for these sweet breakfast treats now that you're trying to eat healthier? Good news! While many ready-made supermarket or bakery muffins may be lightweights when it comes to nutrition (and heavyweights when it comes to calories), the sugar-free muffins in this chapter are tasty and nutritious. Start a queasy morning with a Ginger and Carrot Muffin. Spice up a snack with a Pumpkin Muffin or linger over brunch with a Triple Blueberry Muffin. Whatever flavour you're craving, there's a muffin here for you.

So many muffin cravings, but so little time? Bake a few batches at once, and freeze the extras for munching later on. And don't stop with breakfast. A wholesome muffin (especially when teamed with a piece of cheese) makes the perfect pick-me-up when your blood sugar starts to take a mid-morning or mid-afternoon dive. And, with a glass of milk, there's no better bedtime snack.

Triple Blueberry Muffins

MAKES 12 MUFFINS

Triple the blueberries – preserve, frozen and dried – means triple the taste in these yummy muffins. The addition of porridge oats lends a chewier texture and nuttier taste, plus nets extra fibre.

90 g wholemeal flour
40 g ground linseeds (flaxseeds)
2 teaspoons baking powder
1 teaspoon bicarbonate of soda
135 g porridge oats
325 g honey or maple syrup
160 g all-fruit blueberry preserve or jam
2 medium eggs, lightly beaten
3 tablespoons rapeseed oil
2 teaspoons vanilla extract
115 g frozen blueberries
65 g dried or freeze-dried blueberries

1. Preheat oven to 190°C/gas mark 5. Line a standard-sized 12-hole muffin tin with paper cases.

2. Place the flour, linseeds, baking powder and bicarbonate of soda in a large bowl and stir to mix. Add the oats and stir until well combined. Place the honey, preserve, eggs, oil and vanilla in a medium-sized bowl and stir to mix well. Add the blueberry mixture to the flour mixture and stir gently just until thoroughly blended; take care not to overmix. Gently fold in the frozen and dried blueberries.

3. Spoon the mixture into the prepared muffin tin, dividing it evenly among the muffin holes. Bake for 18–20 minutes until a skewer inserted into the centre of a muffin comes out clean.

4. Transfer the muffins to a wire rack and cool completely. The muffins can be stored in an airtight container for up to 3 days or individually wrapped in cling film and frozen for up to 3 months.

NUTRITION INFO: 1 portion (1 muffin) provides:

Vitamin C: ½ serving

Wholegrains and legumes: 1 serving

Iron: some

Going Fruity? Getting Nutty?

Add an additional 80 g of all-fruit preserve (any flavour) or jam to any muffin mixture, or better still, cut baked muffins in half and slather them with the preserves Are you tired of raisins? Explore other dried fruit options, and chop them as needed – from apricots to mangoes, apples to pears, cherries to blueberries. And don't forget to go nutty – add 60 g of whatever roughly chopped nuts you like (almonds, hazelnuts, pecans, walnuts, to name a few) to the muffin mix. Toast them first for even more flavour (see page 217 for toasting tips). Or toss in 35 g of desiccated coconut.

Gluten-Free Carrot and Almond Muffins

MAKES 8–10 MUFFINS

Ditch the gluten and the dairy without losing the nutrients or the flavour with these moist muffins. The coconut oil supplies a subtle tropical note, but if it's not a shelf staple in your kitchen, rapeseed oil works just as well.

240 g finely ground almond flour
    (available in health-food shops/online)
½ teaspoon salt
½ teaspoon bicarbonate of soda
1 teaspoon ground cinnamon
½ teaspoon ground nutmeg
3 medium eggs, at room temperature
¼ cup coconut oil, melted and cooled
¼ cup maple syrup
110 g peeled carrots, grated

1. Preheat oven to 180°C/gas mark 4. Line 8–10 holes of a standard-sized muffin tin with paper cases.

2. In a large bowl, whisk the almond flour, salt, bicarbonate of soda, cinnamon and nutmeg to combine. In a medium-sized bowl, whisk the eggs, oil and maple syrup. Add the egg mixture to the almond flour mixture and stir until mixed. Stir in the carrots.

3. Spoon 4 tablespoons of the mixture into each muffin case. Bake for about 20 minutes until a skewer inserted into the centre of a muffin comes out clean.

4. Transfer the muffins to a wire rack and cool before serving. Store in an airtight container in the fridge for up to 3 days or wrap individually in cling film and freeze for up to 3 months.

NUTRITION INFO: 1 portion (1 muffin) provides:

Protein: 1 serving

Vitamin A: ½ serving

Omegas: some

Flour Power

Any muffin mixture can benefit from the addition of omega-3-rich (and constipation-combating) ground linseeds (flaxseeds). Substitute 30 g of flaxseed for 30 g of flour. If it's fibre you're looking for, substitute 15 g of wheat bran for 30 g of flour (although linseed will give you the same results, more nutritiously). Want a nuttier flavour, protein boost and some healthy fatty acids? You can use 25 g of ground nuts to take the place of 30 g of flour. For extra nutrients substitute 30 g wheatgerm or 25 g oat bran for 30 g of flour. For more protein use soy flour in place of up to a third of the flour in your recipe. Want to lighten things up? Substitute 60 g of unbleached white flour for 30 g of wholemeal flour.

Savoury Spinach Cheddar Muffins

MAKES 12 MUFFINS

Looking for a savoury spin on a breakfast or snack muffin, or for the perfect sidekick for your lunchtime soup that also kicks up nutrition? Look no further.

240 g wholemeal flour
25 g oat bran
1 tablespoon baking powder
½ teaspoon salt
2 medium eggs
250 ml milk
115 g rapeseed oil
55 g fresh spinach (tough stems removed), roughly chopped
85 g Cheddar cheese, grated
1 tablespoon very finely chopped fresh chives

1. Preheat oven to 200°C/gas mark 6. Line a standard-sized 12-hole muffin tin with paper cases.

2. In a large bowl, mix together the flour, oat bran, baking powder and salt. In a medium-sized bowl, whisk together the eggs, milk and oil. Add the egg mixture to the flour mixture and stir just until blended. Gently stir in the spinach, Cheddar cheese and chives; take care not to over-mix.

3. Spoon the mixture into the prepared muffin tin, dividing it evenly among the muffin cases. Bake for 15–18 minutes until a skewer inserted in the middle comes out clean.

4. Transfer the muffins to a wire rack and cool before serving. Store in an airtight container for up to 5 days or wrap individually in cling film and store in the freezer for up to 3 months.

NUTRITION INFO: 1 portion (1 muffin) provides:

Protein: ½ serving

Vitamin A: ½ serving

Wholegrains and legumes: 1 serving

Iron: some

Fat: ½ serving

Muffins Now, Muffins Later

Are 12 muffins 11 muffins too many? Fortunately, the muffins you bake today can be enjoyed tomorrow and next week – and even for months to come. To store muffins at room temperature, place them in an airtight container or zip-topped bag; they'll keep for up to 3 days. Still haven't polished them off? Wrap each muffin individually in cling film or aluminium foil and freeze them for up to 3 months. To thaw, simply take a muffin out of the freezer and allow it to come to room temperature. Prefer a muffin that tastes fresh out of the oven? Wrap the thawed muffin loosely in foil and place it in a preheated 180°C/gas mark 4 oven for 7–10 minutes until it's warmed through.

Raisin Bran Muffins

MAKES 12–18 MUFFINS

Sure, all that bran will get things going – but these muffins are so delicious, you'll want to eat them on a regular basis even when you're regular.

140 g oat bran
120 g wholemeal flour
90 g porridge oats
2 teaspoons ground cinnamon
60 g toasted nuts such as walnuts,
　　pecans or almonds (see page 217),
　　chopped
2 teaspoons bicarbonate of soda
1 teaspoon baking powder
325 g honey or maple syrup
300 ml buttermilk
2 medium eggs, lightly beaten
3 tablespoons rapeseed oil
2 teaspoons vanilla extract
150 g raisins

1. Preheat the oven to 200°C/gas mark 6. Line a standard-sized 12-hole muffin tin with paper cases.

2. Place the oat bran, flour, oats, cinnamon, nuts, bicarbonate of soda and baking powder in a large bowl and stir to mix. Place the honey, buttermilk, eggs, oil and vanilla in a medium-sized bowl and mix well. Add the honey mixture to the bran mixture and stir gently just until thoroughly blended; take care not to over-mix. Gently fold in the raisins.

3. Spoon the mixture into the prepared muffin cases, dividing it evenly. (You may have extra mixture. If so, just bake a few more muffins.)

4. Bake for 15–18 minutes until a skewer inserted into the centre of a muffin comes out clean.

5. Transfer the muffins to a wire rack and cool completely before serving. The muffins can be stored in an airtight container for up to 3 days or individually wrapped and frozen for up to 3 months.

NUTRITION INFO: 1 portion (1 muffin) provides:

Protein: ½ serving

Vitamin C: 1 serving

Wholegrains and legumes: ½ serving

Iron: some

Omegas: some

Pumpkin Muffins

MAKES 12 MUFFINS

Do you wish every morning had a hint of a crisp winter's day? Here's the sweet taste of pumpkin in a wholesome everyday spice-filled muffin.

120 g wholemeal flour
25 g oat bran
40 g ground linseeds (flaxseeds)
2 teaspoons baking powder
1½ teaspoons bicarbonate of soda
2 teaspoons ground cinnamon
¼ teaspoon ground ginger
¼ teaspoon ground cloves
¼ teaspoon ground nutmeg
185 g tinned pumpkin purée or fresh butternut squash purée
2 medium eggs, lightly beaten
3 tablespoons rapeseed oil
325 g maple syrup
2 teaspoons vanilla extract
60 g walnuts, toasted and chopped (see page 217; optional)

1. Preheat the oven to 200°C/gas mark 6. Line a standard-sized 12-hole muffin tin with paper cases.

2. Place the flour, oat bran, linseeds, baking powder, bicarbonate of soda, cinnamon, ginger, cloves and nutmeg in a large bowl and stir to mix. Place the pumpkin, eggs, oil, maple syrup and vanilla in medium-sized bowl and mix well. Add the pumpkin mixture to the flour mixture and stir gently just until blended; take care not to over-mix. Gently fold in the walnuts, if using.

3. Spoon the mixture into the prepared muffin tin, dividing it evenly among the muffin cases. Bake for 15–18 minutes until a skewer inserted into the centre of a muffin comes out clean.

4. Transfer the muffins to a wire rack and cool completely. The muffins can be stored in an airtight container for up to 3 days or individually wrapped and frozen for up to 3 months.

NUTRITION INFO: 1 portion (1 muffin) provides:

Vitamin C: ½ serving

Vitamin A: ½ serving

Wholegrains and legumes: 1 serving

Iron: some

Omegas: some

Sandwiches

L unchtime boredom sending you out for fast food? Stop filling your lunch box with the same old sandwiches. There's a lot more you can put between two slices of bread than ham and cheese – in fact, sandwiches become even more interesting if you skip traditional bread altogether. So wrap your mouth around a tasty wrap (the perfect take-along lunch, since they're so neat to eat), stuff a pitta or tortilla, layer a bagel or fill a bun – and meet a surprising number of Daily Dozen requirements while you're at it. It's food to go that's good for you.

A Better BLT

MAKES 1 SANDWICH

H ere's a great way to get your BLT without the F (fat). A white bean spread stands in for mayo, adding a tasty fourth dimension. It's a BLT that's built for baby-building – and mum satisfaction.

2 slices wholegrain toast
2 tablespoons White Bean Spread (recipe follows)
30 g red leaf lettuce, sliced
¼ cup carrot, grated
4 slices vegetarian bacon or turkey bacon (about 115 g), cooked
½ medium-sized avocado (preferably Hass), sliced
1 plum tomato, sliced

Spread both slices of toast with the bean spread. Layer the lettuce, carrot, bacon, avocado and tomato on one slice, then top with the other slice.

NUTRITION INFO: 1 portion provides:

Protein: ½ serving

Vitamin C: 1 serving

Vitamin A: 1½ servings

Other fruits and vegetables: 1 serving

Wholegrains and legumes: 2 servings

White Bean Spread

MAKES ABOUT 4 PORTIONS

Hold the mayo, and use this creamy spread on your sandwiches instead. Makes a great dip for crudités and pitta strips, too.

2 tablespoons olive oil
**1 large clove garlic, peeled and crushed
(if raw garlic bothers you, see the box
on page 262; optional)**
**425 g drained and rinsed tinned cannellini
or flageolet beans**
**2 tablespoons roughly chopped fresh
coriander or flat-leaf parsley**
Juice of 1 large lemon
1 teaspoon tahini (optional)
Salt and black pepper

Place the olive oil, garlic, beans, coriander, lemon juice and tahini, if using, in a food processor and process until a smooth purée forms. Season with salt and pepper to taste. Serve at room temperature, or warm in the microwave or on the hob. The bean spread can be refrigerated, covered, for up to 5 days.

From the Test Kitchen

For a spicier spread, swap the white beans for chickpeas in the White Bean Spread, and add 1 teaspoon ground toasted cumin seeds and a pinch of hot paprika and/or cayenne pepper (add both if you you really want to turn up the heat). You can kick it up with more garlic, too.

Prefer a BLT that's tidier to eat? Layer the filling inside a wholegrain bun, pitta or wrap.

NUTRITION INFO: 1 portion
(4 tablespoons) provides:

Wholegrains and legumes: ½ serving

Iron: some

Fat: ½ serving

What a Spread: Not Honey Mustard

Craving a sweet spread on your sandwich? Try this Not Honey Mustard spread. It's sweet like honey mustard, but has a more complex flavour. Yummy on chicken, turkey or meat sandwiches – or anywhere else where you'd enjoy honey mustard. Mix together 4 tablespoons each Dijon mustard and all-fruit apricot preserve. Enjoy!

Chicken Burgers with Mango Relish

MAKES 4 BURGERS

These chicken burgers are cheeseburgers with a twist. Topping the burgers with mango relish as they grill adds an unexpectedly exotic taste. And traditional burgers can't beat this: each chicken burger contains a hefty serving of vitamin A, compliments of the mango.

4 frozen chicken burger patties,
85–115 g each
55 g Cheddar, Gouda or Monterey jack
cheese, grated
Mango Relish (recipe follows)
4 wholegrain buns

1. Prepare the chicken patties according to packet instructions.

2. Preheat the grill to high. Scatter the cheese evenly over the cooked burgers and grill for 1–3 minutes until coloured.

3. Spread a spoonful of the mango relish over each burger. Serve the burgers on wholegrain buns with extra mango relish, if desired.

NUTRITION INFO: 1 portion (1 burger without Mango Relish) provides:

Protein: 1 serving

Calcium: ½ serving

Wholegrains and legumes: 2 servings

Mango Relish

MAKES ABOUT 8 PORTIONS

Scoop up this sweet and spicy salsa with wholegrain tortilla chips, but don't stop there. It'll add a kick to grilled chicken, fish or pork, sass to sandwiches and wraps, and plenty of vitamins A and C to anything you top with it or spread it on. Too much of a kick? Turn the heat down by cutting the amount of jalapeño you add (or cutting it out altogether).

2 ripe medium-sized mangoes, peeled,
stoned and cut into 1-cm pieces
10 g fresh coriander, chopped
2 tablespoons chopped shallot or spring
onions
2 tablespoons fresh lime juice
1 tablespoon white wine vinegar
(or extra lime)
1½ tablespoons deseeded and chopped
jalapeño pepper (about 2 peppers), or
to taste
½ teaspoon coarse salt

Place the mangoes, coriander, shallot, lime juice, vinegar, jalapeño and salt in a small bowl and stir to mix. Or for a finer mixture, pulse everything in a food processor about 5 times until finely chopped. Leftovers will last 2 days refrigerated in an airtight container.

NUTRITION INFO: 1 portion (3 tablespoons) provides:

Vitamin C: 1 serving

Vitamin A: 1 serving

Fill 'Er Up

Tired of the same old sandwich? Add a few of these into your lunch-box rotation. Don't be afraid to mix and match proteins or leave out any ingredient you're not currently feeling or don't have to hand. And, of course, add pickled gherkins or chillies (or anything you're craving). No need to explain – you're pregnant.

- Sliced beef, wholegrain mustard, spinach, fresh basil leaves and tomato slices, on a wholegrain bun

- Sliced beef, Pesto with Sunflower Seeds (page 245), fresh basil leaves, roasted red pepper and roasted red onion, wrapped in a wholemeal tortilla

- Grilled chicken breast, Not Honey Mustard (page 211), Emmental cheese, romaine lettuce and thinly sliced mango, in a pitta

- Sliced chicken, Pesto with Sunflower Seeds (page 245) or wholegrain mustard, shaved Parmesan cheese, fresh basil leaves and roasted red pepper, in a wholegrain wrap

- Sliced turkey breast, mature Cheddar cheese, rocket and cranberry sauce or relish, on a wholegrain roll

- Sliced hard-boiled egg, shaved Parmesan cheese, baby spinach leaves and tomato slices, on a wholemeal muffin

- Egg salad, wholegrain mustard, shaved Parmesan cheese, romaine or rocket, and tomato slices, on a wholemeal bagel

- Cheddar cheese, Not Honey Mustard (page 211), thinly sliced apple or ripe pear, and rocket, on wholegrain bread

- Edam cheese, Creamy Kale Pesto (page 216), tomato slices, fresh basil leaves and rocket in a wholegrain pitta

- Sliced mozzarella cheese, Creamy Kale Pesto (page 216), tomato slices, roasted red pepper and a roasted portobello mushroom, on a wholegrain roll or in a wholegrain wrap

- Grilled aubergine, chopped romaine, hummus and grated Emmental cheese, in a wholemeal pitta

- Smashed ripe avocado on multigrain toast with a squeeze of lime juice (add a layer of sliced hard-boiled egg for a protein boost, hot sauce for a kick)

- Cheddar cheese and mango chutney, on wholegrain toast

- Any cheese and any jam on wholegrain toast

- Hummus, sliced avocado and tomato, and flaky salt, open-faced on wholemeal toast

- Faux tuna salad: 150 g of chickpeas mashed with a fork and mixed with a little mayo, mustard and chopped celery

- Peanut butter and banana on wholemeal bread; dark chocolate chips

- Peanut butter, sriracha and thinly sliced cucumbers on wholegrain toast with a squeeze of lime

- Cottage cheese, sliced avocado, chopped tomato, chopped cucumber, finely chopped chives (optional), on wholegrain bread

Chicken Caesar Wrap

MAKES 1 SANDWICH

Next time you have a craving for chicken Caesar salad, leave the fork behind. Romaine, cheese, roasted red pepper and chicken team up with a creamy dressing to create a salad that's high in flavour but low in fat. And it gets better – rolled up, the tasty salad becomes a super sandwich to go, so you can satisfy those cravings on the road. If you're leaning more plant-based, you can replace the chicken with an equal amount of thinly sliced firm or extra-firm tofu. Smoked tofu would be particularly tasty here.

55 g romaine lettuce, shredded

25 g Edam cheese, grated

2 tablespoons grated Parmesan cheese

1 tablespoon Simple Caesar Dressing
   (page 263), plus more to taste

85 g cooked chicken or turkey,
   sliced thinly

4 strips roasted red pepper (leftovers or
   from a jar)

1 wholegrain tortilla or wrap (30 cm in
   diameter), or wholegrain pitta

1. Place the romaine, Edam cheese, Parmesan cheese and Caesar dressing in a bowl and toss to mix. Add more dressing, if wished.

2. Layer the chicken and roasted pepper strips on the tortilla and top with the romaine salad. If you're using a pitta, trim 1 cm off an edge of the pitta and stuff it into the base of the pitta. Fill the pitta with the chicken and roasted pepper strips, then add the romaine salad.

3. Fold the sides of the tortilla or wrap over the filling.

NUTRITION INFO: 1 portion (without dressing) provides:

Protein: 1 serving

Calcium: 1 serving

Vitamin C: 2 servings

Vitamin A: 2 servings

Wholegrains and legumes: 2 servings

Omegas: some

All Washed Up

Many of these recipes call for salad leaves such as rocket, watercress and romaine lettuce, and herbs including fresh coriander, parsley, dill and basil. As with all fruits and vegetables, you'll need to thoroughly rinse the leaves and herbs and pat them dry before adding them to sandwiches.

If your produce is 'pre-washed', don't wash it again. According to food safety experts, you could actually increase your odds of introducing bacteria by washing it again at home. See page 181 for more tips on washing produce.

Curried Chicken Pitta

MAKES 1 SANDWICH

A healthier version of a favourite, this low-fat, creamy, Indian-inspired chicken salad sandwich really hits the spot when you're looking for something out of the ordinary. A cool combination of tomato, cucumber and salad leaves is tossed with diced chicken spiced up with curry and fresh coriander, stuffed into a pitta, and topped with a scattering of raisins and sunflower seeds.

15 g cooked chicken or turkey, diced
3 tablespoons natural Greek yogurt
    (use low-fat or full-fat milk yogurt for
    a creamier dressing)
2 teaspoons mayonnaise
35 g peeled seedless cucumber, diced
1 plum tomato, diced
1 teaspoon chopped fresh coriander, or
    more, to taste
½ teaspoon curry powder
Pinch of ground cumin
Hot red pepper sauce, such as Tabasco
    (optional)
Salt and black pepper
1 wholemeal pitta
30 g butterhead lettuce or romaine,
    shredded
1 tablespoon raisins (optional)
1 tablespoon toasted sunflower seeds
    (optional; see page 217)

1. Place the chicken, yogurt, mayonnaise, cucumber, tomato, coriander, curry powder and cumin in a mixing bowl and stir to mix. Season with hot sauce, if desired, and salt and pepper to taste.

2. Trim 1 cm off an edge of the pitta and stuff it into the base of the pitta. Fill the pitta with the lettuce, then add the chicken salad. Top with the raisins and sunflower seeds, if using.

NUTRITION INFO: 1 portion provides:

Protein: 1 serving

Vitamin C: 1 serving

Vitamin A: ½ serving

Other fruits and vegetables: ½ serving

Wholegrains and legumes: 2 servings

Fat: ½ serving

Chicken for Days

Prepare and freeze a big batch of chicken breasts so you can put together sandwiches in a flash.

Place chicken in a single layer in a baking dish. Salt and pepper generously. Bake in a 190°C/gas mark 5 oven for 25–30 minutes until the chicken's internal temperature reads 74°C. If you're eating it immediately, cover the chicken with foil and leave to rest for 15 minutes before slicing. If you want to freeze the chicken, leave the breasts to cool completely before wrapping tightly in foil and placing them in a large freezer bag. Leftover chicken can be stored in an airtight container in the fridge for up to 3 days or frozen for up to 2 months.

Salmon Parcel

MAKES 1 SANDWICH

Looking for a home for leftover cooked or tinned salmon? How about this tasty Salmon Parcel? It combines salad leaves, tomato, avocado and pesto with salmon for a lunch or dinner that packs in not only protein but also those baby-friendly omega-3 fatty acids.

1 wholemeal pitta or 2 slices
   wholegrain bread
75 g flaked cooked salmon
   (fresh or tinned)
2 tablespoons Pesto with Sunflower
   Seeds (page 245) or Creamy Kale
   Pesto (recipe follows)
1 small plum tomato, thinly sliced
¼ medium-sized avocado
   (preferably Hass), thinly sliced
10 g rocket or other tender salad leaves

Trim 1 cm off an edge of the pitta and stuff it into the base of the pitta. Fill the pitta with the salmon, then spoon the pesto over it. Top with the tomato, avocado and rocket.

NUTRITION INFO: 1 portion
(without pesto) provides:

Protein: 1 serving

Calcium: 1 serving if made with tinned salmon with bones

Vitamin C: 1 serving

Vitamin A: ½ serving

Other fruits and vegetables: ½ serving

Wholegrains and legumes: 2 servings

Omegas: some

Creamy Kale Pesto

MAKES ABOUT 4 PORTIONS

The kale in this peppy pesto kicks up flavour and nutrition, while the yogurt slims down the fat content of this Mediterranean classic. It's creamy enough to use as a dip for veggies or a spread for sandwiches, but don't forget to use it the traditional way – tossed with pasta and cheese, and maybe some chicken or prawns. Any kale will work, but if kale doesn't work for you at all (or you can't find it), you can switch it for extra spinach. Hungry for even more flavour? Toast the walnuts before adding them (see the box on the opposite page).

135 g rinsed, patted-dry kale leaves with
   ribs removed, torn
60 g baby spinach
45 g grated Parmesan cheese
30 g walnuts
2 cloves garlic, very finely chopped
   (If raw garlic bothers you, see the
   box on page 262; optional)
2 tablespoons natural Greek yogurt,
   plus more as needed
1 tablespoon fresh lemon juice,
   plus more as needed
2 tablespoons olive oil, plus more
   as needed
Salt and coarsely ground black pepper

Place the kale, spinach, Parmesan, walnuts and garlic in a food processor and process until finely minced. Add the yogurt, lemon juice and olive oil and process until well blended. Too thick?

A Toast to Toasted Nuts

Tempted to skip the toasting when a recipe calls for toasted nuts or seeds? You'll be skipping more than you think. Toasting brings out the true nutty flavour, adding a rich dimension to any salad, sandwich, pasta, poultry – you name it. There are several ways to toast 60 g of nuts or 15–30 g seeds.

On the hob: Scatter the nuts or seeds in an ungreased heavy frying pan (don't use a non-stick one). Cook over medium heat, stirring frequently, for 5–7 minutes until the nuts begin to colour.

In the oven: Spread the nuts or seeds in an ungreased shallow tin. Bake uncovered in a 180°C/gas mark 4 oven, stirring frequently, for about 10 minutes until the nuts are lightly coloured.

In the microwave: Spread the nuts or seeds evenly in a flat microwave-safe dish. Cook on high power for 2–3 minutes, stirring halfway through, until they are lightly coloured.

Toasted nuts will continue to darken after you remove them from the heat. A good test for doneness, along with colour, is when you can smell a toasted (not burnt – that's overdone) aroma.

When toasting small seeds in a frying pan, use a splatter screen, if possible. The seeds tend to pop around.

For ground nuts or seeds, you can grind toasted nuts or seeds in a food processor or mini grinder. Just take care not to over-process them, or you'll end up with nut or seed butter.

Add a little more yogurt, olive oil and/or lemon juice. Season with salt and pepper to taste. The pesto can be refrigerated, covered tightly, for up to 5 days.

NUTRITION INFO: 1 portion (4 tablespoons) provides:

Vitamin C: 1 serving

Vitamin A: 1 serving

Iron: some

Fat: ½ serving

Omegas: some

From the Test Kitchen

For a more traditional pesto, substitute 30 g of basil leaves for 65 g of the kale. For a zippier pesto, substitute arugula for the spinach. For a creamier sandwich spread, add a tablespoon or two of mayonnaise to the pesto along with the yogurt.

Black Bean Quesadilla

MAKES 1 QUESADILLA

Quesadillas – Mexican-style cheese toasties – are quick to make and easy to customise. Packed with authentic flavour and an impressive array of nutrients, this Black Bean Quesadilla features cheese, tangy black bean salsa, avocado and tomato. Off to work? Take it cold, then heat it in the office microwave.

1 wholegrain tortilla or wrap
  (30 cm in diameter)
55 g Monterey jack or Cheddar cheese,
  grated
¼ quantity Black Beans in Lime and
  Cumin Vinaigrette (recipe follows)
¼ medium-sized avocado
  (preferably Hass), sliced
½ medium-sized tomato, chopped
½ medium-sized red pepper, chopped
2 tablespoons chopped fresh coriander,
  or to taste (optional)
Lime wedge for serving

1. Line a microwave-safe plate with a sheet of kitchen paper and place the tortilla on top. Scatter half of the cheese over half of the tortilla. Top the cheese with the Black Beans in Lime and Cumin Vinaigrette (page 219), avocado, tomato and bell pepper. Scatter the remaining cheese on top.

2. Fold the bare half of the tortilla over the filling, covering it. Microwave on high power for 1–2 minutes until the cheese melts.

3. Remove and discard the kitchen paper, then cut the quesadilla into wedges. Sprinkle the coriander over it and add a squeeze of lime, if wished, before serving.

From the Test Kitchen

There's more than one way to fill a tortilla – dozens, in fact. Here's one more: Spread 3–4 tablespoons fat-free refried beans over a tortilla. Top with 3 tablespoons of your favourite salsa. Scatter 30 g of your choice of grated cheese over the salsa and microwave the tortilla on high power for 1–2 minutes until the cheese melts. Roll the tortilla and enjoy it immediately, or wrap it to go. Have leftover chicken, pork, steak, fish or prawns? Layer it on the tortilla, too. And that's a wrap!

NUTRITION INFO: 1 portion (without beans) provides:

Protein: 1 serving

Calcium: 2 servings

Vitamin C: 2½ servings

Vitamin A: 1 serving

Other fruits and vegetables: ½ serving

Wholegrains and legumes: 2 servings

Black Beans in Lime and Cumin Vinaigrette

SERVES 4

These marinated black beans show off bold American-style Mexican flavours. Try using them in your next burrito, or on the side of grilled meat, chicken or seafood.

425 g tinned black beans, drained and rinsed
1 medium-sized red pepper, finely chopped
1 medium-sized tomato, finely chopped
4 spring onions (white and light green parts), trimmed and sliced
2 tablespoons chopped fresh coriander
1 tablespoon chopped fresh flat-leaf parsley
2 tablespoons fresh lime juice
1 tablespoon olive oil
½ teaspoon ground cumin, plus more to taste
Salt and black pepper

Place the black beans, red pepper, tomato and green onions in a salad bowl and stir to mix. Add the coriander, parsley, lime juice, olive oil and cumin and toss to mix. Taste for seasoning, adding salt and pepper and more cumin if necessary. The beans can be refrigerated, covered, for up to 2 days.

From the Test Kitchen

B eans are a great source of protein – but they can also be a great source of wind. Keep the protein and skip the wind by substituting cooked edamame.

NUTRITION INFO: 1 portion provides:

Protein: ½ serving

Calcium: ½ serving

Vitamin C: 1½ servings

Vitamin A: ½ serving plus

Wholegrains and legumes: 1 serving

Iron: some

Fruity Turkey Salad

SERVES 2

A chewy (and vitamin-packed) surprise – dried apricots – makes this salad a treat for the taste buds. Nuts add crunch and important omegas. Serve the turkey salad with red leaf lettuce in a pitta or on bread. And chicken can sub for the turkey.

200 g cooked turkey or chicken breast, chopped

1 medium-sized stick celery, thinly sliced

6 dried apricot halves, roughly chopped

2 tablespoons roughly chopped toasted walnuts (see page 217)

2 tablespoons chopped red onion or spring onion (white and light green parts)

3 tablespoons natural Greek yogurt (full-fat milk yogurt makes a creamier dressing)

1 tablespoon mayonnaise

1 tablespoon wholegrain mustard

1 tablespoon all-fruit apricot preserve or jam (finely chop any pieces of fruit)

1 tablespoon fresh lemon juice, plus more to taste

1 tablespoon chopped fresh flat-leaf parsley

Salt and black pepper

1. Place the turkey, celery, apricots, nuts and onion in a bowl and stir to mix.

2. Place the yogurt, mayonnaise, mustard, apricot preserve, lemon juice and parsley in a small bowl and stir to mix. Taste for seasoning, adding more lemon juice as necessary, and salt and pepper to taste.

3. Add the yogurt mixture to the turkey mixture, and stir to coat well.

NUTRITION INFO: 1 portion provides:

Protein: 1 serving

Vitamin A: ½ serving

Other fruits and vegetables: 1 serving

Fat: ½ serving

Iron: some

Omegas: some

Greek Salad Sandwich

SERVES 1

Can't decide between a salad and a sandwich? Here's a Greek salad that eats like a sandwich, neatly tucked into a pitta. It's flexible, too. Keep it veggie or add the protein of your choice.

1 plum tomato, ripe but firm, deseeded and diced

½ small cucumber, deseeded and diced

1 (4-mm-thick) slice red onion, cut in half, rings separated, rinsed and drained

2 tablespoons crumbled pasteurised feta cheese

4 stoned kalamata olives, chopped

1–2 pickled chilli peppers, drained and
   diced
1 teaspoon red wine vinegar
2 teaspoons extra-virgin olive oil
Salt and black pepper
1 small or ½ large wholemeal pitta, lightly
   toasted
1½ teaspoons mayonnaise
2 large leaves of romaine lettuce

1. In a medium bowl, combine half the tomato, the cucumber, onion, feta, olives and pickled chilli peppers. Add more tomato if wished. Toss with the vinegar and olive oil. Scatter with salt and pepper to taste.

2. Cut the pitta in half and gently open. Spread mayonnaise on the inside base of each half, tuck in a lettuce leaf and scoop the salad mixture evenly into each pitta half. Serve immediately.

NUTRITION INFO: 1 portion (1 pitta) provides:

Calcium: ½ serving

Vitamin C: 2 servings

Other fruits and vegetables: 1 serving

Wholegrains and legumes: 2 servings

Fat: 2 servings

Spicy Egg Salad

SERVES 2

This kicked-up classic is perfect on its own or served on toast with lettuce leaves. Other add-ins could be fresh herbs, chopped dill pickle or gherkin, or walnut pieces.

From the
Test Kitchen

- Use omega-3 eggs for even more baby brain-boosting power. For an Asian twist, swap the Tabasco sauce with 1 teaspoon of sriracha and add a squeeze of lemon.

- Fortify your sandwich and score a protein serving by adding diced cooked chicken or chopped cooked prawns.

4 hard-boiled eggs, peeled and
   roughly chopped
2 tablespoons mayonnaise
1 tablespoon finely chopped celery
2 teaspoons Dijon mustard
2 teaspoons hot red pepper sauce,
   such as Tabasco
Salt and black pepper

Place the eggs, mayonnaise, celery, mustard and hot sauce in a medium-sized bowl. Stir gently to combine. Season to taste with salt and pepper.

NUTRITION INFO: 1 portion provides:

Protein: ½ serving

Fat: 1½ servings

Omegas: some

Soups

......

'S oup's on' can mean lots of things. For a cool, elegant start to a summer brunch, think Tomato Soup with Avocado. For a hearty, soul-warming meal in a bowl on a winter's evening, there's Broccoli and Cheese Soup or Turkey Chilli. And for a nourishing pick-me-up in the middle of a long afternoon, pick Vegetable and Edamame Soup or Red Lentil and Tomato Soup. But there's one thing that all these soups and chillies serve up: plenty of delicious nutrients in a soothing form, a definite plus if you're finding sipping easier than chewing on queasy days.

Butternut Squash and Pear Soup

SERVES 4

Creamy and fragrant, this bisque only looks like it took a lot of effort. It's easier and faster to cook than you'd think, and you'll rack up powerful nutritional rewards. The sweet and subtly spiced combination of squash and pears will reward your taste buds, too.

675 g pre-cut diced butternut squash
700 ml low-salt vegetable stock or
    chicken stock
Salt
1 tablespoon butter or rapeseed oil
1 small onion, very thinly sliced
2 red pears, peeled, cored and roughly
    chopped
2 teaspoons curry powder

½ teaspoon ground ginger (optional)
80 g natural full-fat Greek yogurt
White pepper
55 g Cheddar cheese, grated,
    for serving

1. Place the squash, 600 ml of the stock and a pinch of salt in a large saucepan over a medium-high heat and bring to the boil. Reduce the heat and allow it to simmer for about 35 minutes until the squash softens. Set the squash aside with its cooking liquid.

2. While the squash is cooking, melt the butter or heat the oil in a large frying pan over a medium heat. Add the

onion and cook, stirring frequently, for about 5 minutes until softened. Add the pears and cook, stirring frequently, for about 5 minutes until softened. Add the curry powder, turmeric and ginger, if using, and the remaining 100 ml stock and bring it to a simmer. Cover the frying pan and allow the mixture to cook for about 10 minutes until the flavours blend.

3. Add the onion and pear mixture to the cooked squash. Allow the mixture to cool slightly, then working in batches if necessary, transfer it to a blender or food processor and purée until smooth.

4. Return the soup to the saucepan, add the yogurt and season with salt and pepper to taste. Place the pan over a low heat and allow the soup to heat through, stirring frequently, for 2–3 minutes. Do not allow it to boil. Pour the soup into serving bowls and top each with 2 tablespoons Cheddar cheese.

From the Test Kitchen

Only serving two (and a half) for dinner tonight? Make the Butternut Squash and Pear Soup through Step 3, then divide it in half. Continue with Step 4, using 3 tablespoons yogurt and 4 tablespoons Cheddar cheese. The rest of the soup can be refrigerated, covered, for up to 2 days. Reheat it before continuing with Step 4. Want to double up on calcium? Double the cheese you sprinkle.

NUTRITION INFO: 1 portion (1 bowl) provides:

Calcium: ½ serving

Vitamin A: 2 servings

Other fruits and vegetables: 1 serving

The Cream of the Crop

Love cream-based soups but don't love all the calories that come with them? Get creamy the low-fat way.

Say potato: Adding a diced Maris Piper potato to a soup before cooking it will result in a very creamy texture for a puréed soup that's creamless.

Milk it. Light evaporated milk made with semi-skimmed milk is more concentrated than regular milk and will make soup creamier. Buttermilk also adds more creaminess than regular milk, along with a tangier taste. Add evaporated milk or buttermilk just before you are ready to serve; gently bring the soup back to a simmer over very low heat, whisking as it warms.

Go yogurt. Adding yogurt will make soup creamier and thicker. For a richer flavour, use full-fat yogurt, which while higher in fat still has far less than cream. All with a calcium bonus. Whisk yogurt into the hot soup, then serve it immediately.

Try tofu. Adding 115 g well-drained, puréed soft tofu to a warm puréed soup will lend creaminess without the cream, and with no noticeable taste.

Ginger and Carrot Soup
SERVES 4

Ginger and carrot soup makes a soothing way to take your vitamins, especially when morning sickness outlasts the morning.

2 teaspoons olive oil or butter
1 medium-sized sweet onion, chopped
1 clove garlic, very finely chopped
    (optional)
450 g baby carrots
5-cm piece fresh ginger, peeled and
    thinly sliced
950 ml low-salt chicken stock or
    vegetable stock
Fresh lemon juice
Salt and black pepper
Natural low-fat Greek yogurt, for serving

1. Heat the olive oil in a large saucepan over a medium heat. Add the onion and garlic, if using, and cook for about 5 minutes until softened. Add the carrots and ginger and cook, stirring frequently, for about 2 minutes until the ginger is fragrant.

2. Add the stock, increase the heat to medium-high and bring the soup to the boil. Cover the saucepan, reduce the heat and allow the soup to simmer for about 15 minutes until the carrots are very soft.

3. Allow the soup to cool slightly, then working in batches if necessary, transfer it to a blender or food processor and purée it until velvety smooth.

4. Return the soup to the saucepan and season it with lemon juice, salt and

From the Test Kitchen

Don't have the time – or the stomach – to fry the onions and carrots for Ginger and Carrot Soup? Place the carrots, onion (you don't even have to chop it, quartering will do, and you can leave out the garlic) and ginger in a pot with the stock. Bring it to the boil and allow to simmer until the carrots are soft, then purée it. Add a little lemon juice and some salt and pepper and you've got a lighter soup without that lingering onion odour in your kitchen.

pepper to taste. Bring the soup to a simmer over a medium-low heat and cook until heated through. Pour the soup into serving bowls and top each with a large spoonful of yogurt. The soup can be refrigerated, covered, for 2 days.

NUTRITION INFO: 1 portion (1 bowl) provides:

Vitamin C: ½ serving

Vitamin A: 3 servings

Other fruits and vegetables: ½ serving

Sweet Potato Vichyssoise

SERVES 4

With more flavour and nutrition than traditional vichyssoise, making the soup with sweet potatoes is an elegant way to serve up your yellow vegetables.

1 tablespoon butter or olive oil
2 large leeks (white and light green parts), trimmed, rinsed well and thinly sliced
2 medium-sized sweet potatoes, peeled and chopped
700 ml low-salt chicken stock or vegetable stock
4 tablespoons chopped fresh flat-leaf parsley
Salt and black pepper

1. Melt the butter or heat the olive oil in a saucepan over a medium-high heat. Add the leeks and cook for about 3 minutes until they soften. Add the sweet potatoes and cook for about 5 minutes until they begin to soften. Add the stock and parsley and bring the soup to the boil. Reduce the heat and allow it to simmer for about 10 minutes until the sweet potatoes are completely soft.

Make Soup a Meal

Topped with grated cheese and served with a salad and some wholegrain bread, most soups make an easy but sustaining meal at the end of a long day. Or pack a flask of soup, with cheese already melted on top, to take to work with you.

From the Test Kitchen

If you'd like this soup a little more sippable, add some milk or buttermilk after it cools. You'll get a creamier taste and a calcium bonus.

2. Allow the soup to cool slightly, then working in batches if necessary, transfer it to a blender or food processor and purée it until smooth. Season the soup with salt and pepper to taste. The soup can be served either hot or cold. Reheat it over a low heat after puréeing, if wished. The soup can be refrigerated, covered, for up to 4 days.

NUTRITION INFO: 1 portion (1 bowl) provides:

Vitamin C: ½ serving

Vitamin A: 1 serving

Other fruits and vegetables: ½ serving

Spiced-Up Gazpacho

SERVES 6

Like a salad you can sip, this soup is especially easy going down. Easy prepping, too. No cooking means no cooking smell or mess, plus once you make it, you can enjoy it for several days as a starter or a snack. Adding olive oil will make a richer gazpacho, but the soup is refreshing without it.

6 large plum tomatoes or 3 medium-sized
    tomatoes, roughly chopped
1 medium-sized seedless cucumber,
    peeled and roughly chopped
1½ large red peppers, chopped
1 small red onion, chopped
1 clove garlic, very finely chopped
    (if raw garlic bothers you, see the
    box on page 262; optional)
3 tablespoons chopped fresh flat-leaf
    parsley
2 tablespoons chopped fresh basil
950 ml tomato juice or vegetable juice
    such as V8
3 tablespoons red wine vinegar
3 tablespoons olive oil (optional)
1 tablespoon fresh lemon juice,
    plus more to taste
Salt and black pepper
Tabasco sauce

1. Place the tomatoes, cucumber, red peppers, onion, garlic, if using, parsley, basil, tomato juice, vinegar, olive oil, if using, and lemon juice in a food processor and pulse until the vegetables are finely chopped but not puréed.

2. Transfer the gazpacho to a large bowl and season it with salt, black pepper and Tabasco sauce to taste. Add more lemon juice, if wished. Refrigerate the soup, covered, until chilled through, or for at least 2 hours and up to 3 days. Serve in soup bowls or in glasses. The

From the Test Kitchen

There are any number of possible variations on this gazpacho. Here are just a few:

- For a chunkier gazpacho, don't run the vegetables through the food processor. Or process only half the veggies.

- For a little taste of Mexico, swap 2 tablespoons chopped fresh coriander for the basil and fresh lime juice for the lemon juice; garnish the soup with chopped avocado.

- Chop two hard-boiled eggs and add them just before serving.

- For a more substantial soup, cut chilled cooked prawns or scallops in half lengthways and float them on top. Feeling really flush? Add chunks of chilled cooked crab or lobster.

- For a more sippable soup, use a whole 1-litre bottle of juice.

soup can be refrigerated, covered, for up to 4 days.

NUTRITION INFO: 1 portion (1 bowl) provides:

Vitamin C: 3 servings; 3½ if made with vegetable juice

Vitamin A: 2½ servings; 3 if made with vegetable juice

Other fruits and vegetables: 1 serving

Fat: ½ serving if made using olive oil

Tomato Soup with Avocado

SERVES 4

This versatile and vitamin-packed soup is yummy hot and refreshing chilled.

2 teaspoons olive oil
3 spring onions (white and light green
    parts), trimmed and thinly sliced
½ teaspoon roughly chopped garlic
    (from 1 clove)
365 g tinned chopped tomatoes,
    with their juices
950 ml tomato juice or vegetable juice
    such as V8
4 tablespoons thinly sliced fresh basil
    leaves
Salt and black pepper
Diced avocado, for serving
½ red pepper, finely chopped, for serving
4 lime wedges, for serving

1. Heat the olive oil in a saucepan over a medium heat. Add the spring onions and garlic and cook for about 2 minutes until softened.

2. Add the tomatoes, tomato juice and basil, increase the heat to medium-high and bring the soup to the boil. Reduce the heat and allow it to simmer until for about 15 minutes the flavours are well blended. Season with salt and pepper to taste.

From the Test Kitchen

Swap chopped fresh coriander for the basil, add some hot sauce and your soup becomes a *sopa*.

3. Pour the soup into serving bowls, scatter avocado and red pepper on top, and serve the lime wedges alongside. The soup can also be served chilled. It can be refrigerated, covered, for up to 2 days.

NUTRITION INFO:

Vitamin C: 2½ servings if made with tomato juice; 3 if made with vegetable juice

Vitamin A: 1½ servings if made with vegetable juice

Red Lentil and Tomato Soup

SERVES 2

Besides being prettier to look at than green or brown lentils, red lentils have a creamier texture and a milder taste. Teamed with chunky tomatoes, carrot and celery, they make a rich-tasting, nutritious and sustaining soup that's gentle on the stomach.

1 tablespoon olive oil
1 medium-sized onion, chopped
½ teaspoon ground cumin
½ teaspoon ground turmeric
½ teaspoon ground mixed spice
½ tablespoon fresh ginger, peeled and very finely chopped
600 ml low-salt vegetable stock or chicken stock
100 g red lentils
1 large stick celery, chopped
1 medium-sized carrot, peeled and chopped
4 plum tomatoes, roughly chopped (set aside 1 chopped tomato)
Salt and black pepper

1. Heat the olive oil in a large saucepan over a medium heat. Add the onion and cook for about 5 minutes until softened.

2. Add the cumin, turmeric, mixed spice and ginger and cook, stirring frequently, for about 1 minute until fragrant.

3. Add the stock, lentils, celery, carrot and 3 of the chopped tomatoes, increase the heat to medium-high and bring the soup to the boil. Reduce the heat and allow it to simmer for about 30 minutes until the lentils are tender.

From the Test Kitchen

Substitute any lentil for the red (they come in green, black and basic brown) – though simmer time may need to be adjusted. Don't have all those spices on your shelf or fresh ginger to hand? Just substitute 1 teaspoon of any of these: cumin, paprika, curry powder or chilli powder.

4. Add the remaining tomato and season with salt and pepper to taste. Allow the soup to simmer for about 3 minutes until heated through. The soup can be refrigerated, covered, for up to 2 days.

NOTE: If you are serving only half of the soup now, add half of 1 chopped plum tomato at this stage. Add the second half after the rest of the soup has been reheated.

NUTRITION INFO: 1 portion (1 bowl) provides:

Protein: ½ serving

Vitamin C: 1 serving

Vitamin A: 2 servings

Other fruits and vegetables: ½ serving

Wholegrains and legumes: 1½ servings

Iron: some

Fat: ½ serving

Roasted Vegetable Soup

SERVES 4

Thick and rich-tasting, but without a drop of cream, this soup is super satisfying. Add a handful of grated cheese and some crusty wholegrain bread and your soup becomes supper. Just plan ahead for roasting time.

Cooking oil spray
2 medium-sized carrots, cut into 2.5-cm
    chunks
2 medium-sized parsnips, cut into 2.5-cm
    chunks
90 g peeled broccoli stems, cut into
    2.5-cm chunks
1 small red onion, quartered, each quarter
    cut in half
1 tablespoon olive oil
Salt and black pepper
4 teaspoons fresh thyme leaves
700–950 ml low-salt chicken stock
Toasted pumpkin seeds (see page 217),
    for serving
Chopped fresh flat-leaf parsley,
    for serving

1. Preheat the oven to 200°C/gas mark 6. Spray a large baking tray with cooking oil spray, or just line an unsprayed tray with baking paper.

2. Place the carrots, parsnips, broccoli and onion in a large bowl, add the olive oil and toss to coat evenly. Spoon the vegetable mixture in an even layer on to the prepared baking tray. Season with some salt and pepper and scatter 3 teaspoons of the thyme leaves on top.

3. Roast the vegetables, stirring occasionally, for about 45 minutes until tender.

4. Transfer the roasted vegetables to a large saucepan and add 700 ml of the stock and the remaining 1 teaspoon thyme leaves. Bring the soup to the boil over a high heat, then reduce the heat and allow it to simmer for about 15 minutes until the vegetables are very tender.

5. Allow the soup to cool slightly, then working in batches if necessary, transfer it to a blender or food processor and purée it until slightly chunky or smooth, as you prefer. If the soup is too thick, add more stock to thin it. Taste for seasoning, adding more salt and/or pepper as necessary.

6. If the soup has cooled down too much, return it to the saucepan and gently reheat it over a low heat. Scatter pumpkin seeds and parsley on top just before serving. The soup can be refrigerated, covered, for up to 2 days.

NUTRITION INFO: 1 portion (1 bowl) provides:

Vitamin A: 1½ servings

Other fruits and vegetables: 1 serving

Iron: some

Vegetable and Edamame Soup

SERVES 4

This hearty but quick-cooking vegetable soup combines the best in beans – in this case white beans and protein-packed edamame (soya beans). The soup is half puréed, half chunky, so you get an interesting mix of textures, too. Edam or Cheddar cheese – your choice – adds even more flavour and a serving of calcium, too.

1 tablespoon olive oil
1 small onion, chopped
1 clove garlic, very finely chopped
   (optional)
4 plum tomatoes, roughly chopped
2 medium-sized carrots, roughly chopped
700–950 ml low-salt vegetable stock or
   chicken stock
2 teaspoons fresh thyme leaves
4 tablespoons chopped fresh flat-leaf
   parsley
175 g shelled cooked edamame
425 g tinned flageolet beans, drained and
   rinsed
Salt and black pepper
115 g Edam cheese or Cheddar cheese,
   grated, for serving

1. Heat the olive oil in a large saucepan over a medium heat. Add the onion and garlic, if using, and cook for about 5 minutes until softened. Add the tomatoes and carrots and cook, stirring often, for about 10 minutes until the carrots are softened. Set aside about 250 ml of the cooked vegetables.

2. Add 700 ml of the stock, the thyme and the parsley to the saucepan. Increase the heat to medium-high and bring the soup to the boil, then cover the saucepan and reduce the heat to low. Allow the soup to simmer for about 15 minutes until the vegetables are very tender.

3. Allow the soup to cool slightly, then transfer it to a blender or food processor, working in batches if necessary, and purée the soup.

4. Return the soup to the saucepan and add the reserved cooked vegetables, the edamame and beans. If the soup is too thick, add more stock to thin it. Bring the soup to a simmer over a medium heat and cook for about 5 minutes until the beans are heated through. Season the soup with salt and pepper to taste. Scatter the cheese over the soup before serving. The soup can be refrigerated, covered, for up to 2 days.

NUTRITION INFO: 1 portion (1 bowl) provides:

Protein: ½ serving

Calcium: 1 serving

Vitamin C: 1 serving

Vitamin A: 1 serving

Wholegrains and legumes: 1 serving

Iron: some

Broccoli and Cheese Soup

SERVES 2

Broccoli, cheese and potatoes are friends from way back. This velvety-smooth and vitamin-rich soup brings them together for a delicious reunion. You'll never miss the cream – or the calories it would add. Save time by using a package of pre-cut broccoli florets.

1 tablespoon butter or olive oil
½ medium-sized brown onion, chopped
1 clove garlic, very finely chopped
   (optional)
175 g broccoli florets
1 medium-sized Maris Piper potato, diced
600 ml low-salt chicken stock or
   vegetable stock
55 g Cheddar cheese, grated
4 tablespoons buttermilk, or more to taste
Salt and black pepper

1. Melt the butter or heat the oil in a large saucepan over a medium heat. Add the onion and garlic, if using, and cook for about 5 minutes until softened.

2. Add the broccoli, potato and stock, increase the heat to high and bring it to the boil. Reduce the heat, cover the saucepan and allow the soup to simmer for about 7 minutes until the broccoli and potato are softened.

3. Allow the broccoli mixture to cool slightly, then transfer it to a blender or food processor, and working in batches if necessary, purée it until satiny smooth.

4. Return the soup to the saucepan, add half of the cheese and the buttermilk. Cook the soup over a low heat for about 3 minutes until the cheese melts (do not allow it to boil). Season with salt and pepper to taste. Pour the soup into serving bowls and top each with 2 tablespoons of the remaining cheese.

NUTRITION INFO: 1 portion provides:

Protein: ½ serving

Calcium: almost 2 servings

Vitamin C: 2 servings

Vitamin A: 2 servings

Other fruits and vegetables: ½ serving

Fat: ½ serving

Burn, Baby, Burn?

If pregnancy indigestion has you feeling the burn, try omitting garlic and/or onion from your soups, or subbing a sprinkle of garlic granules or onion powder.

Turkey Chilli

SERVES 6

Leaner than your average chilli, but no less flavourful. You can adjust the amount of chilli powder to sound as many – or as few – alarms as you and your heartburn can handle. Substitute lean beef mince for the turkey if you'd like to up your iron. Want to stay away from tummy troubles? Use edamame (soya beans) instead of the black beans.

1 tablespoon olive oil

1 medium-sized onion, chopped

2 cloves garlic, very finely chopped (optional)

675 g turkey breast mince

1 medium-sized red pepper, chopped

1 medium-sized yellow pepper, chopped

1 small jalapeño pepper, deseeded and diced (optional)

2 tablespoons chilli powder, or more or less to taste

1 tablespoon ground cumin

1 tablespoon tomato purée

425 g tinned red kidney beans, drained and rinsed

400 g tinned chopped tomatoes, with their juices

175 g Cheddar cheese, grated for serving

2 tablespoons chopped fresh coriander, for serving

1. Heat the olive oil in a large saucepan over a medium heat. Add the onion and garlic, if using, and cook for about 2 minutes until they begin to soften. Add the turkey, red and green peppers, and jalapeño, if using, and cook, stirring occasionally to break up the turkey, for about 3 minutes until the peppers begin to soften. Stir in the chilli powder, cumin and tomato purée and cook for about 2 minutes until fragrant.

2. Add the beans and tomatoes and bring the chilli to a simmer. Reduce the heat and allow it to simmer for about 10 minutes until the flavours are blended.

3. Spoon the chilli into serving bowls and top with the cheese and coriander. (Garnish just before serving.) The chilli can be refrigerated, covered, for up to 3 days.

NUTRITION INFO: 1 portion (1 bowl) provides:

Protein: 1 serving plus

Calcium: 1 serving

Vitamin C: 2 servings

Vitamin A: 1 serving

Wholegrains and legumes: ½ serving

Iron: some

Wrap It Up, I'll Eat It Here

Wrap leftover turkey or vegetarian chilli, along with a little chopped tomato, avocado, cheese and maybe a spoonful of salsa or low-fat soured cream, in a warm wholemeal tortilla for a quick but satisfying lunch or dinner.

Mexican Tortilla Soup

SERVES 4

This authentically flavoured meal in a bowl will take you to Mexico in 25 minutes or less. Leaving the garlic unpeeled produces a heady flavour without the burn – plus it saves chopping time.

4 wholegrain corn tortillas
  (each about 15 cm in diameter)
1 large head garlic
2 tablespoons olive oil
2 medium-sized onions, finely chopped
450 g skinless, boneless chicken breasts,
  cut into 2.5-cm strips
2 medium-sized carrots, peeled and
  finely chopped
2 bay leaves
1 teaspoon ground cumin
950 ml low-salt chicken stock
400 g tinned chopped tomatoes
4 tablespoons chopped fresh coriander
4 lime wedges, for serving

1. Preheat the oven to 150°C/gas mark 2.

2. Cut the tortillas into 1-cm-wide strips and place them flat on a large baking tray. Bake the tortillas for about 20 minutes until crisp. (The baked tortilla strips can be stored in an airtight container at room temperature for up to 1 week.)

3. Meanwhile, remove and discard the loose papery skin on the outside of the head of garlic. Place the head of garlic on its side on a work surface and, holding it steady, use a sharp knife to cut it in half widthways. Set the garlic aside.

4. Heat the olive oil in a large saucepan over a medium heat. Add the onions and cook for about 2 minutes until they begin to soften. Add the chicken, carrots, bay leaves, cumin and garlic head halves and cook for about 3 minutes

From the Test Kitchen

Add even more flavour, texture and nutrition to the tortilla soup with any of the following:

- Diced avocado
- Diced red pepper
- Chopped pickled jalapeño peppers
- Grated Cheddar cheese

until the chicken colours and the carrots begin to soften.

5. Add the stock and tomatoes, increase the heat to medium-high and bring the soup to the boil. Reduce the heat and allow it to simmer for about 10 minutes until the flavours are well blended.

6. Remove and discard the garlic and bay leaves. If serving only half of the soup, set aside the rest. (It can be refrigerated, covered, for up to 3 days.) Pour the hot soup into bowls and scatter each with coriander and a squeeze of lime. Scatter tortilla strips on top and serve.

NUTRITION INFO: 1 portion (1 bowl) provides:

Protein: 1 serving

Vitamin C: ½ serving

Vitamin A: 1½ servings

Other fruits and vegetables: 1 serving

Wholegrains and legumes: 1 serving

Fat: ½ serving

Hearty Fish and Potato Chowder
SERVES 2

Go ahead – chow down on this creamy-but-creamless chowder. Add a green salad and dinner's a done deal.

1 tablespoon olive oil
1 medium-sized onion, chopped
1 stick celery, chopped
1 medium-sized carrot, chopped
350 ml low-salt chicken stock or
    vegetable stock
250 ml full-fat milk
4 small red potatoes, scrubbed and
    quartered
Salt and black pepper
225 g skinless salmon, sea bream or
    red mullet fillets, cut into 2.5-cm cubes
1 tablespoon chopped fresh dill or
    1 teaspoon dried dill
½ medium-sized red pepper (optional),
    finely diced

1. Heat the olive oil in a large saucepan over a medium heat. Add the onion, celery and carrot and cook for about 5 minutes until the vegetables are softened.

2. Reduce the heat to low, add the stock and milk, and bring the soup to a simmer.

3. Add the potatoes, allow the soup to return to a simmer and cook for about 10 minutes until the potatoes are tender. Season the soup with salt and black pepper to taste. The soup can be prepared up to this point and refrigerated, covered, for 1 day. Reheat the soup gently over a low heat before proceeding with Step 4.

From the Test Kitchen

Like to cover even more Daily Dozen bases in your bowl of fish chowder? Substitute cubes of sweet potato for the red ones and score an extra vitamin A serving. Prefer a seafood chowder? Sub peeled, deveined prawns for the fish.

4. Add the fish and dill and allow the soup to simmer until the fish is just cooked through (don't over-cook it). Pour the soup into serving bowls and top with a scattering of red pepper, if wished.

NUTRITION INFO: 1 portion (1 bowl) provides:

Protein: 1 serving

Calcium: ½ serving

Vitamin C: 1½ servings

Vitamin A: 1½ servings

Other fruits and vegetables: 1 serving

Fat: ½ serving

Omegas: some, if using salmon

Pasta

....

N othing satisfies a carb craving or comforts a tumultuous tummy like a plateful of pasta. And there's good news for pregnant pasta lovers: though pasta of the past was almost always made with refined wheat, you can now find an impressive selection of wholegrain, high-protein and legume-based pasta alongside that white stuff. Not only are these pasta options more nutritious, with more fibre, more trace minerals and more naturally occurring vitamins, their chewier bite and nutty taste bring a new dimension to standard pasta recipes.

You can toss virtually anything – seafood, poultry, vegetables, cheese – with pasta and call it a meal. From Linguine with Prawns and Red Pepper to Chickpea Pasta with Chicken, Tiny Tomatoes and Spinach, you're bound to find the one-bowl dinner of your dreams in the recipes that follow.

Pasta Presto

L ooking for a way to shave time off your pasta prep? Try this trick: add the contents of an entire packet of pasta to a pot of boiling salted water and cook it for 5 minutes. Remove half the pasta (or as much as you want to save for later) from the pot and drain it. Toss this pasta with about 2 tablespoons olive oil (just enough to coat it lightly) and 4 tablespoons chopped fresh flat-leaf parsley. Allow the pasta to cool to room temperature, then refrigerate it in an airtight container until you're ready for another pasta fest – up to 1 week, if you can wait that long. Continue cooking the remaining pasta until it's done and use it for tonight's dinner. When you're next in the mood for pasta, simply heat a sauce or stock in a saucepan and add the partially cooked pasta. Simmer the pasta until it has finished cooking, then serve.

Fettuccine with Turkey and Wild Mushrooms

SERVES 2

Take a walk on the wild side and explore the intriguing texture wild mushrooms add to fettuccine. Yogurt makes the sauce Alfredo-like, without Alfredo's fat. Not feeling wild? Use white button or chestnut mushrooms or portobellos instead.

115 g wholegrain fettuccine

1 tablespoon olive oil

225 g raw turkey breast, thinly sliced
   across the grain

225 g sliced wild mushrooms
   (such as shiitakes)

2 shallots, very finely chopped

1 teaspoon fresh thyme leaves

85 g natural Greek yogurt (full-fat yogurt
   makes a creamier sauce)

3 tablespoons very finely chopped fresh
   flat-leaf parsley

40 g Parmesan cheese, grated

Salt and black pepper

2 tablespoons toasted pine nuts or
   walnuts (see page 217; optional)

1. Bring a large pot of water to the boil over a medium-high heat. Add the fettuccine and cook it according to the instructions on the packet.

2. Meanwhile, heat the olive oil in a large non-stick frying pan over a medium heat. Add the turkey and cook, stirring occasionally, for about 3 minutes until almost cooked through. Add the mushrooms, shallots and thyme and cook for 3–4 minutes until the mushrooms soften. Add the yogurt and parsley and toss to mix. Set the turkey and mushroom mixture aside until the fettuccine is ready, covering it to keep warm.

From the Test Kitchen

Sliced carrots, steamed or microwaved until just tender, would add extra vitamin A, a bit of crunch and a little colour to the Fettuccine with Turkey and Wild Mushrooms. Toss them in after the mushrooms have cooked for about 2 minutes.

3. Drain the fettuccine, shaking off any excess water. Reserve 125 ml pasta water. Toss the fettuccine with the turkey and mushroom mixture and the Parmesan cheese. Add pasta water 2 tablespoons at a time until a sauce forms, then season with salt and pepper to taste. Sprinkle the nuts over the fettuccine, if wished.

NUTRITION INFO: 1 portion provides:

Protein: 1½ servings

Calcium: 1 serving plus

Vitamin C: ½ serving

Vitamin A: ½ serving

Other fruits and vegetables: 3 servings

Wholegrains and legumes: 2 servings

Fat: ½ serving

Omegas: some

Chickpea Pasta with Chicken, Tiny Tomatoes and Spinach

SERVES 2

Chicken, cherry tomatoes and spinach make a colourful and nutritious combo for a light yet zesty sauce that's a flash in the pan to prepare.

115 g chickpea spirals or rotini, such as Banza

1 tablespoon olive oil

225 g skinless, boneless chicken breasts or turkey steaks, thinly sliced

2 shallots, thinly sliced

1 clove garlic, thinly sliced (optional)

150 g cherry or grape tomatoes

175 g baby spinach

2 tablespoons sliced fresh basil leaves (optional)

55 g mozzarella cheese, grated

4 tablespoons grated Parmesan cheese

Coarsely ground black pepper

Grated zest of 1 medium-sized lemon

1. Bring a large pot of water to the boil over a medium-high heat. Add the pasta and cook it according to the instructions on the packet.

2. Meanwhile, heat the olive oil in a large frying pan over a medium-high heat. Add the chicken and cook, stirring occasionally, for 3–5 minutes until it is no longer pink. Remove the chicken from the pan and set aside.

3. Add the shallots and garlic, if using, to the frying pan and cook over a medium heat for about 3 minutes until softened. Add the tomatoes and cook for about 3 minutes until they soften. Return the chicken to the pan, then add the spinach and basil, if using. Cover the pan and cook for about 1 minute until the spinach wilts. Set the chicken mixture aside until the pasta is ready, covering it to keep warm.

4. Drain the pasta, shaking off any excess water. Toss the pasta with the mozzarella, Parmesan cheese and coarsely ground black pepper. Divide the pasta between 2 serving bowls. Spoon the chicken mixture over it, then scatter the lemon zest on top.

NUTRITION INFO: 1 portion provides:

Protein: 2 servings

Calcium: 1½ servings

Vitamin C: 2 servings

Vitamin A: 3 servings

Wholegrains and legumes: 2 servings

Iron: some

Fat: ½ serving

Omegas: some

Alotta Broccoli with Chicken and Penne

SERVES 2

A plateful of broccoli never tasted so good. Not surprising, considering the tasty company it keeps: chicken, cheese and crunchy walnuts. The result is a lightly sauced but flavour-filled pasta dish.

Chickened Out?

You can substitute turkey breast strips, sliced lean beef, scallops, or peeled and deveined prawns in almost any pasta recipe that calls for chicken. Prawns and scallops won't need to cook as long; simmer or sauté them only until they're firm and opaque – don't allow them to over-cook.

For a vegetarian alternative, use vegetable stock and swap chunks of well-drained extra-firm tofu for the chicken. Add the tofu after the other ingredients have cooked through. If you have the time, it will pick up more flavour if you let it cook briefly. Or just get your protein fix by using bean or legume pasta.

For extra spice, add ½ teaspoon (or more) dried chilli flakes to any pasta dish.

---

115 g wholegrain or legume penne
175 g broccoli florets
1 tablespoon olive oil
1 small onion, chopped
1 clove garlic, very finely chopped (optional)
225 g skinless, boneless chicken breast, cut into 1-cm strips
4 tablespoons low-salt chicken stock, plus more if necessary
½ teaspoon dried oregano
55 g Cheddar cheese, grated
40 g Parmesan cheese, grated
1 tablespoon chopped fresh flat-leaf parsley
2 tablespoons roughly chopped toasted walnuts (see page 217)
Coarsely ground black pepper

1. Bring a large pot of water to the boil over a medium-high heat. Add the penne and cook according to the instructions on the packet.

2. Meanwhile, following the instructions on page 315, steam the broccoli for about 5 minutes until crisp-tender.

3. Heat the olive oil in a large non-stick frying pan over a medium-low heat. Add the onion and garlic, if using, and cook, stirring, for about 3 minutes until

they begin to soften. Add the chicken and cook, stirring occasionally, for about 4 minutes until it is no longer pink. Add the stock and oregano and cook for about 1 minute until heated through.

4. Remove the broccoli from the steamer and add it to the chicken. Reduce the heat to low and cook, stirring frequently, for about 2 minutes until the flavours blend. Set the chicken and broccoli mixture aside until the penne is ready, covering it to keep warm.

5. Drain the penne, shaking off any excess water. Add the penne, Cheddar, half of the Parmesan, and the parsley to the chicken and broccoli mixture and toss to mix. If the penne seems too dry, add more stock.

6. Divide the penne among four serving bowls. Top it with the remaining Parmesan and the walnuts. Scatter black pepper over the penne and serve at once.

NUTRITION INFO: 1 portion provides:

Protein: 1½ servings; 2 if made with legume pasta

Calcium: 1½ servings

Vitamin C: 2 servings

Vitamin A: 2 servings

Other fruits and vegetables: 1 serving

Wholegrains and legumes: 2 servings

Fat: ½ serving

Omegas: some

Pasta Primer

Don't know fusilli from fettuccine? Not to worry. Most recipes will work no matter what pasta you pick. Still, some pasta shapes are better suited to certain types of dishes than others. Here's a handy guide:

- Regular spaghetti is typically served with light tomato-based sauces.

- The skinniest pastas, such as capellini (angel hair) and vermicelli, work best in stocks and with thinner sauces.

- Long, flat pastas, such as fettuccine and linguine, stand up to thicker, creamier sauces.

- Specialist pasta shapes, such as farfalle, shells, fusilli, rotelle, radiatori, cavatappi and so on, can trap chunkier sauce and hold it as it travels from plate to mouth (so you won't end up with quite so many stains on your bump). Most are also sturdy enough to use in pasta salads and casserole bakes.

- Tubular pasta, such as penne or ziti, is the pasta of choice for salads, thick sauces and casseroles. Tubes with grooves on the exterior, such as fusilli, penne rigate and rigatoni, do a better job of securing sauces.

Penne with Chicken and Cheesy Tomato Sauce

SERVES 2

Why settle for pasta with tomato sauce from a jar when you can make a healthier and tastier version in just a few minutes? Want an extra serving each of vitamin A and vitamin C? Add 150 g of steamed broccoli florets.

115 g wholegrain or legume penne
1 tablespoon olive oil
225 g skinless, boneless chicken breast,
    thinly sliced
1 clove garlic, thinly sliced (optional)
½ small onion, finely chopped
1 medium-sized red pepper, chopped
475 g tinned chopped tomatoes
1½ teaspoons chopped fresh oregano or
    ½ teaspoon dried oregano
1 tablespoon chopped fresh basil or
    ½ teaspoon dried basil (optional)
40 g Pecorino Romano cheese, grated
40 g Parmesan cheese, grated
2 tablespoons chopped fresh flat-leaf
    parsley

1. Bring a large pot of water to the boil over a medium-high heat. Add the penne and cook according to the instructions on the packet.

2. Meanwhile, heat the olive oil in a large non-stick frying pan over a medium heat. Add the chicken and cook, stirring, for about 4 minutes until it is no longer pink. Add the garlic, if using, and cook for about 1 minute until the flavour is released. Add the onion and red pepper and cook for about 3 minutes until they begin to soften. Add the tomatoes, oregano and basil, if using, and simmer the

From the Test Kitchen

Don't have both kinds of cheese to hand? Just double up on either Parmesan or Pecorino Romano.

sauce for about 4 minutes until the flavours are well blended. Set the chicken sauce aside until the penne is ready, covering it to keep warm.

3. Drain the penne, shaking off any excess water. Toss the penne with the Pecorino Romano, half of the Parmesan and the parsley. Divide the penne between two serving bowls and top it with the chicken sauce and the remaining Parmesan.

NUTRITION INFO: 1 portion provides:

Protein: 1½ servings; 2 if using legume pasta

Calcium: 2 servings

Vitamin C: 3 servings

Vitamin A: 2 servings

Wholegrains and legumes: 2 servings

Fat: ½ serving

Omegas: some

Alfredo Light

SERVES 2

Craving a creamy Alfredo but wish you could dig in without spooning up all that fat? This enlightened alternative to the uber-caloric classic may be your pasta dream come true. Add steamed sugar snap peas, asparagus tips, peas or any of your favourite greens for a veggie-forward meal, or sautéed chicken strips or prawns for a protein boost. Use chickpea pasta for protein plus-plus.

115 g wholegrain or chickpea cavatappi (such as Banza)
1 tablespoon olive oil
1 clove garlic, very finely chopped (about 1 teaspoon; optional)
300 ml skimmed milk
1 teaspoon plain flour
85 g cream cheese
1 teaspoon coarse salt
½ teaspoon black pepper
40 g Pecorino Romano cheese, grated

1. Bring a large pot of water to the boil over a high heat. Add the cavatappi and cook according to the instructions on the packet.

2. Meanwhile, heat the oil in a large frying pan over a medium heat. Add the garlic, if using, and cook, stirring constantly, for about 1 minute until fragrant. Whisk together the milk and flour in a small bowl. Pour the milk mixture into the frying pan, bring to the boil and cook, stirring occasionally, for about 1 minute until slightly thickened. Whisk in the cream cheese, salt and pepper, stirring until the cream cheese melts. Reduce the heat to low and stir in the Pecorino.

3. Drain the cavatappi, shaking off any excess water. Stir into the sauce until well coated. Serve immediately.

NUTRITION INFO: 1 portion provides:

Protein: ½ serving

Calcium: 1 serving

Wholegrains and legumes: 2 servings

Fat: 1 serving

Red Pepper and Edamame Peanut Noodles

SERVES 2

A super-nutritious twist on an Asian favourite that satisfies many of pregnancy's most common cravings, all in one dish: sweet, salty, spicy, crunchy . . . and peanut butter. Double the recipe to double the pleasure later in the week – no heating means speedy, easy eating.

115 g uncooked wholewheat linguine or
    buckwheat soba noodles
150 g frozen shelled edamame, thawed
4 tablespoons low-salt soy sauce
65 g smooth peanut butter
2 tablespoons soft brown sugar
1 tablespoon rapeseed oil
1 tablespoon very finely chopped, peeled
    fresh ginger
1 teaspoon sesame oil (optional)
1 clove garlic, very finely chopped (if raw
    garlic bothers you, see the box on
    page 262)
1 teaspoon sriracha sauce or ½ teaspoon
    hot red pepper sauce, such as
    Tabasco
185 g ready-made coleslaw mix
1 medium-sized red pepper, thinly sliced
2 teaspoon sesame seeds, toasted (see
    page 217; optional)

1. Bring a large pot of water to the boil over a medium-high heat. Add the linguine and cook it according to the instructions on the packet. Drain the linguine in a colander.

From the Test Kitchen

For extra protein, toss in or top with cooked chicken or prawns.

2. Meanwhile, bring another pot of water to the boil and cook the edamame according to the packet instructions. Drain with the linguine.

3. Whisk together the soy sauce, peanut butter, brown sugar, rapeseed oil, ginger, sesame oil, if using, garlic, sriracha and sesame seeds (if using) in a small bowl.

4. Combine the coleslaw mix, red pepper, linguine and edamame in a large bowl. Add the dressing and toss to coat. Serve at room temperature or chilled. Store leftovers in the refrigerator, covered, for up to 3 days.

NUTRITION INFO: 1 portion provides:

Protein: 1 serving

Vitamin C: 2 servings

Vitamin A: 2 servings

Wholegrains and legumes: 2 servings

Fat: 1½ serving

Macaroni and Cheese, Outside the Box

SERVES 4

Comfort food at its most nutritious, this macaroni and cheese is definitely different from the stuff you get in a box or tin. It's a whole lot tastier, too. Four cheeses add flavour and calcium, and kale adds vitamins. Plus you'll love the leftovers – they reheat in the microwave in minutes.

225 g wholegrain or legume elbow macaroni or shells

30 g butter

1½ tablespoons wholemeal flour

250 ml milk

55 g Gouda cheese, grated

55 g mild Cheddar cheese, grated

115 g pasteurised part-skim mozzarella cheese, grated

Hot red pepper sauce, such as Tabasco (optional)

Salt and black pepper

125 g chopped cooked kale

2 tablespoons grated Parmesan cheese

1½ tablespoons wholemeal breadcrumbs

1. Preheat the oven to 180°C/gas mark 4.

2. Bring a large pot of water to the boil over a medium-high heat. Add the pasta and cook it according to the instructions on the packet.

3. Meanwhile, melt the butter in a non-stick saucepan over a medium heat. Add the flour and cook, stirring, for 1–2 minutes until a paste forms. Add the milk and bring it to the boil, stirring constantly. When the sauce thickens slightly, remove it from the heat and add the Gouda, Cheddar and mozzarella. Stir until the cheeses melt. Season the cheese sauce with a dash of hot sauce, if wished, and salt and pepper to taste, then set aside.

From the Test Kitchen

For a bigger protein punch, toss diced tofu, cooked chicken or edamame with the macaroni and cheese. You can also add another vegetable – or more than one. Try 150–175 g chopped roasted red peppers, cooked broccoli florets, sweetcorn kernels, green peas or chopped cooked spinach. To go white-on-white, use 125 g chopped cooked cauliflower instead of the kale. You won't even notice that you're eating your vegetables.

4. Drain the pasta, shaking off any excess water, and return it to the pot. Add the cheese sauce and stir to coat evenly. Add the kale and stir to combine. Place the pasta mixture in a 23 x 33-cm baking dish.

5. Place the Parmesan and breadcrumbs in a small bowl and stir to mix, then scatter over the pasta.

6. Bake the pasta and cheese until hot and bubbly, about 10 minutes.

NUTRITION INFO: 1 portion provides:

Protein: 2 servings

Calcium: 2½ servings

Vitamin C: ½ serving

Vitamin A: 1 serving

Wholegrains and legumes: 2 servings

Fat: ½ serving

Creamy Linguine with Prawns and Red Pepper

SERVES 2

No need to skimp on this seafood, lightened up with chicken stock but rich in flavour. It's easy and cheesy, packing protein not only from the prawns but the chickpea pasta. Red peppers and parsley add a pop of colour and a side of baby-friendly nutrients.

115 g chickpea or other legume-based linguine
1 tablespoon olive oil
1 teaspoon chopped garlic or 2 cloves garlic, thinly sliced (optional)
1 medium-sized red pepper, thinly sliced
225 g shelled and deveined large prawns
500 ml low-salt chicken stock, fish stock or shellfish stock
55 g Edam cheese, grated
40 g Parmesan cheese, grated
150 g courgetti (sprialised courgette)
2 tablespoons chopped fresh flat-leaf parsley
Coarsely ground black pepper
¼ teaspoon dried chilli flakes, or to taste (optional)

1. Bring a large pot of water to the boil over a medium-high heat. Add the linguine and cook according to the instructions on the packet.

2. Meanwhile, heat the olive oil in a frying pan over a medium heat. Add the garlic, if using, and cook for 2 minutes until just golden. Add the red pepper and cook for about 2 minutes until slightly softened. Add the prawns and cook for about 4 minutes until cooked through and opaque. Remove the red pepper and prawns from the skillet and set aside, covered, to keep warm.

3. Add the stock to the frying pan and bring to a simmer. Add the Edam and Parmesan, courgetti, parsley and pepper to taste. Stir to combine.

4. Drain the linguine, shaking off any excess water. Divide the linguine between two serving bowls. Spoon the stock and courgetti over it and top with the prawns and red peppers. If you like a little spice, scatter dried chilli flakes on top.

NUTRITION INFO: 1 portion provides:

Protein: 1½ servings

Calcium: 1½ servings

Vitamin C: 1 serving

Vitamin A: 1 serving

Other fruits and vegetables: 2 servings

Wholegrains and legumes: 2 servings

Iron: some

Fat: ½ serving

Omegas: some

Extra (Pasta) Sauce

At a loss for pasta sauce? You won't be if you make extra-large batches of these sauces. Toss with pasta and whatever veggies and protein you like, and you'll have a meal in minutes!

Pesto with Sunflower Seeds

MAKES ABOUT 2 PORTIONS

Instead of the traditional pine nuts, this pesto gets its rich flavour – and healthy fatty acids – from sunflower seeds (or, if you prefer, pumpkin seeds). Spoon this zesty pesto on pasta, into sandwiches, on poultry or on anything else that could use a pick-me-up.

60 g fresh basil leaves
75 g shelled lightly toasted sunflower or
    pumpkin seeds
1½ teaspoons chopped garlic (if raw
    garlic bothers you, see the box on
    page 262; optional)
2 tablespoons olive oil, plus more for
    storing
Juice of 1 medium-sized lemon
40 g Parmesan cheese, grated
Salt and black pepper

1. Place the basil, sunflower seeds and garlic in a food processor and process until finely chopped.

2. With the motor running, add the olive oil and lemon juice in a steady stream through the feed tube.

From the Test Kitchen

Really want to up the omega-3 ante? Substitute toasted walnuts for the seeds.

3. Transfer the pesto to a small bowl. Fold in the Parmesan cheese, and salt and pepper to taste. To use, toss 55-g servings of hot pasta with several tablespoons of pesto. To store, place the pesto in a small airtight container and float a thin layer of olive oil over the top to keep the basil from turning brown. The pesto can be refrigerated for 2 weeks.

NUTRITION INFO: 1 portion (8 tablespoons) provides:

Calcium: ½ serving

Vitamin C: 1 serving

Vitamin A: 1 serving

Fat: ½ serving

Omegas: some

Turkey Bolognese Sauce

MAKES ABOUT 2½ PINTS

Have a beef with greasy meat sauce? This Bolognese swaps out the beef with turkey, for a leaner profile and a light taste. Miss the beef but not the grease? Use extra-lean beef mince.

1 tablespoon olive oil
1 medium-sized onion, chopped
3 medium-sized carrots, peeled and
  chopped
2 sticks celery, chopped
2 cloves garlic, peeled and crushed, or
  1 teaspoon chopped garlic (optional)
1½ pounds turkey mince
2 x 400-g tins chopped tomatoes,
  with their juices
800 g tomato passata
1½ teaspoons dried oregano
2 bay leaves
4 tablespoons chopped fresh flat-leaf
  (Italian) parsley
Salt and black pepper

1. Heat the olive oil in a saucepan over a medium heat. Add the onion and cook for about 1 minute until slightly softened. Add the carrots, celery and garlic, if using, and cook for about 2 minutes until the carrots and celery start to soften.

2. Add the turkey and cook, chopping up the pieces with a wooden spoon, for about 10 minutes until the turkey is cooked through.

3. Add the chopped tomatoes, passata, oregano, bay leaves and parsley. Bring the sauce to a simmer and cook for about 15 minutes until the flavours blend. Allow it to cool to room temperature, add salt and pepper to taste, then remove and discard the bay leaves. Spoon the sauce into three 500-ml containers. The sauce can be refrigerated for 3 days or frozen for up to 2 months. Thaw it in the refrigerator overnight before reheating.

NUTRITION INFO: 1 portion (250 ml) provides:

Protein: 1 serving

Vitamin C: 2 servings

Vitamin A: 2 servings

Saucy Secrets

Feel like you can't look at another carrot or red pepper or another piece of broccoli or cauliflower? Don't look at them – hide them in tomato sauce. Tomato sauces, or tomato-and-meat sauces, can camouflage just about any vegetable, which is why you'll want to keep this trick up your sleeve when you start feeding a picky toddler. And what you can't see or smell won't be off-putting to you. If you're making sauce from scratch, add the finely chopped vegetable or vegetables when you fry the onion and garlic. If you're opening up a jar, just simmer the vegetables in the sauce until they're tender enough to be inconspicuous. If you're adding meat mince to ready-prepared sauce, add the veggies when you cook the meat.

Salads

....

S ure, you can fill a bowl with lettuce and tomato, douse it with bottled dressing and call it a salad. But why settle for that when there are so many exciting salad combinations just waiting to be tossed your way? Whether a salad's a side dish or the main event, all the varieties you'll find here deserve a starring role on the table. There's a salad in here for everybody (and any of the salads that serve two can easily be doubled).

Side Salads

W ant a little salad with your dinner? Try one of these tasty side salads. Each crunchy serving will satisfy your taste buds and your nutritional requirements. Don't have room on the side, or don't want to overload your tummy with too much at a time? Serve your salad first. Starting with a salad can also help you pace yourself, so you don't get too full too fast (slow and steady always wins the pregnancy eating race).

Enough Is Like a Feast

S alad eaters come in all kinds of packages, including the kind who can eat their way through a whole bag of salad leaves – and the kind who can barely make it through leaf one. The salad servings in this section are geared to that salad eater in the middle: the one who can happily manage about 75 g of salad leaves (which, when dressed, wilt down to considerably less). If the recipe makes too much salad for you, cut the servings by half. If the recipe doesn't make enough salad, double the recipe – and double the nutrients you'll be able to score.

Spicy Watermelon, Cucumber and Feta Salad

SERVES 2

Watermelon makes your mouth water? Wait until your mouth gets a load of a mum-to-be's favourite melon tossed with salty feta, zesty lime and a kick of mint. Add grilled prawns or scallops, and it's dinner. Or top with cottage cheese for a yummy meatless meal.

4 tablespoons freshly squeezed lime
  juice (about 3 limes)
2 teaspoons honey
¼ teaspoon coarse salt
¼ teaspoon dried chilli flakes
2 tablespoons extra-virgin olive oil
750 g seedless watermelon flesh, cut into
  2-cm cubes
275 g seedless cucumber, chopped
75 g pasteurised feta cheese, crumbled
40 g red onion, thinly sliced (optional)
2 tablespoons chopped fresh mint leaves

1. Whisk together the lime juice, honey, salt and chilli flakes in a small bowl. Gradually whisk in the oil until completely incorporated.

2. Stir together the watermelon, cucumber, feta and onion in a large bowl to combine. Gently stir in 2 tablespoons of the dressing. Chill for at least 20 minutes or up to 2 hours.

3. Just before serving, gently stir in the mint. Whisk the dressing to recombine it and drizzle over the salad.

NUTRITION INFO: 1 portion provides:

Calcium: 1 serving

Vitamin C: 2 servings

Other fruits and vegetables: 2 servings

Fat: 1 serving

Ginger Melon Salad

SERVES 2

Always save your fruit salad for dessert? This melon mix makes a refreshing first course or side for grilled chicken or fish. Best of all, it's a comforting way to tuck away vitamins – without vegetables.

1 tablespoon honey
½ tablespoon very finely chopped,
  peeled fresh ginger
½ tablespoon chopped fresh mint
½ teaspoon grated lime zest
2 tablespoons fresh lime juice
150 g watermelon flesh, cut into 2.5-cm
  cubes
150 g cantaloupe flesh, cut into 2.5-cm
  cubes

From the Test Kitchen

For a calcium bonus and a salty contrast to the sweet melon, toss in or top the salad with 75 g pasteurised feta or goat cheese.

1. Place the honey, ginger, mint, lime zest and lime juice in a small bowl and stir to mix.

2. Place the watermelon and cantaloupe cubes in a large salad bowl, pour the lime and ginger mixture over them, and toss to coat evenly. Cover the salad and refrigerate for at least 1 hour before serving.

NUTRITION INFO: 1 portion provides:

Vitamin C: 1½ servings

Vitamin A: 1 serving

Other fruits and vegetables: 1 serving

Mucho Mango Salad

SERVES 2

Few fruits – or even vegetables – bring as many vitamins to the table as the sweet mango. This salad doubles the mango, and the nutrients, by using it in the dressing, too.

1½ large ripe mangoes, cubed
2 tablespoons natural full-fat yogurt
1½ tablespoons fresh lime juice
1½ tablespoons fresh orange juice
2 teaspoons grated peeled fresh ginger
½ teaspoon ground coriander (optional)
Salt and black pepper
85 g peeled kiwi fruit, cubed
75 g fresh blueberries
75 g mild baby salad leaves
2 tablespoons chopped macadamia nuts
Lime wedges, for serving

1. Place about one third of the mango cubes, the yogurt, lime juice, orange juice, ginger and coriander, if using, in a food processor and process until smooth. Season the dressing with salt and pepper to taste.

2. Place the remaining mango cubes, kiwi and blueberries in a large salad bowl, pour the dressing on top and toss to coat evenly. Divide the salad leaves between two salad plates, top each with half of the mango salad, then scatter the nuts on top. Serve with lime wedges.

NUTRITION INFO: 1 portion provides:

Vitamin C: 3½ servings

Vitamin A: 2 servings

Mango and Orange Salad

SERVES 2

Mango, orange and mint mingle with a red wine vinegar dressing in a refreshing salad that's just about bursting with flavour.

1 ripe mango, peeled and stoned
1 medium-sized seedless orange, peeled
　　and white pith removed
1 tablespoon red wine vinegar
1 teaspoon chopped fresh mint leaves
Coarse salt, to taste (optional)

Cut the mango into thin slices and place in a bowl. Segment the orange and add to the bowl. Add the vinegar and mint and toss to mix. Sprinkle with salt if desired.

NUTRITION INFO: 1 portion provides:

Vitamin C: 2 servings

Vitamin A: 1 serving

Crunchy Pear Salad

SERVES 2

Pick a pear that's ripe enough to be fragrant, yet firm enough to lend crunch to this lovely autumn salad.

1 ripe pear, halved, cored, peeled and
　　thinly sliced
125 g baby spinach or rocket
2 tablespoons balsamic vinegar
2 tablespoons olive oil
1 teaspoon Dijon mustard
1 teaspoon very finely chopped shallot
　　(optional)
Salt and black pepper
55 g Parmesan cheese shavings
　　(see page 251)
30 g toasted walnut pieces (see page 217)

1. Place the pear and spinach in a salad bowl and stir to mix.

2. Place the balsamic vinegar, olive oil, mustard and shallot in a small bowl

and whisk to mix, then season with salt and pepper to taste. Toss the salad with enough dressing to coat it evenly. Divide the salad between two smaller salad bowls and top with the Parmesan shavings and walnut pieces.

NUTRITION INFO: 1 portion provides:

Protein: ½ serving

Calcium: 1 serving

Vitamin C: 1 serving if made with spinach; ½ serving if made with rocket

Vitamin A: 2 servings

Other fruits and vegetables: ½ serving

Iron: some

Fat: 1 serving

Omegas: some

Pomegranate Salad

SERVES 2

In this sassy spin on a standard salad, pomegranate seeds add crunch and a tangy sweetness to the salad leaves, while pomegranate juice lends a rich flavour to the dressing. Both are great sources of vitamins and anti-oxidants. Parmesan cheese adds a salty component.

125 ml pomegranate juice
1 tablespoon balsamic vinegar
1 tablespoon olive oil
1 teaspoon wholegrain mustard
1 shallot, very finely chopped (optional)
Fresh lemon juice
Salt and black pepper
125 g baby salad leaves, such as baby
**   spinach or spring mix**
Seeds from ½ pomegranate (see Note)
55 g Parmesan cheese shavings
**   (see A Quick Shave)**

1. Place the pomegranate juice in a small saucepan and bring to the boil over a medium heat. Reduce the heat and simmer for about 10 minutes until the juice is reduced to about 2 tablespoons. Remove from the heat and allow to cool.

A Quick Shave

Those fancy curls of Parmesan cheese only look like they take forever – and a culinary degree – to create. They're actually as easy as this: let a chunk of Parmesan soften slightly at room temperature, then use a potato peeler to peel off thin shavings. That's all there is to it!

From the Test Kitchen

Turn Pomegranate Salad into a main dish by doubling the recipe and topping it with grilled prawns or chicken.

2. Add the balsamic vinegar, olive oil, mustard and shallot, if using, to the reduced juice and whisk to mix. Season with lemon juice, salt and pepper to taste.

3. Place the salad leaves and pomegranate seeds in a large salad bowl. Toss with enough dressing to coat evenly. Divide the salad between two smaller salad bowls, scatter the Parmesan shavings on top and serve immediately.

NOTE: Some stores carry ready-prepared pomegranate seeds in the refrigerated aisle of the produce department.

NUTRITION INFO: 1 portion provides:

Calcium: 1 serving

Vitamin C: 1 serving

Vitamin A: 2 servings

Other fruits and vegetables: 1 serving

Iron: some

Fat: ½ serving

Fig and Rocket Salad with Parmesan Shavings

SERVES 2

Fresh figs make this a very sexy salad. Can't get fresh (figs, that is)? Use sliced dried figs instead.

1 teaspoon very finely chopped shallot

2 tablespoons balsamic vinegar

2 tablespoons extra-virgin olive oil

1 teaspoon wholegrain mustard

Salt

8 fresh figs, cut in half vertically

125 g rocket

Black pepper

55 g Parmesan cheese shavings
(see the box on page 251)

1. Place the shallot, balsamic vinegar, olive oil, mustard and a pinch of salt in a large salad bowl and whisk to mix. Add the figs, toss to coat them evenly and allow them to stand, covered with cling film, for 20 minutes.

2. Add the rocket to the figs and toss to mix. Season with salt and pepper to taste, then toss well. Divide the fig salad between 2 smaller salad bowls and top with the Parmesan shavings.

NUTRITION INFO: 1 portion provides:

Calcium: 1 serving

Vitamin C: 1 serving

Vitamin A: 2 servings

Fat: 1 serving

Omegas: some

Move Over, Croutons

Crave a crunch on your salad? Think outside the crouton box to these tasty toppings:

Parmesan Crisps: Preheat the oven to 160°C/gas mark 3. Coat a baking tray with olive oil cooking spray. Mound heaped tablespoons of freshly grated Parmesan cheese on the baking tray. Using the back of a spoon, pat each mound into a 7.5-cm circle. Bake for 6–8 minutes until the cheese is bubbling. Let the crisps cool slightly, then transfer them to kitchen paper to finish cooling and crisping. Serve on top of any cheese-friendly salad. They also make a super soup-topper. Or just snack on them.

Crunchy Chickpeas: Preheat the oven to 190°C/gas mark 5. Drain a tin of chickpeas and pat them dry thoroughly with kitchen paper. Spread the chickpeas out on a baking tray, spray them with olive oil cooking spray and scatter grated Parmesan cheese over them. Bake the chickpeas for about 30 minutes until crunchy. Use the chickpeas to top salads or soups or just enjoy them by the handful. Experiment with other yummy flavour combos: Parmesan and garlic powder, paprika and cumin, lime juice and chilli powder, even cinnamon and a sprinkle of sugar.

Rocket, Shaved Fennel, and Roasted Pepper Salad

SERVES 2

Serve this classic Italian salad alongside or as a tasty bed for grilled meat, chicken, salmon or prawns – or as a first stop on the way to a pasta dinner. For a milder salad, substitute baby spinach or mixed baby salad leaves for the rocket. Or kick it up a notch with baby kale.

125 g rocket
2 tablespoons chopped fresh flat-leaf parsley
1 small fennel bulb, trimmed, halved and very thinly sliced widthways
2– 4 tablespoons Lemon Vinaigrette (recipe follows)
1 roasted red pepper (leftover or from a jar), sliced into strips
55 g Parmesan cheese shavings (see the box on page 251)

1. Place the rocket, parsley and fennel in a salad bowl and toss to mix. Toss with enough Lemon Vinaigrette to coat the salad evenly.

2. Divide the salad between 2 salad plates, then top it with the roasted peppers and Parmesan shavings.

From the Test Kitchen

Cheese up the Lemon Vinaigrette by adding 4 tablespoons of grated Parmesan cheese. Add extra Italian flavour with a sprinkling of dried oregano.

NUTRITION INFO: 1 portion (without dressing) provides:

Protein: 1 serving

Calcium: 1 serving

Vitamin C: 2½ servings

Vitamin A: 3 servings

Lemon Vinaigrette

MAKES ABOUT 125 ML

This simple dressing can zest up almost any salad leaves. It's also delicious on grilled veggies.

4 tablespoons fresh lemon juice
4 tablespoons olive oil
Grated zest of 1 lemon
1 clove garlic, very finely chopped (if raw garlic bothers you, see the box on page 262; optional)
Salt and black pepper

Combine the lemon juice, olive oil, lemon zest and garlic in a small bowl and whisk to mix. Season the vinaigrette with salt and pepper to taste. The dressing can be stored in an airtight container or jar for up to 1 week. Whisk or shake to recombine before using.

NUTRITION INFO: 1 portion (2 tablespoons) provides:

Vitamin C: ½ serving

Fat: 1 serving

Omegas: some

It's Mediterranean to Me Salad

SERVES 2

This salad combines the best of Greece and Italy for a delicious Mediterranean hybrid.

110 g romaine lettuce, chopped
½ small red pepper, diced
½ medium-sized avocado
(preferably Hass), diced
¼ seedless cucumber, peeled and diced
¼ medium-sized red onion, chopped
(optional)
2 plum tomatoes, deseeded and diced
75 g Italian provolone cheese (available
from cheese specialists) or halloumi
cheese, cubed
50 g drained tinned chickpeas, rinsed
1 tablespoon chopped fresh flat-leaf
parsley
1 teaspoon chopped fresh oregano
leaves or ¼ teaspoon dried oregano
1 teaspoon chopped fresh mint leaves or
¼ teaspoon dried mint (optional)
25 g pitted kalamata olives, sliced
2 tablespoons balsamic vinegar
2 tablespoons olive oil
1½ teaspoons fresh lemon juice, plus
more to taste
1 small clove garlic, very finely chopped
(if raw garlic bothers you, see the box
on page 262; optional)
Salt and black pepper

1. Place the romaine, red pepper, avocado, cucumber, onion if using, tomatoes, cheese, chickpeas, parsley, oregano, mint, if using, and olives, if using, in a large salad bowl and stir to mix.

From the Test Kitchen

Here's a time-saving hint: chop everything except the avocado early in the day and store the ingredients separately in the fridge. Toss the salad right before serving. Make it a meal by adding cubes of cooked chicken or turkey, chilled grilled prawns, chunks of cold leftover salmon or even tinned tuna or salmon.

2. Place the balsamic vinegar, olive oil, lemon juice and garlic, if using, in a small bowl and whisk to mix. Season with salt and black pepper to taste. Toss the salad with enough dressing to coat evenly. Taste for seasoning, adding more lemon juice, salt and/or black pepper if desired. Divide the salad between 2 smaller salad bowls and serve.

NUTRITION INFO: 1 portion provides:

Calcium: 1 serving

Vitamin C: 1½ servings

Vitamin A: 1½ servings

Other fruits and vegetables: 1 serving

Iron: some

Fat: 1 serving

Broccoli, Tomato and Mozzarella Salad

SERVES 2

Sure, tomato and mozzarella are made for each other – especially when fresh basil joins the party. But did you ever think of adding crunchy broccoli to the mix? You should – your taste buds will thank you.

100 g small broccoli florets

2 ripe plum tomatoes, deseeded and roughly chopped

55 g pasteurised part-skimmed mozzarella, cubed

3 tablespoons sliced fresh basil leaves

2 tablespoons balsamic vinegar

1–2 tablespoons olive oil

Fresh lemon juice

Salt and black pepper

2 tablespoons toasted pine nuts (see page 217)

1. Steam the broccoli, following the instructions on page 315, for 3– 5 minutes until crisp-tender. Set the broccoli aside in a large salad bowl and allow it to cool completely. Add the tomatoes, mozzarella and basil, and toss to mix.

2. Place the balsamic vinegar and olive oil in a small bowl and whisk to mix.

From the Test Kitchen

Not feeling the love for broccoli? Leave it out and substitute 2 sliced medium-sized tomatoes.

Pour the dressing over the salad and toss well to coat evenly. Squeeze a little lemon juice on top, season with salt and pepper to taste, and toss again. Divide the salad between 2 smaller salad bowls, then sprinkle the pine nuts on top.

NUTRITION INFO: 1 portion provides:

Calcium: 1 serving

Vitamin C: 2 servings

Vitamin A: 1½ servings

Fat: ½ serving if made with 1 tablespoon oil; 1 serving if made with 2

Spicy Salad Leaves with Ginger Dressing

SERVES 2

The salad leaves may be wilted, but the flavour will be lively. Add a dash of dried chilli flakes if you'd like it livelier still.

3 tablespoons seasoned rice vinegar
1 tablespoon low-salt soy sauce
1 tablespoon sesame oil
2 teaspoons very finely chopped peeled
    fresh ginger
2 tablespoons chopped fresh coriander
    (optional)
3 spring onions (white and light green
    parts), trimmed and sliced
1 x 150 g bag peppery salad mix
    (see Note) or baby spinach
1 tablespoon toasted sesame seeds
    (see page 217)

1. Place the rice vinegar, soy sauce, sesame oil and ginger in a small saucepan over a low heat and cook, stirring, for about 3 minutes until hot but not boiling. Stir in the coriander, if using.

2. Place the spring onions and salad mix in a heatproof bowl and toss to mix. Pour the hot dressing over the leaves, sprinkle the sesame seeds on top and toss well. Serve immediately.

NOTE: Look in the produce section for a peppery salad mix with a spicy combination of salad leaves such as spinach, mizuna, chard and red mustard.

NUTRITION INFO: 1 portion provides:

Vitamin C: 1 serving

Vitamin A: 3 servings

Iron: some

Fat: ½ serving

Ginger Cucumber Salad

SERVES 2

This crunchy salad pulls double duty as either a snack or a side dish. Pair it with your favourite Chinese-style chicken, fish or pork main.

300 g seedless cucumber, thinly sliced
    (peeling optional)
55 g thinly sliced red onion (optional)
1½ teaspoons grated peeled fresh ginger
¼ cup roughly chopped fresh coriander
    leaves (or mint)
3 tablespoons unseasoned rice vinegar
2 teaspoons low-salt soy sauce
1 tablespoon sesame oil
Thinly sliced spring onions (optional)

Place the cucumber, onion, ginger, coriander, vinegar, soy sauce and sesame oil in a medium bowl. Toss to combine. Allow to stand for 5 minutes. Scatter with spring onions, if desired, and serve.

NUTRITION INFO: 1 portion provides:

Other fruits and vegetables: 2 servings

Fat: ½ serving

Oriental Slaw

SERVES 2

Move over, bland ready-prepared coleslaw. Rice vinegar, sesame oil, ginger and coriander give this tangy slaw an oriental kick.

200 g ready-prepared coleslaw mix (or 50 g each white and red cabbage, shredded, plus 100 g carrots, shredded)
½ medium-sized red pepper, thinly sliced
3 tablespoons seasoned rice vinegar
1 tablespoon fresh lime juice
1 tablespoon sesame oil
1 tablespoon olive oil (optional)
1 tablespoon grated peeled fresh ginger
1 tablespoon honey, or to taste
Pinch of dried chilli flakes
3 tablespoons chopped fresh coriander
1 tablespoon toasted sesame seeds (see page 217)

1. Place the coleslaw mix (or white and green cabbages and carrots) and red pepper in a large salad bowl and toss to mix.

2. Place the rice vinegar, lime juice, sesame oil, olive oil, if using, ginger, honey, chilli flakes and coriander in a small bowl and whisk to mix.

From the Test Kitchen

For a crunchy and extra-nutritious slaw, you can substitute 100 g shredded broccoli stalks for the cabbages or use a combination of both.

3. Just before serving, pour the dressing over the slaw mixture and toss to coat evenly. Sprinkle with sesame seeds and serve.

NUTRITION INFO: 1 portion provides:

Vitamin C: 2 servings

Vitamin A: 3½ servings

Fat: ½ serving without olive oil; 1 serving with it

Curtido

SERVES 4

This Mexican-style slaw takes only moments to prep, but it's a dish that keeps on giving – unlike most slaws, it actually tastes even better the day after. Top tacos with curtido or serve it alongside sandwiches.

200 g white cabbage, very thinly sliced
55 g red onion, very thinly sliced
55 g peeled carrot, shredded
1 small jalapeño pepper, deseeded and
    very finely chopped (optional)
4 tablespoons cider vinegar
2 teaspoons sugar
1 teaspoon coase salt

Place the cabbage, onion, carrot and jalapeño, if using, in a large bowl and stir to mix. Place the vinegar, sugar and salt in a small saucepan and cook over medium a heat, stirring, until the salt and sugar are dissolved. Pour the dressing over the vegetables and stir to mix. Cover and refrigerate for at least 1 hour before serving.

From the Test Kitchen

Not only does curtido have staying power (you can store it in the fridge in an airtight container for about a week), but the flavour actually improves with age.

NUTRITION INFO: 1 portion (scant 1 cup) provides:

Vitamin C: ½ serving

Vitamin A: 1 serving

Carrots Only

Can't stomach cabbage? Try a vitamin-packed all-carrot slaw instead: Mix 150 g drained, tinned crushed pineapple (packed in juice) with 225 g shredded carrots, 75 g raisins and 120 g natural full-fat Greek yogurt. Add 2 teaspoons fresh lemon juice, honey to taste, a pinch of ground cinnamon and 1 teaspoon grated peeled fresh ginger or ¼ teaspoon ground ginger. Chill the slaw. Just before serving, stir in 2 tablespoons chopped toasted walnuts (see page 217). The slaw can be refrigerated for up to 3 days.

Dinner Salads

Looking for a light and easy way to end a long day? Turn off the oven and chill out with a dinner salad. Pretty much any salad (from Caesar to Greek) can be turned into a meal when you top it with your choice of protein (fish, seafood, beef, poultry, eggs or cheese). To keep things really cool, use last night's leftovers for your salad topper – you'll save yourself time and effort. Serve dinner salads with crusty wholegrain bread or buns. And, of course, don't forget to take them to lunch, too.

Curried Chicken Salad

SERVES 4

Have some leftovers from last night's chicken dinner? Chop them up to make this yummy salad. Or simply simmer a couple of chicken breasts in stock until cooked through, allow them to cool and you're ready to start. Serve the salad on top of salad leaves or in a cantaloupe half (don't forget to count them in your Daily Dozen). Any leftover chicken salad you have will make a great sandwich for tomorrow – and the day after. Just pile into a pitta and you're good to go.

120 g natural low-fat Greek yogurt
2 tablespoons mayonnaise
2–3 teaspoons curry powder
1 tablespoon fresh lime juice
2 teaspoons grated peeled fresh ginger
Salt and black pepper
450 g cooked skinless, boneless chicken
    breasts or turkey breast, cut into 1-cm
    pieces
4 spring onions (white and light green
    parts), trimmed and sliced

1 firm but ripe mango, chopped
60 g chopped Granny Smith apple
½ red pepper, very finely chopped
40 g toasted cashews (see page 217),
    roughly chopped

Place the yogurt, mayonnaise, curry powder, lime juice and ginger in a large salad bowl and stir to mix. Season with salt and pepper to taste. Add the chicken, spring onions, mango, apple, red pepper and cashews and toss gently to combine. The salad can be refrigerated, covered, for up to 3 days.

NUTRITION INFO: 1 portion provides:

Protein: 1 serving

Vitamin C: 1 serving

Vitamin A: ½ serving

Fat: ½ serving

Omegas: some

Taco Salad

SERVES 2

Unlike most taco salads, which tend to be off the charts in fat and calories, this one's extra lean. Luckily, it's also extra tasty.

1 tablespoon olive oil

2 cloves garlic, very finely chopped

1 medium-sized red pepper, chopped

½ medium-sized yellow pepper, chopped

½ small onion, chopped

225 g lean beef mince

2 teaspoons chilli powder

1 teaspoon ground cumin

75 g drained tinned pinto or kidney beans, rinsed

375 g ready-prepared tomato-based salsa

2 tablespoons chopped fresh coriander (optional)

Hot red pepper sauce, such as Tabasco (optional)

200 g romaine lettuce, shredded

2 large plum tomatoes, deseeded and chopped

55 g Cheddar or Monterey jack cheese, grated

30 g wholegrain or bean tortilla chips, slightly crumbled

1. Heat the olive oil in a large frying pan over a medium heat. Add the garlic, red and yellow peppers, and onion, and cook for about 5 minutes until softened.

From the Test Kitchen

Add a dollop of low-fat Greek yogurt and maybe a squeeze of lime for a little tang.

---

2. Add the beef, chilli powder and cumin and cook, stirring frequently, for 3–4 minutes until the meat is crumbly and cooked through. Add the beans and salsa, bring to the boil, reduce the heat and allow to simmer for about 2 minutes until the beans are heated through and the flavours are blended. Add the coriander and Tabasco to taste, if using.

3. Divide the lettuce between two large plates or bowls, then top each with half of the meat mixture. Scatter half of the chopped tomato, cheese and tortilla chips over each salad and serve immediately.

NUTRITION INFO: 1 portion provides:

Protein: 1½ servings

Calcium: 1 serving

Vitamin C: 4 servings

Vitamin A: 3 servings

Wholegrains and legumes: ½ serving

Iron: some

Fat: ½ serving

Steak Salad

SERVES 2

No need to trek over to your local steakhouse. Here are steak and salad all on the same plate. You can substitute sliced grilled or roasted portobello mushrooms for the raw mushrooms.

1 x 350 g sirloin steak or tenderloin steak (about 3 cm thick), trimmed of fat
Salt and coarsely ground black pepper
1 teaspoon finely grated lemon zest
2 tablespoons fresh lemon juice
2 tablespoons mayonnaise
Black pepper
1 medium-sized red onion, cut into 5-mm-thick slices
125 g rocket
75 g button mushrooms, thinly sliced
1 roasted red pepper (leftover or from a jar), thinly sliced
55 g Parmesan cheese shavings (see page 251)

1. Preheat the grill or set up the barbecue and preheat it to high.

2. Season the steak all over with salt and coarsely ground pepper. Grill the steak for 3–5 minutes per side until the internal temperature taken with an instant-read meat thermometer is 70°C.

3. Meanwhile, place the lemon zest, lemon juice and mayonnaise in a small bowl and whisk to mix. Season with salt and pepper to taste. Set the dressing aside.

4. Transfer the steak to a chopping board, leaving the grill on. Allow the steak to rest for 5 minutes. Slice it into 5-mm-thick strips. Reserve the meat juices.

5. Grill the onion for about 3 minutes per side until cooked through and slightly charred. Place the cooked onions, rocket, mushrooms and roasted pepper in a large salad bowl and stir to mix. Add the dressing and toss to coat evenly.

6. Divide the rocket mixture between 2 plates. Arrange the steak slices on top and drizzle any meat juice over them. Scatter the Parmesan cheese over the salads and serve.

NUTRITION INFO: 1 portion provides:

Protein: 1½ servings

Calcium: 1 serving

Vitamin C: 2½ servings

Vitamin A: 3 servings

Other fruits and vegetables: 2 servings

Iron: some

Fat: 1 serving

Prawn Caesar Salad

SERVES 2

Is chicken your go-to topper when you're making a a meal out of Caesar salad? It's time to go prawns.

12 large prawns, shelled and deveined
Salt, black pepper and garlic granules
   (optional)
2 teaspoons olive oil
200 g romaine lettuce, shredded
1 medium-sized red pepper,
   thinly sliced
150 g small cherry or grape tomatoes
3 tablespoons Simple Caesar Dressing
   or Tangy Caesar Dressing
   (for both, see facing page)
55 g Parmesan cheese, grated,
   plus more for serving
2 lemon wedges, for serving

1. Preheat the grill. Line a large baking tray with foil.

2. Place the prawns in a bowl and toss with olive oil. Season with salt, pepper and garlic granules, if using.

The Heart of the Matter

Love a good Caesar salad, but not so crazy about your post-Caesar breath? Removing the central core of the garlic before using it raw makes it easier on your breath – and your tummy. Or just substitute ⅛ teaspoon of garlic granules. Or skip the garlic altogether.

From the Test Kitchen

There's always room at the top of a Caesar for the old standard – grilled chicken breast. Grilled salmon's another tasty possibility – or sliced steak.

3. Transfer the prawns to the baking tray and arrange in a single layer without overlapping.

4. Grill the prawns for about 4 minutes until cooked through and opaque. Set aside.

5. Place the lettuce, red pepper, tomatoes, salad dressing and Parmesan cheese in a salad bowl and toss to mix.

6. Divide the salad between 2 salad plates and top each with 6 prawns. Serve with lemon wedges and more Parmesan, if desired.

NUTRITION INFO: 1 portion (without dressing) provides:

Protein: 1 serving

Calcium: 1 serving

Vitamin C: 4 servings

Vitamin A: 3 servings

Omegas: some

Simple Caesar Dressing

MAKES ABOUT 125 ML

A traditional Caesar dressing made with raw or barely cooked egg could be off the menu when you're expecting (unless the eggs have the British Lion stamp or are pasteurised). What's a pregnant Caesar-craver to do? Toss your salad with this creamy dressing, which swaps mayo for the eggs and oil. Not sold on anchovies? Add just a little at a time, or substitute a splash of Worcestershire sauce, which approximates the salty, briny flavour.

1 teaspoon chopped garlic (if raw garlic
    bothers you, see the box on page 262)
Salt
4 tablespoons fresh lemon juice
4 tablespoons mayonnaise
1 anchovy fillet, drained and roughly
    chopped, plus more to taste (optional)
4 tablespoons grated Parmesan cheese,
    plus more to taste
Coarsely ground black pepper

Place the garlic and ¼ teaspoon salt in a small bowl and mash with a fork to form a paste. Transfer to a blender or food processor, add the lemon juice, mayonnaise, anchovy and Parmesan, and purée to form a smooth dressing. Season with more salt, Parmesan and coarsely ground pepper to taste.

NUTRITION INFO: 1 portion
(4 tablespoons) provides:

Calcium: ½ serving

Vitamin C: ½ serving

Fat: 2 servings

Tangy Caesar Dressing

MAKES ABOUT 250 ML

Here's a dressing that's full of flavour but not full of fat.

4 tablespoons buttermilk
4 tablespoons natural full-fat yogurt
4 tablespoons grated Parmesan cheese,
    plus more to taste
2 tablespoons fresh lemon juice, plus
    more to taste
2 tablespoons mayonnaise or olive oil,
    plus more mayonnaise to taste
1 clove garlic, very finely chopped
    (if raw garlic bothers you, see the
    box on page 262)
1 teaspoon chopped shallot
2 anchovy fillets, drained (optional)
½ teaspoon Worcestershire sauce,
    plus more to taste
Salt and black pepper

Place the buttermilk, yogurt, Parmesan cheese, lemon juice, mayonnaise or oil, garlic, shallot, anchovies, if using, and Worcestershire in a blender or food processor and pulse until combined. Taste for seasoning, adding more Parmesan, lemon juice, mayonnaise and/or Worcestershire as necessary, and salt and pepper to taste. If you prefer, you can toss more Parmesan with the salad rather than add it to the dressing.

NUTRITION INFO: 1 portion
(4 tablespoons) provides:

Calcium: almost 1 serving

Fat: ½ serving

Salmon Salad Niçoise

SERVES 2

Have leftovers from last night's grilled salmon feast? Use them to top this delicious dinner (or lunchtime) salad.

12 asparagus stalks, cut into
    7.5-cm pieces
200 g romaine lettuce, shredded
2 x 115-g cooked skinless salmon fillets
4 small red potatoes, cooked and
    quartered
2 plum tomatoes, quartered
2 large hard-boiled eggs, quartered
25 g pitted kalamata olives, sliced
2 teaspoons drained capers
3 tablespoons fresh lemon juice
3 tablespoons olive oil
2 teaspoons Dijon mustard
1½ teaspoons fresh tarragon leaves,
    chopped or ½ teaspoon dried
Salt and black pepper

1. Steam the asparagus, following the instructions on page 315, for 4–6 minutes until crisp-tender, depending on thickness. Pat dry with kitchen paper.

2. Divide the lettuce between 2 plates and place a salmon fillet on top of each. Surround the salmon with the asparagus, potatoes, tomatoes, eggs and olives, dividing them equally between the plates. Top the salmon with the capers, dividing them equally.

3. Place the lemon juice, olive oil, mustard and tarragon in a small bowl and whisk to mix. Season with salt and pepper to taste. Spoon the dressing over the salads, then serve.

NUTRITION INFO: 1 portion provides:

Protein: 1 serving plus

Vitamin C: 2 servings

Vitamin A: 2 servings

Fat: 1½ servings

Omegas: some

From the Test Kitchen

No leftover salmon in the fridge? Just open up a tin. Can't find asparagus this time of year? Crisp-tender whole green beans make a classic substitute.

Prawn and Mango Salad with Sesame Ginger Vinaigrette

SERVES 2

Do the dog days of summer have you panting for something refreshing? Chill out with this salad – super simple if you buy the prawns already cooked. It's equally yummy with cubes of cooked chicken or turkey.

12 large prawns, shelled and deveined
140 g baby salad leaves
1 pickling cucumber, peeled and thinly
    sliced (you can substitute ¼ of a
    regular cucumber)
Sesame Ginger Vinaigrette
    (recipe follows)
1 ripe mango, thinly sliced
1 medium-sized red pepper, thinly sliced

1. If the prawns are not already cooked, steam them, following the instructions on page 315, for 4–5 minutes until they are cooked through and turn opaque. Transfer to a bowl and refrigerate until chilled. (You can also use grilled prawns.)

2. Place the salad leaves and cucumber in a salad bowl. Add 4 tablespoons of the Sesame Ginger Vinaigrette and toss to mix. Divide the salad leaves between 2 salad plates.

3. Place the prawns, mango and red pepper in the salad bowl. Toss with enough of the remaining vinaigrette to coat evenly. Top the salad leaves with the prawn mixture and serve.

NUTRITION INFO: 1 portion
(without dressing) provides:

Protein: 1 serving

Vitamin C: 3 servings

Vitamin A: 3 servings

Other fruits and vegetables: ½ serving

Sesame Ginger Vinaigrette

MAKES ABOUT 125 ML

The sweet and tangy punch of this Oriental-inspired dressing comes from seasoned rice vinegar.

2 spring onions (white and light green
    parts), trimmed and thinly sliced
1 tablespoon grated peeled fresh ginger
1 tablespoon chopped fresh coriander
¼ teaspoon chopped garlic (if raw garlic
    bothers you, see the box on page 262;
    optional)
75 ml seasoned rice vinegar
1 tablespoon extra virgin olive oil
1 tablespoon low-salt soy sauce
1 tablespoon sesame oil
Black pepper

Place the spring onions, ginger, coriander, garlic, if using, rice vinegar, olive oil, soy sauce and sesame oil in a small bowl and whisk to mix. Add black pepper to taste.

NUTRITION INFO: 1 portion
(4 tablespoons) provides:

Fat: 1 serving

From the Test Kitchen

Open, sesame: if you have sesame seeds to hand (preferably toasted), toss a couple of tablespoons with the leaves for a nutty crunch.

Pregnant Cobb Salad

SERVES 2

Craving a Cobb salad but concerned about how it fits into your pregnancy profile? It's easy. Just opt for freshly cooked chicken or turkey instead of cold meats, and reach for pasteurised blue cheese (with the other fixings). Serve it with the American Southwest Russian Dressing (recipe follows) or Yogurt Ranch (or Yogurt Blue cheese); see page 291.

200 g romaine lettuce, shredded
225 g cooked chicken or turkey breast, cubed
2 small tomatoes, chopped, or
   150 g cherry tomatoes, halved
1 small ripe avocado, thinly sliced
55 g blue cheese, crumbled
4 rashers turkey bacon, cooked until crisp
   and crumbled (optional)
2 hard-boiled eggs, chopped

1. Divide the lettuce between 2 large bowls or plates.

2. Place half the chicken in each bowl, arranged in the centre in a straight line.

3. Place half the tomatoes and avocado in a line on either side of the chicken, then distribute the blue cheese

crumbles, bacon, if using, and egg in lines across the top of the salad, in whatever order you'd like.

4. Serve with the dressing on the side.

NUTRITION INFO: 1 portion provides:

Protein: 1 serving plus

Calcium: 1 serving

Vitamin A: 2 servings

Omegas: some

Other fruits and vegetables: 1 serving

American Southwest Russian Dressing

MAKES ABOUT 250 ML

Pair your Pregnant Cobb Salad with this Russian dressing, which has a zippy taste of the American Southwest and the tangy taste of buttermilk. It's also good with a simple chopped lettuce and tomato salad. Use any left over as a dip for veggies or a spread on sandwiches.

125 ml buttermilk
4 tablespoons ready-prepared mild salsa
   (preferably a chunky tomato one)
2 tablespoons mayonnaise
1 tablespoon chopped fresh flat-leaf
   parsley
2 teaspoons fresh lemon juice
¼ teaspoon mustard powder
1 tablespoon sweet pickle relish
Salt and black pepper

From the Test Kitchen

Like your Russian dressing sweet? Add honey to taste. Like it spicy? Spike it with hot red pepper sauce.

Place the buttermilk, salsa, mayonnaise, parsley, lemon juice and mustard in a blender and blend at a low speed until smooth. Transfer the dressing to a bowl and stir in the pickle relish. Season with salt and pepper to taste. The dressing can be stored in the refrigerator, covered, for 2 days.

NUTRITION INFO: 1 portion (4 tablespoons) provides:

Fat: ½ serving

Building a Salad in a Jar

L ove a good salad for lunch – but not one that's good and soggy by the time you get around to eating it? Had one too many leaky dressing incidents in your car or on your clothes? Take your salad to work in a jar. That's right – a salad in a preserving jar makes the perfect take-along lunch. No sog, no spills – just crunchy, fresh-tasting, perfectly dressed salad to go.

Think complicated pickling techniques (and your great-grandmother) when you think of preserving jars, aka 'putting up'? Don't be put off. You're not sealing your salad for the winter – just for lunch. All you need to know is how hungry you'll be when lunch rolls around. A 450-ml (1-lb) jar will satisfy most salad cravings, but to fill a larger appetite, go for the 950-ml (2-lb) size. Then get ready to layer.

Layer 1: Dressing. This ALWAYS goes on the bottom.

Layer 2: Proteins and grains. Grains such as quinoa and farro, along with proteins such as chicken, steak, chickpeas or edamame (basically anything large and chunky) go next. This allows your grains and proteins to marinate while protecting your more delicate top layers from getting soggy.

Layer 3: Everything else except salad leaves. Combinations, such as cucumbers, halved cherry tomatoes and grated Cheddar cheese, can be packed atop cooked proteins.

Layer 4: Top your jar with salad leaves: mixed lettuce, chopped romaine hearts, baby spinach, rocket, baby kale, etc.

How to eat: Simply turn your salad in a jar upside down and gently shake to distribute your dressing. Remove the top and eat right out of the jar. Or pour the ingredients into a bowl and stir to coat.

Winning Combinations:

1. Lemon-oregano vinaigrette, chopped grilled chicken breast, cucumber, cherry tomatoes, pecorino cheese and chopped romaine hearts

2. Balsamic dressing, farro, edamame, cubed cooked beetroot or cooked sweet potato, and baby spinach

3. Creamy dressing, chickpeas, thinly sliced steak, quinoa, diced peppers, shaved Parmesan and baby kale

Pickled Vegetables

SERVES 10

Already polished off that jar of pickles and still craving more? How about pickles that satisfy more than your cravings? Just about any veggie can be pickled, but picking ones that pack in nutrients (say, carrots or cauliflower) gives you that pickled pleasure with a vitamin boost. Feeling fruity? Pickle some mango.

250 ml unseasoned rice vinegar

1 tablespoon salt

1 tablespoon sugar

2 bay leaves

2 teaspoons mustard seeds

2 teaspoons black peppercorns

2 teaspoons coriander seeds

4 thin slices fresh ginger, peeled

450 g vegetables, such as topped and
    tailed green beans, cauliflower florets,
    quartered carrots, thinly sliced red
    onions or cucumbers

1. Wash two wide-mouthed 450-ml (1-lb) preserving jars and their lids well with warm, soapy water; dry completely.

2. Place the vinegar, 250 ml water, the salt and sugar in a medium-sized nonreactive saucepan and bring to the boil over a medium-high heat, stirring to dissolve the salt and sugar.

3. Divide the bay leaves, mustard seeds, peppercorns, coriander seeds and ginger between the two jars. Tightly pack the vegetables into the jars. Carefully pour the vinegar mixture over the vegetables, filling to within 1 cm from the top. Seal tightly and allow to cool to room temperature. Refrigerate for 24 hours before serving. Pickled vegetables will keep refrigerated, tightly closed, for up to 2 months.

Meat

. . . .

H as red meat always been your guilty pleasure? Well, lose the guilt – and bring on the pleasure. Red meat gets a green light when you're expecting for a couple of reasons. First, cholesterol's not a concern for the pregnant set. Secondly, red meat is among the best sources of dietary iron, plus it packs plenty of protein and other pregnancy-friendly nutrients (such as the B vitamins) into every bite (omega-3s, too, if you use grass-fed beef or buffalo). Whether you're looking for comfort food (in a perfect winter warmer such as Tomato-Layered Mini Meat Loaves or a good old-fashioned Slow-Cooker Roast Beef), or you're craving contemporary (such as Pork Medallions with Rocket and Tomatoes or Beef Kebabs with Cumin Marinade), or you'd like to put an international spin on supper (with Ginger Beef Stir-Fry or Mexican Lasagne), there's a meat recipe for everyone in this section. So dig in like the carnivore you've always wanted to be.

Ginger Beef Stir-Fry

SERVES 2

P robably quicker than a takeaway, this stir-fry can be on your table in less than 20 minutes – without those leaky cardboard containers. A boldly sauced and delicious combination of rump steak, red pepper, carrots and broccoli cooks up in no time flat, and packs in both protein and vitamins. A bonus: the ginger is great for queasy days. Sniff some while you cook. The stir-fry is just as tasty prepared with chicken, turkey, lean pork, firm tofu or prawns. Have leftovers? Mix them with soba (buckwheat) or other wholegrain noodles and toss in another tablespoon or so of ginger sauce.

Cooking oil spray

3 teaspoons sesame oil

225 g lean boneless beef (such as rump
    steak), thinly sliced

1 clove garlic, very finely chopped

1 medium-sized red pepper, sliced

100 g small broccoli florets

75 g baby carrots

2 spring onions (white and light green
    parts), trimmed and thinly sliced

4 tablespoons low-salt beef stock

Ginger Sauce (recipe follows)

1 tablespoon chopped fresh coriander

200 g cooked brown rice, for serving
    (optional)

Cook It Once, Eat It All Week

If you cook 450 g of brown rice or other wholegrain once a week, you can simply reheat smaller portions in the microwave. It will take only a minute or two to reheat 100 g rice.

1. Coat a large frying pan with cooking oil spray. Add 1 teaspoon of the sesame oil and heat over a medium-high heat. Add the beef and stir-fry for about 5 minutes until coloured and cooked through. Remove the beef and set aside.

Want to Beef Up?

Most of the recipes in this section call for 115 g of meat per serving, not only because that's all you need to net a protein serving, but also because smaller portions are easier for a pregnant tummy to handle. But if you've got the appetite for a bigger slab, knock yourself out with it – eat a 175-g portion and tally up 1½ protein servings . . . or on a really hungry day, tackle 225 g and count out 2 servings. Score omega-3s whenever you choose grass-fed beef.

2. Add the remaining 2 teaspoons sesame oil to the skillet and heat over a medium-high heat. Add the garlic and cook for about 1 minute until its flavour is released. Add the red pepper, broccoli, carrots and spring onions and cook for about 2 minutes until slightly softened. Add the beef stock. Turn the heat down to medium, cover and allow to cook, stirring occasionally, for about 3 minutes until the vegetables are tender but still slightly crunchy.

3. Return the beef to the pan. Turn the heat to high, add the Ginger Sauce and cook, stirring frequently, for about 2 minutes until heated through. Sprinkle the coriander over the stir-fry. Serve over brown rice.

NUTRITION INFO: 1 portion (with sauce) provides:

Protein: 1 serving

Vitamin C: 3½ servings

Vitamin A: 3½ servings

Wholegrains and legumes: 1 serving

Iron: some

Fat: ½ serving

Ginger Sauce

MAKES ABOUT 75 ML

This assertive ginger-flavoured sauce can be tossed with just about any stir-fry. If you like a little heat, include a dash or two of your favourite hot sauce.

**1 tablespoon grated peeled fresh ginger
or ½ teaspoon ground ginger**
2 tablespoons rice vinegar
1 tablespoon low-salt beef stock
2 teaspoons honey or soft brown sugar
2 tablespoons low-salt soy sauce
2 teaspoons sesame oil

Place the ginger, rice vinegar, beef stock, honey, soy sauce and sesame oil in a small bowl and whisk to mix.

Stir-Fry Made Even Easier

Stir-frying is probably one of the quickest ways to get dinner on the table. The only time-consuming part is the chopping, grating and slicing involved in prepping the ingredients for the wok or frying pan. Fortunately for the perpetually time challenged, there's good news on that front: almost everything you'd want to toss into a stir-fry can be bought ready-prepared. Check your supermarket's meat section for pre-sliced beef, lamb, pork, chicken or turkey. Scan the produce aisles for chopped, sliced, shredded or peeled fresh onions, garlic, broccoli, cauliflower, cabbage, carrots and peppers. And if the produce section is running on empty, head to the frozen food aisle for some ready-to-use veggies.

Slow Cooker Beef Stew

SERVES 6

Entered the pregnancy hunger zone and trying to eat your way out? A big bowl of this hearty stew will get the job done, guaranteed. Let the slow cooker do the heavy lifting while you're at work or on the run, then get busy chowing down. Table for 2 (and a baby) tonight? You'll have plenty of leftovers to look forward to.

2 teaspoons olive oil, divided

900 g boneless braising steak, trimmed and cut into 4-cm pieces

2 teaspoon coarse salt

½ teaspoon black pepper

2 teaspoon fresh thyme leaves

700 ml low-salt beef stock

1 cup sliced celery

2 cups chopped carrots

5 cloves garlic, peeled and crushed

175 g uncooked farro

1 x 400 g tin chopped tomatoes, drained

2 tablespoons wholegrain mustard

1 tablespoon red wine vinegar

150 g frozen green peas, thawed

1. Heat 1 teaspoon oil in a large heavy frying pan over a high heat. Season the beef with salt and pepper and place half of it in the pan. Sear the beef on all sides until well coloured. Remove the beef from the pan and set aside on a plate. Repeat with remaining oil and beef.

2. Pour the stock into the frying pan and bring to the boil, scraping up any brown bits from the bottom of the pan.

3. Pour the stock into a 5–5.5-litre slow cooker. Stir in thyme, celery, carrots, garlic, farro, tomatoes and seared meat. Cook on LOW for 7 hours until beef and farro are tender. Stir in mustard, vinegar and peas. The stew can be refrigerated, covered, for up to 2 days.

NUTRITION INFO: 1 portion provides:

Protein: 1½ servings

Vitamin C: ½ serving

Vitamin A: 1 serving

Other fruits and vegetables: 1 serving

Wholegrains and legumes: 1 serving

Iron: from the beef

Many Peppers Steak Bake

SERVES 2

Many peppers plus one baking tray make for a super-healthy version of a classic Chinese dish that's almost as easy as ordering in. A variety of veggies add both colour and nutrients, while the cashews add crunch. Serve over brown rice.

225 g boneless lean beef such as rump
   steak, thinly sliced
1 medium-sized red pepper,
   cut into 5-mm-wide strips
1 medium-sized yellow pepper,
   cut into 5-mm-wide strips
1 medium-sized orange pepper,
   cut into 5-mm-wide strips
1 medium-sized green pepper,
   cut into 5-mm-wide strips
55 g carrots, grated
½ large red onion, thinly sliced
2 tablespoons olive oil
½ teaspoon coarse salt
¼ teaspoon black pepper
¼ teaspoon garlic granules
1 teaspoon ground ginger
¼ teaspoon dried chilli flakes (optional)
2 tablespoons low-salt soy sauce
1 tablespoons soft brown sugar
75 ml low-salt beef stock
30 g toasted cashews (see page 217)
200 g cooked brown rice (optional)

1. Place a baking tray in the oven and preheat the grill. (Do not remove the baking tray while the grill preheats.)

2. Place the steak, peppers, carrots, onion, olive oil, salt, pepper, garlic granules, ginger and chilli flakes, if using, in a large bowl, stirring until well mixed. Transfer the meat to a separate bowl. Spread the vegetables in a single layer on the hot baking tray. Grill for about 10 minutes until the vegetables are charred and mostly tender. Push the vegetables to the ends of the tray and spread the steak slices and any juices from the meat in a single layer in the centre. Grill until the meat is charred and your desired degree of doneness – about 3 minutes for medium-rare.

3. Meanwhile, combine the soy sauce, sugar and beef stock in a small saucepan and whisk to mix. Bring to the boil over a high heat and cook for 2 minutes until the sugar has dissolved and the sauce has slightly thickened. Stir in the cashews. Serve the steak and peppers over rice, if wished, pouring the sauce on top.

NUTRITION INFO: 1 portion provides:

Protein: 1 serving

Vitamin C: 4 servings

Vitamin A: 3 servings

Other fruits and vegetables: ½ serving

Wholegrains and legumes: 1 serving

Iron: some

Fat: 1 serving

Beef Kebabs with Cumin Marinade

SERVES 2

Here's a meal on a stick – once you've placed the stick over some couscous, quinoa, brown rice or other grain. You'll need to plan ahead a bit: the beef marinates for at least 3 hours (marinate in the morning, enjoy at night). If you are using wooden skewers, soak them in water first for 30 minutes.

225 g lean beef such as top sirloin, well
    trimmed and cut into 1-inch pieces
2 tablespoons low-salt soy sauce
2 tablespoons fresh lemon juice
1 tablespoon olive oil
1 teaspoon ground cumin
1 large red pepper, cut into 5-cm pieces
½ medium-sized red onion, cut into 5-cm
    pieces
8 button mushrooms, caps only, wiped
    clean
8 cherry or grape tomatoes

1. Place the beef, soy sauce, lemon juice, olive oil and cumin in a bowl and stir to coat the beef evenly with the marinade. Cover the bowl with cling film and refrigerate for at least 3 hours or as long as overnight.

2. Preheat the grill or set up the barbecue and preheat it to high.

From the Test Kitchen

If you want sweet beef kebabs instead, substitute 2 tablespoons of pineapple juice for the lemon juice, and use pineapple and mango chunks instead of the mushroom caps and tomatoes.

3. Remove the beef from the marinade and thread it on to 4 skewers, alternating peppers, pieces of onion, mushrooms and tomatoes between the pieces of meat. Discard any remaining marinade.

4. Grill the kebabs, turning occasionally, for 8–10 minutes until the beef is tender.

NUTRITION INFO: 1 portion provides:

Protein: 1 serving

Vitamin C: 2½ servings

Vitamin A: 1 serving

Other fruits and vegetables: 1½ servings

Iron: some

Tomato-Layered Mini Meat Loaves

SERVES 6

Comfort food for colder days, served up in mini form for maximum convenience. Leftovers can be easily rewarmed one mini loaf at a time, or sliced for a cold meat loaf sandwich.

900 g lean beef mince
115 g Cheddar cheese, grated
2 tablespoons ketchup
1 medium egg, lightly beaten
3 tablespoons porridge oats
½ teaspoon dried oregano
¼ teaspoon garlic granules
¼ teaspoon salt
¼ teaspoon black pepper
2 medium-sized ripe tomatoes,
    thinly sliced

1. Preheat the oven to 190°C/gas mark 5.

2. Place the beef, Cheddar, ketchup, egg, oats, oregano, garlic granules, salt and pepper in a large bowl and mix them together with a fork. Press half of the beef mixture into six holes of a muffin tin, dividing it evenly among them. Top each meat loaf with a slice of tomato, then press the remaining beef mixture into the holes.

3. Bake the mini meat loaves for about 20 minutes until cooked through.

4. Remove the meat loaves from the tin straight away and serve. Wrap any leftover meat loaves in aluminium foil and refrigerate them. The baked meat

From the Test Kitchen

Not in the mood for beef? Make the meat loaves with 900 g turkey breast mince or lean pork mince instead. Want to A-list your meat loaf? Mix in finely grated carrot.

loaves can be refrigerated for 2 days or frozen for up to 2 weeks. Defrost before reheating. To reheat the defrosted loaves, pop them, still wrapped in foil, in a preheated 180°C/gas mark 4 oven for 10 minutes, or remove the foil and heat in the microwave for 1 minute on high power. The meat loaves can also be frozen uncooked, wrapped in cling film, for up to 1 month. To thaw before cooking, leave the meat loaves in the refrigerator overnight.

NUTRITION INFO: 1 portion provides:

Protein: 1½ servings

Calcium: almost 1 serving

Vitamin C: almost ½ serving

Iron: some

Mexican Lasagne

SERVES 6

Enchiladas, meet lasagne. This Mexican take on the traditional Italian favourite is like a fiesta for your eyes and taste buds – plus, it layers on the nutrients.

2 teaspoons olive oil

1 medium-sized onion, chopped

1 medium-sized red pepper, chopped

2 cloves garlic, very finely chopped

450 g extra-lean ground beef

75 g carrots, grated

1 tablespoon chilli powder

1½ teaspoons ground cumin

1 teaspoon dried oregano

150 g fresh or frozen sweetcorn kernels

240 g enchilada sauce (in the Mexican section in supermarkets or available online)

425 g passata

450 g low-fat cottage cheese

2 medium eggs, lightly beaten

4 tablespoons grated Parmesan cheese

Black pepper

Cooking oil spray

12 small wholegrain corn or flour tortillas

175 g Cheddar cheese, grated

Natural yogurt or soured cream, chopped fresh coriander, chopped fresh tomato and/or chopped black olives, for serving (optional)

1. Preheat the oven to 190°C/gas mark 5.

2. Heat the olive oil in a large non-stick frying pan over a medium heat. Add the onion, red pepper and garlic and cook for about 5 minutes until softened. Add the beef, carrots, chilli powder, cumin and oregano and cook, chopping up the meat with a wooden spoon, for about 10 minutes until the meat cooks through. Stir in the sweetcorn, enchilada sauce and passata and allow to simmer, stirring frequently, for about 5 minutes until the flavours blend.

3. Place the cottage cheese, eggs and Parmesan in a bowl and stir to mix. Season lightly with black pepper. Set aside.

4. Coat a 23 x 33-cm baking dish with cooking oil spray. Place 6 of the tortillas on the bottom (they'll overlap slightly). Spread half of the meat mixture over the tortillas. Spread the cottage cheese mixture over the meat mixture. Arrange the remaining 6 tortillas on top of the cottage cheese mixture. Top the tortillas with the remaining meat mixture.

5. Bake the lasagne for 20 minutes. Remove it from the oven and scatter the Cheddar evenly over the top. Return the lasagne to the oven and bake for about 10 minutes longer until the cheese is melted.

6. Allow the lasagne to stand for 10 minutes before serving. Top with yogurt, coriander, tomato and/or olives, if wished. The lasagne can be refrigerated, covered, for up to 3 days. Reheat leftovers in the microwave.

NUTRITION INFO: 1 portion provides:

Protein: 1½ servings

Calcium: 1 serving

Vitamin C: 1 serving

Vitamin A: 1 serving

Other fruits and vegetables: 1 serving

Wholegrains and legumes: 2 servings

Iron: some

Pork Medallions
with Rocket and Tomatoes

SERVES 2

Here's a very quick dish that's impressive enough for company but easy enough for the busiest weekday. Cook extra pork while you're at it – leftovers make a yummy sandwich with fresh rocket and tomatoes.

Olive oil cooking spray
3 teaspoons olive oil
2 cloves garlic, very finely chopped
   (optional)
225 g pork fillet, cut into 2.5-cm-thick
   slices
Salt and black pepper
2 tablespoons balsamic vinegar
4 ripe plum tomatoes, deseeded and
   chopped
1 x 150–175-g bag rocket or baby spinach
20 g Parmesan cheese, roughly grated

1. Coat a large non-stick frying pan with cooking spray. Add 2 teaspoons of the olive oil and heat over a medium heat. Add the garlic, if using, and cook, stirring, for about 4 minutes until golden.

2. Season the pork slices with salt and pepper and add them to the pan. Increase the heat to medium-high and cook for about 5 minutes per side until the pork is well coloured and cooked through. Transfer the pork to a plate and cover it with aluminium foil to keep warm.

3. Allow the pan to cool for a minute, off the heat. Then heat the pan over a low heat and add the remaining 1 teaspoon oil and the balsamic vinegar, stirring to scrape up any brown bits. Add the tomatoes and stir for 1 minute until the tomatoes are warmed through. Remove from the heat. Add the rocket and toss until wilted. Season with salt and pepper to taste.

4. Spoon the rocket and tomato mixture over the pork, scatter the Parmesan on top and serve immediately.

NUTRITION INFO: 1 portion provides:

Protein: 1 serving

Calcium: ½ serving

Vitamin C: 2 servings

Vitamin A: 3 servings

Iron: some (if using spinach)

Fat: ½ serving

Omegas: some

Pacific Rim Pork Kebabs

SERVES 4

Looking for a super-easy dish with Hawaiian punch? These sweet and tangy pork kebabs are heady with grated ginger and zesty with lime. If using wooden skewers, soak them in water first for 30 minutes. And try subbing chicken or prawns for the pork.

450 g lean pork fillet, cut into 2.5-cm
    cubes

2 medium-sized red peppers, cut into
    2.5-cm pieces

1 x 565-g tin pineapple chunks in juice,
    drained, reserving 4 tablespoons
    of the juice

2 tablespoons fresh lime juice

2 teaspoons rapeseed oil

2 teaspoons grated peeled fresh ginger

1 teaspoon curry powder

1 teaspoon very finely chopped garlic
    (optional)

400 g cooked brown rice, quinoa or
    another wholegrain, for serving

1. Thread the pork, red peppers and pineapple on to 8 skewers, alternating pieces of each. Set the kebabs aside.

2. Place the pineapple juice, lime juice, oil, ginger, curry powder and garlic, if using, in a large resealable plastic bag and squeeze the bag to blend the marinade. Add the kebabs, seal the bag and gently shake and turn the bag to coat the kebabs evenly. Allow the kebabs to marinate for about 30 minutes.

3. Preheat the grill or set up the barbecue and preheat it to high.

4. Remove the kebabs from the marinade and grill, turning occasionally, for about 10 minutes until the pork is cooked through. Discard any remaining marinade. Unskewer the kebabs and serve on top of the brown rice or quinoa.

NUTRITION INFO: 1 portion provides:

Protein: 1 serving

Vitamin C: 3 servings

Vitamin A: 1 serving

Wholegrains and legumes: 1 serving

Pork Fillet with Sweet Potato and Apple Bake

SERVES 2

This one-dish meal is ready for the oven in minutes – the only hard part will be resisting the aroma of the sweet, savoury, deliciously caramelised pork while you're waiting for it to rest after roasting.

Cooking oil spray
225 g pork fillet
2 teaspoons olive oil
1 teaspoon coarse salt
½ teaspoon black pepper
1 medium-sized sweet potato, peeled and cut into 4-mm-thick slices
1 medium-sized apple, cored and cut into 1-cm-thick slices
1½ tablespoons wholegrain mustard
2 teaspoons honey
Grated zest and juice of 1 lemon
1 teaspoon chopped fresh thyme leaves

1. Preheat the oven to 230°C/gas mark 8. Coat a baking tray with cooking oil spray.

2. Pat the pork dry with kitchen paper; rub evenly with 1 teaspoon of the oil. Sprinkle evenly with ½ teaspoon of the salt and ¼ teaspoon of the pepper. Place in the centre of the baking tray.

3. Toss together the sweet potato, apple and the remaining 1 teaspoon oil, ½ teaspoon salt and ¼ teaspoon pepper in a large bowl. Arrange the mixture evenly around the pork on the baking tray.

4. Whisk together the mustard, honey, lemon zest and juice, and thyme in a small bowl. Brush the glaze evenly over the pork, sweet potato and apple.

5. Bake for 15 minutes. Turn on the grill to high and grill for about 5 minutes until the pork is browned on top and the internal temperature taken with an instant-read meat thermometer is 62.8°C. Remove from the oven and allow to rest for about 10 minutes.

6. Transfer the pork to a chopping board and slice. Serve with the sweet potato-apple mixture.

NUTRITION INFO: 1 portion provides:

Protein: 1 serving
Vitamin C: ½ serving
Vitamin A: 1 serving
Other fruits and vegetables: 1 serving

Poultry

....

T ired of the same old chicken that tastes, well, like chicken? Here's a flock of recipes that'll shake (and bake and fry and grill) the way you feel about the UK's favourite bird. Want to fill your plate with something healthy and crunchy? Try Oven-Fried Chicken Breasts. Take your bird on a round-the-world tour with Basque Chicken. Or play it safe – and soothing – with Apricot Ginger Glazed Chicken. Talking turkey? You will be once you try Turkey with Corn and Edamame Salsa and Turkey Steaks in Mushroom Sauce. What's more, since most of these recipes serve 4, you can get 2 meals for half the cooking effort. Serve leftovers on salads or in sandwiches.

Rosemary Lemon Chicken

SERVES 4

A simple vinaigrette of fragrant fresh rosemary and tangy lemon brightens this super-simple chicken dish, making it perfect for a quick meal or leisurely dinner. Serve it hot the first night, and serve the leftovers (if there are any) cold the next night, perhaps sliced over a salad. Or make a tasty sandwich or wrap for lunch.

1 tablespoon chopped fresh rosemary
1 tablespoon drained capers
1 teaspoon chopped garlic (optional)

1 teaspoon olive oil
Juice of 1 medium-sized lemon, plus
    1 lemon, very thinly sliced
1 tablespoon pine nuts
4 x 115-g skinless, boneless chicken
    breast halves
Salt and black pepper

1. Preheat the oven to 180°C/gas mark 4.

2. Place the rosemary, capers, garlic, if using, olive oil, lemon juice and pine nuts in a small bowl and stir to mix. Set aside.

3. Place the lemon slices in a single layer in a baking dish large enough to hold the chicken breasts in a single layer. Season the chicken breasts with a pinch each of salt and pepper, then place them on top of the lemon slices. Spoon about a tablespoon of the rosemary mixture over each chicken breast. Bake the chicken for 20–25 minutes until it is no longer pink inside.

NUTRITION INFO: 1 portion provides:

Protein: 1 serving

Omegas: some

Oven-Fried Chicken Breasts

SERVES 2

Who needs a takeaway? These chicken breasts are crunchy on the outside, moist on the inside, completely greaseless – and still finger-licking good.

50 g dried wholemeal breadcrumbs
4 tablespoons grated Parmesan cheese
1 teaspoon paprika
½ teaspoon garlic granules
Salt and black pepper
75 ml buttermilk (or add 1 teaspoon lemon juice to 75 ml milk; rest for 5 minutes)
1 tablespoon Dijon mustard (optional)
1 tablespoon mayonnaise
Olive oil cooking spray
2 x 115-g skinless, boneless chicken breast halves

1. Preheat the oven to 200°C/gas mark 6.

2. Place the breadcrumbs, Parmesan, paprika and garlic granules in a large shallow bowl and stir to mix. Season with salt and pepper to taste.

3. Place the buttermilk, mustard, if using, and mayonnaise in another shallow bowl and stir to mix.

4. Coat a baking sheet with olive oil cooking spray. Dip the chicken breasts in the buttermilk mixture, then dredge them in the breadcrumb mixture. Place the breasts on the baking tray. Spray the breasts with a little olive oil, too. Bake the chicken for about 25 minutes until it is no longer pink inside.

NUTRITION INFO: 1 portion provides:

Protein: 1 serving

Calcium: ½ serving

Wholegrains and legumes: 1 serving

Fat: ½ serving

Omegas: some

Bigger Breasts?

The recipes in this section call for 115 g of chicken or turkey per person – because that's all you need for 1 portion. Plus, petite portions are easier on pregnant digestion. But if you've got the appetite – and larger breasts in your refrigerator – go right ahead and enjoy. If you use 175-g breasts, count yourself in for 1½ protein servings. Or go for a full 225 g and score 2 full servings. Score extra omega-3s by choosing free-range or organic chicken that enjoy access to the outdoors.

Chunky Tomato Chicken Parmesan

SERVES 2

Mamma mia! Baby's going to love this dish because it's nutritious – but you're going to love it because it's super easy and super yummy. Vitamin-packed roasted peppers, rich tomato sauce, chopped fresh tomatoes and a blanket of cheese top chicken breasts in a healthy remake of an old Italian favourite. Extra-hungry? Serve the chicken on pasta. Sandwich any leftovers into your favourite roll for a filling lunch.

4 tablespoons wholemeal breadcrumbs

2 tablespoons grated Parmesan cheese

2 x 115-g skinless, boneless chicken
   breast halves

Salt and coarsely ground black pepper

½ teaspoon dried oregano

½ roasted red pepper (leftover or from
   a jar), cut into 4 strips

125 g good-quality ready-prepared
   tomato-based pasta sauce

90 g deseeded ripe tomatoes, chopped

2 x 25-g slices provolone cheese (available
   from cheese specialists) or halloumi
   cheese, or 50 g grated mozzarella

1. Preheat the oven to 180°C/gas mark 4.

2. Place the breadcrumbs and Parmesan cheese in a small bowl and stir to mix, then set aside.

3. Season the chicken breasts lightly with salt and pepper and the oregano. Place them in a baking dish. Scatter the breadcrumb mixture evenly over the chicken. Top each chicken breast with 2 strips roasted pepper, half of the pasta sauce and half of the tomatoes. Place half the cheese on top of each breast. Bake the chicken for about 25 minutes until it is no longer pink inside.

NUTRITION INFO: 1 portion provides:

Protein: 1 serving

Calcium: 1 serving

Vitamin C: 1½ servings

Vitamin A: ½ serving

Wholegrains and legumes: ½ serving

Omegas: some

Apricot Ginger Glazed Chicken

SERVES 2

Craving something sweet but in the market for dinner, not dessert? Here's the ticket. An added bonus for queasy mums: The ginger is sure to soothe. Serve the chicken with a wild rice or quinoa pilau tossed with dried apricots and toasted slivered almonds.

1 tablespoon all-fruit apricot preserve

½ tablespoon low-salt soy sauce

½ teaspoon ground ginger

⅛ teaspoon cayenne pepper (optional)

2 x 115-g skinless, boneless chicken
   breast halves

Salt and black pepper (optional)

1. Place the apricot preserve, soy sauce, ginger and cayenne, if using, in a small bowl and stir to mix. Divide the apricot and ginger glaze in half and set aside.

2. Preheat the grill or set up the barbecue and preheat it to high.

3. Lightly season the chicken breast halves with salt and pepper, if desired, then brush one side of each with half of the glaze. Grill the chicken glazed side up for 5–6 minutes. Turn the chicken over, brush the second side with the other portion of the glaze and grill for a further 5–6 minutes until it is no longer pink inside.

NUTRITION INFO: 1 portion provides:

Protein: 1 serving

Omegas: some

Teriyaki Chicken

SERVES 2

Just about anything you're cooking – from turkey, beef or pork to salmon, from firm tofu to portobello mushrooms – tastes better prepared teriyaki style. Serve the chicken with brown rice and a veggie stir-fry. Turn leftovers into a sandwich: layer chicken with salad leaves, grated carrot and sliced cucumber on your favourite bread or wrap with a touch of mayo.

2 tablespoons low-salt soy sauce
1 tablespoon honey
1½ teaspoons grated peeled fresh ginger
   or ½ teaspoon ground ginger
1 teaspoon sesame oil
1 tablespoon chopped fresh coriander or
   ½ teaspoon ground coriander
2 x 115-g skinless, boneless chicken
   breast halves

1. Place the soy sauce, honey, ginger, sesame oil and coriander in a small bowl and whisk to mix.

2. Place the chicken in a baking dish and pour the teriyaki marinade over it, turning the breasts to coat them evenly. The chicken can marinate, covered, in the refrigerator for up to 8 hours.

3. Preheat the grill or set up the barbecue and preheat it to high.

4. Grill the chicken for 5–6 minutes per side until it is no longer pink inside.

NUTRITION INFO: 1 portion provides:

Protein: 1 serving

Omegas: some

Cooking in a Parcel

Love a home-cooked meal but hate the clean-up that comes after? Skip the pots and pans, and cook your dinner in a parcel! Most any combination of poultry, meat or fish with vegetables and seasonings can be adapted to pouch cooking. All you need is a lot of aluminium foil and a little imagination. (You can also cook parcels in baking paper or parchment roasting bags. Don't overstuff, to allow the parchment to expand.) Here are some tips:

- Choose ingredients that cook quickly – boneless chicken breasts instead of legs; grated carrots, not chunks; and courgette rather than squash. Extra-firm tofu also works well in a parcel.

- Tear off a square of heavy-duty aluminium foil large enough to completely enclose one portion of meat or fish and veggies and place it on a work surface.

- Layer the ingredients you want to cook on the foil, starting with the heaviest, such as sliced onions and strips of beef and ending with the lightest ones such as mushrooms. Top everything with herbs and other seasonings.

- Season aggressively, using generous amounts of spices and fresh herbs – more than you would ordinarily. They'll have to stand up to the steam created in the parcel.

- If the ingredients aren't likely to form a sauce (tomatoes will, cabbage won't), pour a couple of tablespoons of stock, a little soy sauce or a few squeezes of lemon, lime or orange juice over everything. Citrus slices make an ideal addition to many fish and poultry parcels.

- Fold the foil over the ingredients and crimp the edges all around to seal the parcel very tightly. This will seal in the steam and those very intense flavours and aromas.

- Bake the parcel on a baking tray in a hot oven, 200°C/gas mark 6. Cooking times vary, depending on the ingredients you use, but will usually be between 15 and 25 minutes.

- For a dramatic and aromatic presentation, open the foil parcel at the table, but do it carefully. The escaping steam is very hot, so keep your face and hands out of harm's way.

Chicken Enchiladas

SERVES 4

In this case, the whole enchilada offers a whole lot of nutrition – and flavour – but very little fat. Plus, leftovers reheat deliciously.

450 g skinless, boneless chicken breasts, cut into 1-cm cubes

1 medium-sized red pepper, cut into small dice

1–2 mild green chillies, chopped, or to taste

2 teaspoons chilli powder

½ teaspoon dried oregano

Pinch of salt

1 tablespoon plus 2 teaspoons olive oil

1 x 400-g tin chopped tomatoes, with their juices

425 g tinned black beans, drained and rinsed

285 g enchilada sauce (in the Mexican section in supermarkets or available online)

4 large wholegrain corn tortillas (30 cm in diameter)

55 g each Cheddar and Monterey jack cheese or 115 g Cheddar cheese only, grated

1. Preheat the oven to 150°C/gas mark 2.

2. Place the chicken, red pepper, chillies, chilli powder, oregano, salt and 1 tablespoon of the olive oil in a large bowl and toss to mix.

3. Heat the remaining 2 teaspoons olive oil in a large non-stick frying pan over a medium heat. Add the chicken mixture and cook 5–7 minutes until the

chicken is no longer pink inside. Add the tomatoes with their juices and the black beans and cook for about 3 minutes until heated through.

4. Place the enchilada sauce in a small saucepan over a medium heat and cook for 3–5 minutes until heated through.

5. Brush a tortilla with a little of the enchilada sauce. Spoon one-quarter of the chicken mixture into the centre of a tortilla and roll it up. Place the filled tortilla in a 23 x 33-cm baking dish, join side down. Repeat with the remaining tortillas and chicken mixture. Pour the remaining enchilada sauce over the filled tortillas and scatter the cheese on top.

6. Bake the enchiladas for 15–20 minutes until the cheese melts. If you are not ready to serve the enchiladas immediately, reduce the oven temperature to 110°C/gas mark ¼; the enchiladas will keep warm until you're ready to eat.

NUTRITION INFO: 1 portion provides:

Protein: 1½ servings

Calcium: 1 serving

Vitamin C: 2 servings

Vitamin A: 1 serving

Wholegrains and legumes: 2 servings

Iron: some

Fat: ½ serving

Omegas: some

Basque Chicken

SERVES 2

In this rustic dish, the combination of tomatoes, kalamata olives and peppers that have practically melted through slow cooking gives the chicken a distinctively Spanish flavour. Serve it over a bed of wholegrain rice or quinoa.

2 teaspoons olive oil
225 g skinless, boneless chicken breasts,
   sliced into 1-cm-long strips
½ medium-sized Spanish onion,
   thinly sliced
2 cloves garlic, thinly sliced
1 small red pepper, cut into julienne strips
1 small green pepper, cut into
   julienne strips
1 small yellow or orange pepper,
   cut into julienne strips
240 g drained tinned chopped tomatoes
25 g pitted kalamata olives, halved
2 teaspoons fresh thyme leaves
1 teaspoon smoked paprika and a pinch
   of dried chilli flakes, plus more to taste
4 tablespoons chopped fresh flat-leaf
   parsley
Salt and black pepper

1. Heat 1 teaspoon of the olive oil in a large non-stick frying pan over a medium heat. Add the chicken and cook for 5–7 minutes until it is no longer pink inside. Remove the chicken from the pan and set aside.

From the Test Kitchen

Not a fan of a smoky flavour? Swap the smoked paprika for hot paprika or sweet paprika. For a salty tang, top the chicken with crumbled pasteurised feta.

2. Add the remaining teaspoon of olive oil to the pan along with the onion, garlic and peppers, reduce the heat to medium-low and cook for about 8 minutes until softened. Stir in the tomatoes, olives, thyme, paprika and 2 tablespoons of the parsley. Cook, stirring frequently, for about 5 minutes until the flavours have blended. Season with salt, pepper and additional paprika to taste. Add the cooked chicken, toss to coat with the sauce and cook until heated through. Scatter the remaining 2 tablespoons parsley over the top.

NUTRITION INFO: 1 portion provides:

Protein: 1 serving

Vitamin C: 5 servings

Vitamin A: 1½ servings

Other fruits and vegetables: 1 serving

Fat: ½ serving

Omegas: some

Turkey Steaks in Mushroom Sauce

SERVES 2

Love mushrooms? You're in for a treat in just minutes. This colourful and flavourful one-pot dish teams turkey with lots of mushrooms (use wild for even more flavour), peas, carrots and fresh herbs. Complement this earthy main – or stretch any leftovers into a meal – by serving it on a bed of wholegrain noodles.

Wholemeal flour
2 x 175-g turkey steaks (1 cm thick; see Note)
Salt and black pepper
Olive oil cooking spray
1 teaspoon olive oil
2 teaspoons butter
2 shallots, very finely chopped
225 g sliced wild or cultivated mushrooms
75 g carrot matchsticks
75 g frozen green peas
1 teaspoon very finely chopped fresh tarragon leaves or ¼ teaspoon dried
2 tablespoons chopped fresh flat-leaf parsley, plus more for garnish
2 tablespoons very finely chopped fresh chives, plus more for garnish
175 ml low-salt chicken stock or mushroom stock

1. Place some flour in a shallow bowl. Season the turkey steaks with salt and pepper, then lightly dredge both sides of each steak in the flour.

2. Coat a large, heavy non-stick frying pan with olive oil spray. Place 1 teaspoon of the olive oil in the pan and heat over a medium heat. Cook the turkey for about 2 minutes per side until coloured but not cooked through. Remove the turkey from the pan and set aside.

3. Coat the frying pan again with olive oil spray, add the butter and melt it over a medium-low heat. Add the shallots and cook for about 2 minutes until slightly softened. Increase the heat to medium-high, add the mushrooms and cook for 2 minutes.

4. Add the carrots, peas, tarragon, parsley, chives and stock and bring to the boil, then lower the heat and simmer for 2 minutes. Return the turkey to the pan. Allow to simmer, stirring frequently, for about 2 minutes until the sauce is slightly reduced and the turkey is cooked through and no longer pink inside. Season with salt and pepper to taste, and garnish with more parsley and chives.

NOTE: If your turkey steaks are more than 1 cm thick, pound them until they are an even 1 cm.

NUTRITION INFO: 1 portion provides:

Protein: 1½ servings

Vitamin C: ½ serving

Vitamin A: 2 servings

Other fruits and vegetables: 3 servings

Fat: ½ serving

Turkey with Corn and Edamame Salsa

SERVES 2

No need to wait until Christmas for this turkey dish – and no need to wait hours for your bird to be ready. Make summer turkey season, too, with a tasty, quick-grilled turkey breast topped with a crisp, cool salsa. New to edamame? This will be a delicious introduction to chewy, nutritious soya beans.

4 plum tomatoes, deseeded and chopped
150 g cooked fresh sweetcorn kernels
(or frozen sweetcorn, thawed)
180 g cooked shelled edamame (soya
beans)
1 teaspoon chilli powder
2 tablespoons chopped fresh coriander,
plus more to taste
2 tablespoons olive oil
2 tablespoons fresh lime juice
Salt and black pepper
225 g turkey steaks
Garlic granules
Olive oil cooking spray
1 medium-sized avocado (preferably
Hass), sliced
4 lime wedges, for serving

1. Place the tomatoes, sweetcorn, edamame, chilli powder, 1 tablespoon of the coriander, 1 tablespoon of the olive oil and the lime juice in a bowl and stir to mix. Season with salt and pepper to taste. Add additional coriander, if wished. Set the salsa aside.

2. Brush the remaining tablespoon of olive oil on the turkey and season it with salt, pepper and garlic granules.

From the Test Kitchen

Here's a time-saving tip: grill double the quantity of turkey steaks while you're at it, then have the leftovers in a sandwich (or in Fruity Turkey Salad, page 220).

3. Coat a large frying pan with olive oil cooking spray and heat over a medium-high heat. Add the turkey and cook for 2–4 minutes per side until completely cooked through and no longer pink inside.

4. To serve, place the turkey on top of the salsa. Sprinkle the remaining tablespoon of coriander over the turkey, then garnish with avocado slices and lime wedges.

NUTRITION INFO: 1 portion provides:

Protein: 1½ servings

Vitamin C: 1 serving

Other fruits and vegetables: 1½ servings

Wholegrains and legumes: 1 serving

Fat: 1 serving

Slow-Cooker Chicken Mole

SERVES 4

A ny day can be Taco Tuesday if you plan ahead. Don't be fooled by the long list of ingredients – the mole sauce blends together in moments. Then, once the slow cooker takes the wheel, the only fingers you'll have to lift are the ones that bring those tacos to your mouth. Double the recipe for double the dinners or lunch leftovers. You can also serve them cold on a salad.

1 dried ancho chilli
4 x 175-g boneless, skinless chicken
    thighs
1 teaspoon coarse salt
425 g tinned whole tomatoes,
    with their juices
1 medium-sized onion, chopped
1 chipotle pepper with 1 tablespoon
    adobo sauce
50 g toasted slivered almonds
    (see page 217)
85 g dark chocolate chips
35 g raisins
4 tablespoons low-salt chicken stock
3 cloves garlic, peeled and crushed
1 tablespoon ground cumin
1 teaspoon ground cinnamon
4 medium (20–25-cm) corn or wholegrain
    flour tortillas, toasted, for serving
Fresh coriander leaves, for serving
55 g Monterey jack cheese or Cheddar
    cheese, grated, for serving
1 lime, cut into wedges, for serving

1. Soak the ancho chilli in hot water for 10 minutes. Drain, discarding the soaking water. Remove the stalk and seeds; set aside the chilli.

2. Place the chicken in a 5.5-litre slow cooker and sprinkle with the salt.

3. Combine the tomatoes, onion, ancho chilli, chipotle, adobo sauce, almonds, chocolate, raisins, chicken stock, garlic, cumin and cinnamon in a food processor or blender; process until smooth.

4. Pour the sauce over the chicken. Cover and cook on LOW for about 8 hours until the chicken is tender.

5. Serve the chicken and sauce, scattered with coriander, with the tortillas, cheese and lime.

NUTRITION INFO: 1 portion provides:

Protein: 1½ servings

Vitamin C: 1 serving

Wholegrains and legumes: 1½ servings

Omegas: some

Chicken Satay Lettuce Wraps

SERVES 2

Chicken breast can easily substitute for the dark meat chicken in this super-fresh, multi-textured wrap. The delicious peanut satay sauce makes enough to toss with your favourite noodles for a yummy chilled noodle salad lunch.

55 g uncooked wholegrain rice vermicelli
noodles
2 x 175-gskinless, boneless chicken
thighs
¼ teaspoon coarse salt
¼ teaspoon black pepper
65 g smooth peanut butter
4 tablespoons well-shaken or stirred
tinned coconut milk
1½ tablespoons fresh lime juice
1 tablespoon low-salt soy sauce
1½ teaspoons sriracha
6 medium Bibb lettuce leaves
75 g red pepper, thinly sliced
Thinly sliced spring onions; chopped
fresh basil leaves; chopped roasted,
salted peanuts, for topping

1. Soak the rice noodles according to packet instructions.

2. Meanwhile, heat a griddle pan over a high heat. Season the chicken with the salt and pepper. Cook for 4–5 minutes per side until charred and no longer pink inside. Transfer to a chopping board and allow to rest for 5 minutes. Thinly slice the chicken across the grain.

3. Whisk together the peanut butter, coconut milk, lime juice, soy sauce and sriracha.

4. Drain the rice noodles. Divide the noodles and chicken slices among the lettuce leaves. Top each with red peppers and drizzle with 1 tablespoon of sauce (or more to taste). Top with spring onions, basil and peanuts; roll up and serve. Extra sauce can be refrigerated, tightly covered, for up to 3 days.

NUTRITION INFO: 1 portion provides:

Protein: 1½ servings

Vitamin C: 1 serving

Vitamin A: 1 serving

Wholegrains and legumes: 1 serving

Fat: 2 servings

Omegas: some

Instant Pot Buffalo Chicken Lettuce Wraps

SERVES 4

Here's how to earn wings for your buffalo chicken – use breasts instead, and wrap them up in lettuce. Add crunch (and tradition) with celery and carrots, and a side of ranch.

125 ml low-salt chicken stock
4 tablespoons Buffalo-style hot sauce
4 x 115-g skinless, boneless chicken
    breasts
¼ teaspoon coarse salt
6 medium-sized butte lettuce leaves
175 g carrots, grated
175 g celery, chopped
250 ml ranch dressing, recipe follows

1. Combine the chicken stock and hot sauce in a programmable pressure multicooker (such as an Instant Pot). Place the chicken in the liquid and sprinkle it with the salt. Cover the cooker with its lid and lock it in place. Turn the steam release handle to the SEALING position. Select the MANUAL/PRESSURE COOK setting. Select HIGH pressure for 4 minutes. (It will take about 5 minutes for the cooker to come up to pressure before cooking begins.)

2. Carefully turn the steam release handle to the VENTING position and let the steam fully escape. (This will take about 3 minutes.) Remove the lid from the cooker.

3. Remove the chicken from the sauce and use two forks to shred it. Stir the chicken back into the sauce. Serve the chicken and sauce on the lettuce leaves, topped with the carrots, celery and ranch dressing.

NUTRITION INFO: 1 portion (1 wrap) provides:

Protein: 1 serving

Vitamin A: 1 serving

Other fruits and vegetables: 1 serving

Omegas: some

Yummy Yogurt Ranch Dressing
SERVES 4

Creamy, tangy and super low-fat, this ranch salad dressing doubles as a dip.

125 ml whole buttermilk
6 tablespoons full-fat Greek yogurt
2 teaspoons cider vinegar
1 teaspoon Dijon mustard
1 tablespoon mayo (optional)
1½ teaspoons coarse salt
1 teaspoon onion powder
1 teaspoon garlic granules
½ teaspoon black pepper
4 teaspoons chopped fresh parsley
4 teaspoons chopped fresh chives

Whisk together all ingredients. Store in an airtight container in the refrigerator for up to 2 weeks.

NUTRITION INFO: 1 portion (250 ml) provides:

Calcium: 1 serving

From the Test Kitchen

Feeling blue? Add crumbled pasteurised blue cheese to the dressing.

Easy Tandoori Chicken

SERVES 4

This trimmed-down take on the Indian classic doesn't require a traditional clay oven or a long list of spices, so it translates well in any kitchen. Just marinate the chicken the night before, then bake before grilling so that it's juicy and tender on the inside, slightly crispy and charred on the outside.

240 g natural full-fat yogurt
1 tablespoon very finely garlic (optional)
1 tablespoon ground cumin
2 teaspoons paprika
2 teaspoons ground ginger
Grated zest of 1 lime
2 teaspoons coarse salt
1½ teaspoons ground coriander
½ teaspoon ground turmeric
2 x 225-g skinless, boneless chicken
    breasts
Cooking oil spray
4 tablespoons chopped fresh coriander
Lime wedges, for serving

1. Combine the yogurt, garlic, if using, cumin, paprika, ginger, lime zest, salt, coriander and turmeric in a small bowl. Place all but 4 tablespoons in a large resealable plastic freezer bag; cover the bowl containing the remainder and place in the refrigerator. Add the chicken to the marinade in the bag, seal the bag and massage to coat the chicken. Marinate in the refrigerator for 8–24 hours, turning occasionally.

2. Preheat the oven to 200°C/gas mark 6. Line a baking tray with aluminium foil and place a wire rack on the foil. Coat the rack with cooking oil spray.

From the Test Kitchen

For an earthier flavour (and even simpler prep), swap the cumin, paprika, ginger, coriander and tumeric for 3 tablespoons of curry powder.

3. Place the chicken on the rack. Discard any marinade in the bag. Bake the chicken for 12–15 minutes until the internal temperature taken with an instant-read meat thermometer is 54.5°C.

4. Turn on the grill to high. Grill the chicken for 6–7 minutes, basting with the reserved marinade every 2 minutes, until the thermometer registers 74°C. (There should be char after each basting.) Remove the chicken from the oven and allow it to rest for 5–10 minutes. Cut the chicken into large chunks. Sprinkle with the coriander and serve with lime wedges.

NUTRITION INFO: 1 portion provides:

Protein: 1 serving

Omegas: some

Coconut Chicken

SERVES 4

This simple poached chicken is the perfect make-ahead meal. Delicious either cold or at room temperature with crunchy veggies and bright herbs, this is the opposite of Sad Desk Lunch. The 'dressing' from the cooking liquid, along with the chicken, will keep in the refrigerator for up to 3 days.

2 cloves garlic, peeled and crushed
1 x 5-cm piece peeled fresh ginger, sliced
1 x 5-cm piece lemongrass stalk, thinly sliced
20 g fresh coriander, chopped
1 x 400-g tin full-fat coconut milk
½ teaspoon coarse salt
¼ teaspoon black pepper
2 x 225-g skinless, boneless chicken breasts
¼ teaspoon red curry powder
Juice of 1 lime
225 g romaine hearts, chopped
50 g seedless cucumber, thinly sliced
50 g peeled carrots, grated
20 g mixed fresh mint and basil leaves

1. Place the garlic, ginger, lemongrass, coriander, coconut milk, salt and pepper in a medium-sized saucepan. Bring to the boil over a medium-high heat. Add the chicken and reduce the heat to medium-low; keep the cooking liquid at 70–80°C.

2. Cook the chicken for about 25 minutes until the internal temperature taken with an instant-read meat thermometer is 70°C. Remove the chicken from the cooking liquid and set aside to cool for 15 minutes. Shred the chicken.

3. Meanwhile, pour the cooking liquid through a fine-mesh sieve into a bowl; discard the solids. Return the cooking liquid to the saucepan. Stir in the curry powder and simmer for 5 minutes. Pour into a bowl, add the lime juice, cover with cling film and refrigerate for at least 30 minutes.

4. Combine the chicken, romaine, cucumbers and carrots in a large bowl and toss with enough of the dressing to coat evenly. Gently stir in the mint and basil. Serve with any remaining dressing.

NUTRITION INFO: 1 portion provides:

Protein: 1 serving

Vitamin C: 2½ servings

Vitamin A: 2 servings

Other fruits and vegetables: 1 serving

Omegas: some

Fish and Seafood

M aybe you're a fish fan from way back. Or maybe you feel lukewarm about seafood – don't mind it, but you probably wouldn't make it your main course of choice. Or maybe you know you should embrace the seafood side of life (for its high-protein, low-fat benefits), but fish is a taste you're still waiting to acquire. No matter how you feel about fish and seafood, these recipes will win you over.

Looking for something exotic? Try Salmon Poached in Thai Carrot Broth. Going gourmet? How about Prawns with Feta or Seared Scallops on White Beans and Kale. Fishing for a quick yet memorable meal? You'll find it here.

Ginger-Steamed Halibut

SERVES 2

A luminium foil parcels enclose an intensely flavoured meal-in-one, steaming not only the halibut but also the couscous and a delicious mix of vegetables.

4 tablespoons uncooked wholewheat couscous
½ large red pepper, thinly sliced
65 g sugar snap peas, topped and tailed

30 g shiitake mushroom caps, sliced
30 g baby spinach leaves
2 teaspoons grated peeled fresh ginger
Salt and black pepper
4 tablespoons low-salt vegetable stock or fish stock
2 x 175-g halibut or salmon fillets
4 fresh basil leaves (optional)

1. Preheat the oven to 230°C/gas mark 8.

2. Tear off two pieces of heavy-duty aluminium foil, each 30 cm long. Place the pieces of foil on a work surface and put 2 tablespoons couscous in the centre of each.

3. Place the red pepper, sugar snap peas, mushrooms, spinach and ginger in a bowl and stir to mix. Season the vegetable mix lightly with salt and black pepper, then place half in the centre of each piece of foil.

4. Fold up the edges of each piece of foil slightly, then spoon 2 tablespoons stock into each.

5. Lightly season the fish fillets with salt and black pepper and place one on top of each mound of vegetables. Top each fish fillet with 2 basil leaves, if using.

6. Seal a parcel by bringing together the two longest edges of the foil and double folding them, leaving room for air circulation inside. Crimp the edge to make a tight seal. Double fold and crimp the remaining 2 edges to finish sealing the parcel. (There should be no gaps where juices can leak out.) Repeat with the remaining parcel.

7. Transfer the foil parcels to a baking tray and bake for 12–15 minutes, depending upon the thickness of the fillets, until the fish is cooked through. To test for doneness, carefully open a parcel; when the fish is cooked through it will flake easily when pierced with a fork.

8. To serve, place the parcels on serving plates and open them at the table, taking care to avoid the escaping hot steam.

Cucumber Sauce

This sauce is delish on any fish, whether it's roasted, poached or grilled. Serve it as a dip for veggies, too, or in sandwiches or wraps.

120 g natural full-fat Greek yogurt
2 pickling cucumbers, peeled,
cut in half lengthways and
deseeded
1 tablespoon chopped fresh dill or
½ teaspoon dried dill
1 ripe tomato, deseeded and diced
Salt and black pepper

Place the yogurt, cucumbers and dill in a food processor and process until just chunky. Fold in the tomato and season the sauce with salt and pepper to taste. Like a little bite? Add a teaspoon or two of well-drained prepared horseradish, and/or Dijon mustard. Very finely chopped fresh chives would also be a welcomed tasty addition.

NUTRITION INFO: 1 portion provides:

Protein: 1½ servings

Vitamin C: 2 servings

Vitamin A: 1 serving

Other fruits and vegetables: ½ serving

Wholegrains and legumes: ½ serving

Iron: some

Omegas: some, if using salmon

Red Snapper with Mango Salsa

SERVES 2

Topping grilled red snapper with a snappy mango salsa gives the fish an authentic island kick. The mango salsa also goes well with turkey, beef, pork or chicken and will keep nicely in the refrigerator for 1–2 days.

1 medium-sized ripe mango,
    cut into small dice
½ medium-sized red pepper,
    cut into small dice
2 spring onions (white and light green
    parts), trimmed and thinly sliced
1 teaspoon very finely chopped fresh
    jalapeño pepper (optional)
2 tablespoons fresh lime juice
2 tablespoons chopped fresh coriander
1 tablespoon olive oil
2 x 175-g red snapper fillets or other
    white fish fillets
Salt and black pepper

1. Preheat the grill.

2. Place the mango, red pepper, spring onions, jalapeño, if using, lime juice, coriander and 1 teaspoon of the oil in a bowl and stir to mix. Set the mango salsa aside.

From the Test Kitchen

Heartburn getting you down? Skip the heat: substitute 1 teaspoon ground cumin for the jalapeño pepper.

3. Brush the fish with the remaining oil and season with salt and black pepper. Grill for 4–5 minutes per side (or less for more delicate fish) until cooked through, opaque and they flake easily with a fork.

4. Serve the fish with large spoonfuls of the mango salsa.

NUTRITION INFO: 1 portion provides:

Protein: 1½ servings

Vitamin C: 2 servings

Vitamin A: 1½ servings

Fat: ½ serving

Full of Fish?

Most recipes in this chapter call for 175-g fish fillets – because that's about the size most commonly encountered at fish markets. That means you'll be racking up 1½ protein servings in each portion. But if that's too much fish for you, scale it back to 115-g portions, and you'll cut your protein serving down to 1. On the other hand, if you can never get your fill of fish, you can occasionally feast on 225g – a portion that will yield 2 full protein servings.

Greek Salad Snapper

SERVES 2

Bake snapper in a snap with a delicious sauce that combines all of your favourite Greek salad ingredients – tomatoes, red pepper, capers, kalamata olives, oregano and feta cheese.

1 tablespoon olive oil
2 spring onions (white and light green parts), trimmed and thinly sliced
2 ripe plum tomatoes, cut into 1-cm pieces
½ large red pepper, cut into 1-cm pieces
1 teaspoon very finely chopped fresh oregano or ½ teaspoon dried oregano
1 teaspoon drained capers, or more to taste
6 pitted kalamata olives, chopped
40 g pasteurised feta cheese, crumbled
2 tablespoons chopped fresh flat-leaf parsley
Black pepper
Fresh lemon juice
Olive oil cooking spray
2 x 175-g red snapper fillets
½ teaspoon chopped fresh dill
Salt

1. Preheat the oven to 200°C/gas mark 6.

2. Heat the olive oil in a small frying pan over a medium-high heat. Add the spring onions and cook for about 1 minute until softened slightly. Add the tomatoes, red pepper, oregano and capers and cook for about 4 minutes until the vegetables soften. Remove from the heat and add the olives and feta, then sprinkle parsley on top and season with black pepper and lemon juice to taste.

From the Test Kitchen

Not a red snapper fan? You can substitute haddock, sea bass, cod or plaice for any recipe that calls for red snapper.

3. Coat a 20-cm-square baking dish with olive oil spray. Place the fish fillets in the centre of the baking dish, sprinkle the dill over them, and season with salt and black pepper. Spoon the vegetable and feta mixture on top. Cover the baking dish with aluminium foil and bake for 8–10 minutes until the fish is cooked through and flakes easily when pierced with a fork. Serve the fish with the vegetable and feta mixture.

NUTRITION INFO: 1 portion provides:

Protein: ½ serving

Calcium: ½ serving

Vitamin C: 1½ servings

Vitamin A: ½ serving

Fat: ½ serving

Roasted Mediterranean Sea Bass with Red Pepper and White Beans

SERVES 2

Here's a quick and easy way to bring the flavours of the Mediterranean to your table. White beans and red pepper pair up to provide a simple yet satisfying base for the bass.

4 spring onions (white and light green parts), trimmed and chopped
30 g loosely packed fresh flat-leaf parsley leaves
4 tablespoons low-salt vegetable stock
1 tablespoon olive oil
1 medium-sized red pepper, thinly sliced
425 g tinned flageolet beans, drained and rinsed
2 x 175-g skinless sea bass or halibut fillets
1 lemon, halved and deseeded (thinly slice 1 half)

1. Preheat the oven to 190°C/gas mark 5.

2. Place the spring onions, parsley, vegetable stock and olive oil in a blender or food processor and purée them.

3. Place the red pepper and beans in a 20-cm-square baking dish. Set aside 3 tablespoons of the spring onion and parsley purée, then spoon the rest over the red pepper and beans. Arrange the fish fillets on top and spoon the remaining spring onion and parsley purée over the fish. Scatter the lemon slices on top.

4. Bake the fish for about 15 minutes until it is cooked through and flakes easily with a fork. Squeeze the remaining lemon half over the fish just before serving.

NUTRITION INFO: 1 portion provides:

Protein: 2 servings

Calcium: ½ serving

Vitamin C: 3 servings

Vitamin A: 2 servings

Wholegrains and legumes: 2½ servings

Iron: some

Fat: ½ serving

Marinated Salmon Fillets with Ginger and Lime

SERVES 4

Simple grilled or barbecued salmon is easy to prepare but much tastier – and just as easy – in this Pacific Rim– inspired dish. The lime and ginger marinade makes it fragrant and flavourful. (It's sassy on prawns, too.) The recipe is easy to cut in half – or enjoy as leftovers the next day, perhaps over a bed of your favourite salad leaves or grains.

Grated zest and juice of 2 limes

2 teaspoons olive oil

2 teaspoons low-salt soy sauce

1 teaspoon sesame oil

1 teaspoon grated peeled fresh ginger

4 x 175-g skinless salmon fillets

3 spring onions (white and light green parts), trimmed and thinly sliced

1. Place the lime zest and juice, olive oil, soy sauce, sesame oil and ginger in a small bowl and stir to mix.

2. Place the salmon in a 23 x 33-cm glass baking dish. Pour half of the lime and ginger mixture over the salmon; set the rest aside. Turn the salmon fillets to coat them evenly with the marinade.

3. Preheat the grill or set up the barbecue and preheat it to high.

4. Grill the salmon for 3–5 minutes per side until it is cooked through and flakes easily with a fork.

Minute Meals

For a fish dinner without any fuss (or unpleasant smells), turn to the microwave. Place a fish fillet (no more than 1 cm thick) in a microwave-safe baking dish. Season the fish with a combination of any of the following: grated lemon or orange zest, a sprinkling of chopped fresh herbs (such as tarragon and dill), and a coating of equal parts wholegrain mustard and mayonnaise. Cover the baking dish with cling film, folding back one corner to allow the steam to escape. Microwave the fish on high power for 2–3 minutes until it's cooked through. Presto! With a squeeze of lemon or lime juice, dinner is ready.

5. Place the salmon fillets on serving plates and spoon the reserved lime and ginger marinade over them. Top the fillets with the spring onions.

NUTRITION INFO: 1 portion provides:

Protein: 1½ servings

Fat: ½ serving

Omegas: some

Instant Pot Lemony Salmon with Sweet Potatoes and Kale

SERVES 2

Ready in an instant, but you'll want to sit down and savour this hearty, healthy, savoury salmon dinner (it's a winner).

450 g peeled sweet potatoes,
    cut in 5-cm pieces
1¼ teaspoons coarse salt
½ teaspoon black pepper
2 x 175-g skinless centre-cut
    salmon fillets)
Grated zest of 1 lemon
1 tablespoon fresh lemon juice
335 g kale (thick stalks removed),
    chopped
1 tablespoon olive oil
2 teaspoons very finely chopped garlic
2 teaspoons unsalted butter

1. Place the sweet potatoes, 250 ml water, ¾ teaspoon of the salt and ¼ teaspoon of the pepper in a programmable pressure multicooker (such as an Instant Pot).

2. Sprinkle the salmon on both sides with the lemon zest and the remaining ½ teaspoon salt and ¼ teaspoon pepper. Place the salmon on top of the potatoes. Cover the cooker with its lid and lock it in place. Turn the steam release handle to the SEALING position. Select the MANUAL/PRESSURE COOK setting. Select HIGH pressure for 4 minutes. (It will take about 5 minutes for the cooker to come up to pressure before cooking begins.)

3. Carefully turn the steam release handle to the VENTING position and let the steam fully escape. (This will take about 3 minutes.) Remove the lid from the cooker.

4. While the cooker is venting, massage the kale with the lemon juice and oil in a large bowl until the kale is softened.

5. Remove the salmon from the cooker and set aside. Select the SAUTÉ setting. Select the HIGH temperature setting and allow the cooker to preheat. Add the kale and garlic to the potatoes. Cook, stirring occasionally, for 4–5 minutes until most of the liquid has evaporated. Add the butter and cook for about 1 minute, stirring and smashing the potatoes with a wooden spoon. Serve immediately with the fish.

NUTRITION INFO: 1 portion provides:

Protein: 1½ serving

Vitamin C: 3 servings

Vitamin A: 5 servings

Fat: ½ serving

Iron: some

Omegas: some

Roast Salmon on a Bed of Lentils

SERVES 2

Earthy lentils provide a nutritious bed for roast salmon. The result is a hearty dish that's sure to satisfy.

2 x 175-g skinless salmon fillets
2 teaspoons olive oil
2 teaspoons fresh thyme leaves
Pinch each of salt and black pepper
Warm Lentil Ragout (recipe follows)
1 tablespoon very finely chopped fresh
    flat-leaf parsley

1. Preheat the oven to 230°C/gas mark 8.

2. Place the salmon fillets in a 20-cm-square baking dish and rub the olive oil all over them. Sprinkle the thyme, salt and pepper on top of the salmon.

3. Bake the salmon for 10–15 minutes until it is cooked through and flakes easily with a fork.

4. Spoon a serving of lentils on to each of two serving plates and place a salmon fillet on top. Sprinkle parsley over each fillet and serve.

NUTRITION INFO: 1 portion salmon (without lentils) provides:

Protein: 1½ servings

Warm Lentil Ragout

SERVES 4

This recipe makes twice as much as you'll need for the salmon. So tomorrow you can serve a grilled chicken breast over the leftovers.

2 teaspoons olive oil
1 medium-sized onion, chopped
2 cloves garlic, very finely chopped
2 medium-sized carrots, diced
200 g green lentils
1 sprig fresh thyme
1 bay leaf
700 g low-salt chicken stock or vegetable
    stock
Salt and black pepper

1. Heat the olive oil in a medium-sized saucepan over a medium-low heat. Add the onion and garlic and cook for 3 minutes until they just begin to soften.

2. Add the carrots and cook, stirring frequently, for about 3 minutes until they soften slightly. Add the lentils, thyme and bay leaf and cook, stirring to mix well, for about 1 minute.

3. Stir in the chicken stock, raise the heat to medium-high and bring to the boil. Reduce the heat and allow to simmer for about 20 minutes until the lentils are tender. Season with salt and pepper to taste. Remove and discard the thyme sprig and bay leaf before serving. The lentils can be refrigerated, covered, for up to 5 days.

NUTRITION INFO: 1 portion provides:

Protein: ½ serving

Vitamin A: 1 serving

Other fruits and vegetables: ½ serving

Wholegrains and legumes: 1½ servings

Iron: some

Omegas: some

Mustard Glazed Salmon

SERVES 2

Fishing for an easy dinner? Serve this salmon: it's sweet, salty, a little spicy and ready to savour in a matter of minutes. Pair it with quickly fried leafy green veggies and brown rice (always keep a stash in your freezer). Leftovers make a scrumptious salad topper.

2 tablespoons maple syrup
1½ teaspoons low-salt soy sauce
1½ teaspoons spicy wholegrain mustard
½ teaspoon rice vinegar
Pinch of dried chilli flakes
2 x 175-g skin-on salmon fillets
2 x 5-mm-thick unpeeled orange slices,
  cut into half-moons
2 teaspoons olive oil
¼ teaspoon coarse salt
1 teaspoon toasted sesame seeds
  (see page 217)

1. Preheat the grill to high. Line a baking tray with a sheet of heavy-duty aluminium foil.

2. Whisk together the maple syrup, soy sauce, mustard, vinegar and chilli flakes in a small bowl. Arrange the salmon skin side down in the centre of the baking tray; brush evenly with 2 tablespoons of the glaze. Place 2 orange pieces on each salmon fillet; brush evenly with the remaining glaze.

3. Grill the salmon for about 8 minutes until it is cooked through and flakes easily with a fork. Scatter with sesame seeds evenly over the fillets and serve immediately.

NUTRITION INFO: 1 portion provides:

Protein: 1½ servings

Omegas: some

Roasted Salmon with a Mild Mustard Crust

SERVES 2

Salmon's rich taste stands up beautifully to this flavourful mustard coating. But don't shy away from trying this crust on a milder fish such as halibut. For that matter, try it on chicken breasts.

Olive oil cooking spray
2 x 175-g skinless salmon fillets
Salt and black pepper

1½ tablespoons wholegrain mustard
2 teaspoons mayonnaise
2 teaspoons chopped fresh dill

1. Preheat the oven to 190°C/gas mark 5.

2. Coat the bottom of a 20-cm-square baking dish with olive oil cooking spray. Place the salmon fillets in the baking dish and lightly season them with salt and pepper.

3. Place the mustard, mayonnaise and dill in a small bowl and stir to mix.

4. Spread the mustard mixture on the salmon fillets.

5. Bake the salmon for about 10 minutes until it is cooked through and flakes easily with a fork.

NUTRITION INFO: 1 portion provides:

Protein: 1½ servings

Omegas: some

From the Test Kitchen

For a sweet-and-pungent taste, skip the dill and add 2 teaspoons all-fruit apricot preserve or jam to the mustard mixture.

Roast This

When fish is so fresh you can taste it, don't cover it up with fancy sauces or coatings. Instead, try the simplest and most satisfying way to prepare fish – roast it. Arrange fish fillets on a bed of fresh herbs, such as sprigs of rosemary, thyme or sage, in a baking dish and sprinkle more herbs on top. Fennel seeds are a nice addition, too. Brush the fish with some olive oil, season with sea salt and coarsely ground pepper, and scatter thin lemon slices over and around the fish. Bake the fish at 230°C/gas mark 8 until it is cooked through and flakes easily with a fork.

Another delicious way to roast fish is on a bed of vegetables. Toss slices or chunks of carrots, beetroot, butternut squash, potatoes (white or sweet) and/or fennel with a little olive oil, fresh thyme leaves, and a little salt and pepper. Spread the vegetables out in a baking dish and roast them in a 230°C/gas mark 8 oven for about 20 minutes until tender. Spoon the roasted vegetables into the centre of the baking dish so they can act as a bed for the fish. Place fillets on top, sprinkle them with herbs and lemon as above, and bake until the fish is done for a rustic fish dinner.

Salmon with Basil and Tomatoes

SERVES 2

Tomatoes and basil, a classic combo, make these salmon fillets moist, fragrant and flavourful. How can so little effort result in something so tasty? Take a few minutes to get these parcels ready for the oven, and you'll find out.

Olive oil cooking spray
2 x 175-g skinless salmon fillets
12 ripe cherry tomatoes, halved
12 fresh basil leaves
1 tablespoon olive oil
Salt and black pepper

1. Preheat the oven to 230°C/gas mark 8.

2. Tear off two pieces of heavy-duty aluminium foil, each 30 cm long. Place the pieces of foil on a work surface and coat them with olive oil spray.

3. Place a salmon fillet in the centre of each piece of foil. Top each fillet with 12 cherry tomato halves and 6 basil leaves. Drizzle 1½ teaspoons olive oil over each fillet, then season with salt and pepper.

4. Seal a parcel by bringing together the two longest edges of the foil and double folding them, leaving room for air circulation inside. Crimp the edge to make a tight seal. Double fold and crimp the remaining 2 edges to finish sealing the parcel. (There should be no gaps where juices can leak out.) Repeat with the remaining parcel.

From the Test Kitchen

Make a double batch and you'll have tomorrow's pasta dinner, too. Flake the salmon into penne, then fold in the cooked cherry tomatoes along with a jar of tomato-based pasta sauce and top with a scattering of Parmesan cheese.

5. Transfer the foil parcels to a baking tray and bake for 15–20 minutes, depending upon the thickness of the fillets, until the salmon is cooked through. To test for doneness, carefully open a parcel; when the salmon is cooked through it will flake easily with a fork and will have turned light pink inside.

6. To serve, place the parcels on serving plates and open them at the table, taking care to avoid the escaping hot steam.

NUTRITION INFO: 1 portion provides:

Protein: 1½ servings

Vitamin C: 1 serving

Fat: ½ serving

Omegas: some

Salmon Poached in Thai Carrot Broth

SERVES 2

Intensely and intriguingly flavoured with sweet carrots, pungent ginger, fresh coriander and tangy lime, this light-as-air salmon dish gives spa food a good name.

500 ml carrot juice

140 g carrots, diced

1 tablespoon very finely chopped, peeled fresh ginger

2 teaspoons grated lemon zest

1 teaspoon grated lime zest

2 tablespoons fresh lime juice, plus more to taste

3 spring onions (white and light green parts), trimmed and sliced

2 x 175-g skinless salmon fillets

2 tablespoons chopped fresh coriander, plus more for garnish

Salt and black pepper

1. Place the carrot juice, carrots and ginger in a medium-sized saucepan that is large enough to hold the salmon fillets without crowding and bring to the boil over a medium-high heat. Reduce the heat and allow to simmer for about 5 minutes until the carrots are tender. Add the lemon and lime zests, lime juice and spring onions and allow to simmer for about 1 minute until heated through.

2. Add the salmon fillets, return to a simmer, cover and cook for about 10 minutes until the salmon is just cooked through and flakes easily with a fork. Spoon the carrot broth over the fillets periodically.

From the Test Kitchen

The carrot broth is too good to save for just salmon. Try poaching halibut, sea bass, prawns, scallops or skinless, boneless chicken breast halves in it, too. Not sold on the taste of coriander? Substitute basil or flat-leaf parsley.

3. Place the salmon fillets in shallow bowls. Add the coriander to the carrot broth, then season it with salt and pepper to taste and add more lime juice, if wished. Pour the carrot broth and carrots over the salmon, garnish with coriander and serve.

NUTRITION INFO: 1 portion provides:

Protein: 1½ servings

Vitamin A: 2 servings; plus 4 more if you sip half the carrot broth

Omegas: some

Salmon Cakes with Tropical Salsa

MAKES 6 CAKES; SERVES 3

Don't have the time (or the stomach) to stop by the fish market for fresh fillets? No harm in fishing some salmon out of a tin. In fact, the soft bones in tinned salmon provide a calcium bonus – and you'll never notice them once they're mashed up. If there are any salmon cakes left over, you can have them cold for lunch.

420 g tinned pink salmon, drained, mashed with a fork

1 medium-sized red pepper, cut into small dice

55 g carrot, grated

1 tablespoon drained capers

1 medium egg

Grated zest of ½ lemon

4 tablespoons wholemeal breadcrumbs

2 tablespoons ground linseeds (flaxseeds)

¼ teaspoon black pepper

2 teaspoons olive oil

165 g pineapple chunks, fresh or drained from a tin

1 large ripe mango, peeled, stoned and cut into chunks

2 tablespoons balsamic vinegar

Pinch of dried chilli flakes

1. Place the salmon, half of the red pepper, the carrot, capers, egg and lemon zest in a bowl and stir to mix.

2. Place the breadcrumbs and linseeds in a small bowl and whisk to mix. Add half of the breadcrumb mixture to the salmon mixture and mix well. Season with black pepper, then stir well to combine.

3. Divide the salmon mixture into 6 equal portions and pat into cakes, each about 1 cm thick. Dredge both sides of the salmon cakes in the remaining breadcrumb mixture.

4. Heat the oil in a large frying pan over a medium-high heat. Add the salmon cakes and cook for about 4 minutes per side until golden brown and heated through. To check for doneness, insert a knife into the centre of a salmon cake; if the knife feels hot when removed, the cake is done.

5. Meanwhile, place the remaining red pepper and the pineapple, mango, balsamic vinegar and chilli flakes in a bowl and stir to mix.

6. Spoon the salsa on to serving plates and top with the salmon cakes.

NUTRITION INFO: 1 portion (2 cakes) provides:

Protein: 1 serving

Vitamin C: 2 servings plus

Calcium: 1 serving if made with bones

Vitamin A: 1 serving

Wholegrains and legumes: ½ serving

Omegas: some

Speedy Salsas

Looking for a way to dress up protein? Try any of these salsas on grilled fish, meat or poultry:

- Chopped deseeded ripe tomato, olives, basil, red onion, garlic and lemon juice

- Chopped deseeded ripe tomato, fresh yellow peaches or nectarines, fresh mint, balsamic vinegar and olive oil

- Chopped fresh or tinned, drained pineapple, red pepper, jalapeño pepper and fresh coriander

- Chopped deseeded ripe tomato, roasted sweetcorn kernels, chopped roasted red pepper, red onion, fresh coriander and lime juice

- Diced mango, yellow pepper, jalapeño pepper, ground cumin, lime juice and olive oil

- Black beans (drained and rinsed), chopped ripe tomato, yellow pepper, coriander, spring onions, lime juice, and olive oil

Seared Sea Scallops on Succotash

SERVES 2

Silken sea scallops love nothing more than a good bed, and crunchy succotash makes a beautiful one.

225 g sea scallops
2 teaspoons fresh lemon juice
2 teaspoons olive oil
¾ teaspoon very finely chopped fresh tarragon, or ¼ teaspoon dried tarragon
Edamame Succotash (page 331)
Grated zest of ½ lemon
½ teaspoon very finely chopped fresh dill
½ teaspoon very finely chopped fresh flat-leaf parsley
Salt and coarsely ground black pepper

1. Place the scallops in a mixing bowl. Add the lemon juice, olive oil and tarragon and stir to coat the scallops evenly. Marinate the scallops in the refrigerator, covered, for up to 30 minutes.

2. Preheat the grill or set up the barbecue and preheat it to high.

3. Grill the scallops for 2–3 minutes per side until they are just cooked through, springy to the touch and have a golden coloured edge.

4. Toss the succotash with the lemon zest, dill and parsley and divide it evenly between 2 serving plates. Season the cooked scallops lightly with salt and pepper. Divide them between the plates and serve at once.

NUTRITION INFO: 1 portion (without the succotash) provides:

Protein: 1 serving

Seared Scallops on White Beans and Kale

SERVES 2

This Spanish-influenced dish marries delicate scallops with a robust ragout of beans, tomatoes and leafy green veggies. The result is hearty, satisfying and speedy to prepare, thanks to the tinned beans and tomatoes.

2 teaspoons olive oil

1 small onion, chopped

2 cloves garlic, very finely chopped (optional)

1 bay leaf

1 x 400-g tin chopped tomatoes, drained

125 g kale (thick stalks removed), chopped

155 g drained tinned navy or cannellini beans, rinsed

1 tablespoon chopped fresh flat-leaf parsley, plus more to garnish (optional)

Salt and black pepper

2 teaspoons fresh lemon juice, plus more to season the beans

1 teaspoon butter

225 g sea scallops

1. Heat the olive oil in a large non-stick frying pan over a medium-low heat. Add the onion, garlic, if using, and bay leaf and cook, stirring frequently, for about 10 minutes until the onion is softened and golden in colour. Add the tomatoes and kale and cook, stirring frequently, for about 10 minutes until they soften. Add the beans and parsley, stir to mix and season to taste with salt, pepper and fresh lemon juice, if wished. Set the bean mixture aside, covered, to keep warm.

2. Preheat the grill.

3. Melt the butter in a small saucepan over a low heat. Stir in the lemon juice.

From the Test Kitchen

Make the white beans again, or cook extra – just about any roasted or grilled fish (halibut, salmon, sea bass), seafood (prawns, calamari), poultry (chicken, turkey) or meat (pork, beef, lamb) will be tasty served on top.

Place the scallops in a grill pan and brush the tops with half of the lemon butter. Grill the scallops close to the heat for 2–3 minutes until coloured. Turn the scallops and brush them with the remaining lemon butter. Grill the second side for 2–3 minutes until the scallops are just cooked through and springy to the touch.

4. Divide the bean mixture between 2 serving plates. Lightly season the scallops with salt and pepper, then arrange them on top of the beans. Scatter chopped parsley on top, if wished.

NUTRITION INFO: 1 portion provides:

Protein: 1½ servings

Vitamin C: 1½ servings

Vitamin A: 2 servings

Other fruits and vegetables: ½ serving

Wholegrains and legumes: 1 serving

Iron: some

Fat: ½ serving

Prawns and Watermelon Kebabs

SERVES 4

When watermelon meets heat, its texture softens and its sweetness deepens, making this expectant-mum favourite fruit an unexpectedly complementary companion for savoury prawns – especially when sriracha adds spice to the mix. Serve the kebabs over brown rice, farro or wholegrain couscous, or toss with rocket and pasteurised feta for a satisfying dinner salad.

450 g shelled and deveined large prawns
2 tablespoons sriracha
1 tablespoon olive oil
1 tablespoon orange juice
1 tablespoon low-salt soy sauce
1 tablespoon honey
1 teaspoon very finely chopped garlic
600 g seedless watermelon flesh,
    cut into 2.5-cm pieces
½ medium-sized red onion, cut into
    2.5-cm pieces
1 teaspoon coarse salt
1 tablespoon chopped fresh basil

1. If you are using wooden or bamboo skewers, soak them in water for 10 minutes so they don't burn.

2. Place the prawns, sriracha, olive oil, orange juice, soy sauce, honey and garlic in a large bowl. Stir to coat the prawns evenly with the marinade. Cover the bowl with cling film and refrigerate for up to 30 minutes.

3. Preheat the grill or heat a barbecue to high. Remove the prawns from the marinade and thread them on to 8 skewers, alternating pieces of watermelon and red onion between the prawns. Discard any leftover marinade. Sprinkle the kebabs with the salt.

4. Grill the prawns, turning them occasionally, for 3–4 minutes in total until they turn pink and are cooked through. Scatter evenly with the basil before serving.

NUTRITION INFO: 1 portion provides:

Protein: 1 serving

Vitamin C: 1 serving

Iron: some

Omegas: some

Prawns with Feta

SERVES 2

Here's a traditional Greek dish that's bound to become a tradition in your home, too – especially when you see how easy it is to make. Serve the prawns over wholewheat orzo, farro, quinoa, brown rice or the wholegrain of your choice.

1 tablespoon olive oil
1 medium-sized red pepper, chopped
1 small fennel bulb, trimmed, halved and
    thinly sliced widthways
3 cloves garlic, very finely chopped
    (optional)
4 ripe plum tomatoes, deseeded and
    chopped
1 tablespoon very finely chopped fresh
    oregano or 1 teaspoon dried oregano
350 g shelled and deveined large prawns
Fresh lemon juice
Black pepper
75 g pasteurised feta cheese, crumbled
35 g toasted pine nuts (see page 217;
    optional)
Salt
2 tablespoons chopped fresh flat-leaf
    parsley

1. Heat the olive oil in a large frying pan over a medium-high heat. Add the red pepper, fennel and garlic, if using, and cook, stirring frequently, for about 5 minutes until the vegetables are softened. Add the tomatoes and oregano and cook, stirring frequently, for about 2 minutes until the tomatoes are slightly softened. Stir in the prawns and cook for about 4 minutes until they are cooked through and turn opaque.

From the Test Kitchen

Don't feel like splurging on prawns? Try substituting an equal amount of cubed skinless, boneless chicken breast or turkey breast strips – or cubed firm tofu for a good vegetarian alternative. Just cook the chicken or turkey until it's cooked through before adding it to the sauce. Add the tofu after the tomatoes and oregano.

2. Season the prawns and vegetables to taste with lemon juice and black pepper. Add the feta, stir well and simmer for about 30 seconds until the cheese begins to melt. Stir in the pine nuts, if using, and season with salt to taste (you may not need any since the feta is salty). Sprinkle the parsley on top and serve.

NUTRITION INFO: 1 portion provides:

Protein: 1½ servings

Calcium: 1 serving

Vitamin C: 3 servings

Vitamin A: 1 serving

Fat: ½ serving

Iron: some

Omegas: some

Prawn Remoulade Toast

SERVES 2

The 'Big Easy' classic that has long been a New Orleans staple made, well, easy. And this prawn remoulade isn't just a lighter lift, it's lighter, too. Top your toast first with a little shredded romaine for some extra nutrition.

225 g shelled and deveined medium-sized
  prawns
2 teaspoons olive oil
2 tablespoons mayonnaise
110 g romaine lettuce, shredded
  (optional)
4 tablespoons natural low-fat Greek
  yogurt
4 tablespoons buttermilk
1½ tablespoons chopped fresh flat-leaf
  (Italian) parsley
1½ teaspoons prepared horseradish,
  drained
1½ teaspoons fresh lemon juice
1½ teaspoons chopped drained capers
½ teaspoon paprika
¼ teaspoon black pepper
4 slices wholegrain bread, toasted
110 g romaine lettuce, shredded
  (optional)

1. Preheat the grill to high.

2. Toss the prawns with the olive oil in a bowl. Arrange the prawns in a single layer on a baking tray. Grill the prawns for about 3 minutes, turning them after 2 minutes, until they are cooked through and turn opaque. Remove from the grill and cool completely.

3. Whisk together the mayonnaise, yogurt, buttermilk, parsley, horseradish, lemon juice, capers, paprika and pepper in a medium-sized bowl. Set aside.

4. Stir the prawns into the remoulade. To serve, top the toast with romaine, if desired, dividing it evenly among the slices. Spoon the prawns and sauce on top of the toast and serve.

NUTRITION INFO: 1 portion provides:

Protein: 1 serving

Vitamin C: 1 serving if using romaine

Vitamin A: 1 serving if using romaine

Wholegrains and legumes: 2 servings

Fat: 1 serving

Iron: some

Omegas: some

Pan-Fried Trout with Tomatoes and Spinach

SERVES 2

A delicious American-style 'cornmeal', aka polenta, crust adds crunch to trout. Then it's topped with a warm salad of tomato and spinach. This is what happens when fish leaves the Southern campfire and goes uptown on the hob. If you can't find buttermilk, add ¾ teaspoon of lemon juice to 4 tablespoons of regular milk, stir and allow to stand for 5 minutes.

65 g wholegrain (non-degerminated) cornmeal or polenta

2 tablespoons grated Parmesan cheese (optional)

1 teaspoon grated lemon zest

Salt and black pepper

Garlic granules

1 medium egg

4 tablespoons buttermilk

2 x 175-g boneless trout fillets

Olive oil cooking spray

1½ tablespoons olive oil

1 tablespoon fresh lemon juice

4 ripe plum tomatoes, deseeded and chopped

2 teaspoons chopped fresh tarragon, or ½ teaspoon dried

1 x 150–175-g bag baby spinach

2 teaspoons very finely chopped fresh chives

Lemon wedges, for serving

1. Place the cornmeal, Parmesan cheese, if using, lemon zest and a pinch each of salt, pepper and garlic granules in a shallow dish and stir to mix. Place the egg and the buttermilk in another shallow dish and gently whisk to combine.

2. Dip each trout fillet in the egg mixture, then in the cornmeal mixture, turning it to coat evenly and thoroughly.

3. Coat a large frying pan with olive oil cooking spray, then heat 1½ teaspoons of the olive oil in it over a medium heat. Add the trout and cook for about 4 minutes per side until the coating is well coloured and the fish is cooked through. Transfer the trout to a platter and cover with aluminium foil to keep warm.

4. Add the remaining 1 tablespoon olive oil and the lemon juice to the pan and scrape up the browned bits. Add the tomatoes and tarragon, reduce the heat to low and cook for about 2 minutes until the tomatoes soften slightly. Add the spinach and cook, stirring, for about 2 minutes until barely wilted. Season with salt and pepper to taste. Top the trout with the tomato and spinach mixture, sprinkle with chives and serve with lemon wedges.

NUTRITION INFO: 1 portion provides:

Protein: 1½ servings

Vitamin C: 2 servings

Vitamin A: 3 servings

Wholegrains and legumes: 1 serving

Iron: some

Fat: ½ serving plus

From the Test Kitchen

The combination of trout and nuts goes way back. To ring the changes, replace the cornmeal coating for the pan-fried trout with a combination of 30 g ground toasted pecans or hazelnuts (see page 217), 30 g dried wholemeal breadcrumbs, 15 g very finely chopped fresh flat-leaf parsley, 1 teaspoon grated lemon zest and a pinch each of salt and black pepper. Skip the egg and buttermilk bath; just moisten the trout fillets with milk before dredging them in the nut mixture. Pan-fry the fish in a combination of 1½ teaspoons butter and 1½ teaspoons olive oil. Scatter the trout with very finely chopped chives and lemon juice, and serve with lemon wedges and a pilau instead of the tomato and spinach mixture.

Veggies,
Beans and Grains

....

S eeking sweet potato chips with that white fish? Broccoli with that beef? A pilau bed for your chicken? Or a meatless main that highlights grains – or legumes (aka pulses such as beans and peas), or veggies? Whether you're searching for the perfect side for your meat, poultry, fish or seafood or planning plant-focused meals, you'll find just what you're looking for in this batch of veggie, bean and grain recipes. Side dishes that aren't besides the point, instead standing out in nutrition and taste – such as Smoky Roasted Carrots with Lime Cream, Cheesy Roasted Cauliflower, Kale and Shiitake Mushroom Salad, and Farro Risotto with Mushrooms. And easy, tasty meatless meals that could satisfy even confirmed carnivores, such as Baked Tofu with Sprouting Broccoli and Sweet Potatoes. Add an egg, some cheese, and any of these veggie sides can become a light meal, too.

Broccoli Vinaigrette

SERVES 4

As much a salad as a veggie side, this delicious hybrid tops steamed broccoli with a zesty vinaigrette. Roughly chopped nuts add a crunchy crowning touch. Want to crown your broccoli twice? Add a scattering of grated Parmesan. The broccoli is delicious the next day, too.

225 g broccoli florets

1 teaspoon very finely chopped shallot

2 tablespoons fresh lemon juice, plus more to taste

2 tablespoons extra-virgin olive oil

2 teaspoons Dijon mustard (optional)

2 teaspoons very finely chopped fresh chives

Salt and black pepper

4 tablespoons coarsely chopped toasted pistachios or walnuts (see page 217)

1. Steam the broccoli following the instructions given in the box below, for 4–5 minutes until crisp-tender. Place the broccoli in a large bowl.

2. Place the shallots, lemon juice, olive oil, mustard, if using, and chives in a small bowl and whisk to mix, then season with salt and pepper to taste. Pour the vinaigrette over the broccoli and toss well to coat. Sprinkle the pistachios over the broccoli just before serving.

NUTRITION INFO: 1 portion provides:

Vitamin C: 1 serving

Vitamin A: 1½ servings

Fat: ½ serving

Omegas: some

Steaming Savvy

When it comes to vegetables, steaming beats boiling hands down. First, it retains far more nutrients. When you boil vegetables, the nutrients end up in the cooking water; that's fine if you're going to drink the cooking water – as in a soup – but not so fine if you'll be pouring the water down the drain. Secondly, steaming eliminates 2 steps: there's no waiting for a big pot of water to boil; and there's no draining afterwards. Thirdly, and possibly most importantly, steaming preserves flavour and texture.

If those aren't enough reasons to switch to steaming, here's one more: it couldn't be easier. Just pour water to a depth of 2.5 cm into a large pot with a tight-fitting cover and bring it to a boil. Season the veggies now if you won't later. Place the veggies in a steamer basket, lower the basket into the pot, cover the pot and steam the vegetables until they are just tender. Serve them as is with just a squeeze of lemon, or toss them into any recipe that calls for cooked veggies. (Steaming is also an easy way to cook prawns.) For microwave steaming tips, see page 322.

Asparagus and Parmesan Curls

SERVES 2

Serve this asparagus alongside a fish, chicken or meat dish or as an elegant start to any meal.

225 g asparagus stalks
2 teaspoons olive oil
Juice and grated zest of ½ lemon
Salt and black pepper
25 g Parmesan shavings (see page 251)

1. Trim off and discard the tough woody ends of the asparagus stalks.

2. Steam the asparagus following the instructions in the box on page 315 for 4–6 minutes, depending on the thickness of the asparagus, until just tende.

3. Pat the asparagus dry and divide them evenly between 2 serving plates. Drizzle the olive oil and lemon juice over the asparagus, and top it with the lemon zest. Season with salt and pepper to taste, then top with the cheese shavings.

From the Test Kitchen

Steam twice as much asparagus as you want to serve, then chill the leftovers for the next day's salad. It's delicious tossed with a little lemon vinaigrette, as in Broccoli Vinaigrette (page 315). Or skip the steaming, and roast the asparagus in a hot oven (see the box on the next page). Like a green leafy option? Substitute broccoli or sprouting broccoli for the asparagus.

NUTRITION INFO: 1 portion provides:

Calcium: ½ serving

Vitamin C: 1 serving

For Veggies with the Most, Just Roast

So long, steaming! To get the most from your veggies, roast them. From Brussels sprouts to cauliflower, carrots to butternut squash, broccoli to mushrooms, pretty much every vegetable takes on a deeper, sweeter, more complex taste and earthy, almost meaty texture when roasted. Plus, the prep and clean-up couldn't be easier. Just preheat the oven to 220°C/gas mark7 and line a large baking tray with baking paper. Then place your veggies, cut into bite-sized pieces (small florets for cauliflower and broccoli, halved Brussels sprouts, small chunks of squash; asparagus can be roasted whole) in one layer on the tray. Spray or drizzle with olive oil and sprinkle with salt, coarse black pepper and, if desired, fresh herbs (say, thyme leaves or rosemary springs, chopped flat-leaf parsley or sage), then toss to coat. Roast the veggies, stirring once during baking, until tender and golden, even a little charred around the edges. Roasting times will vary, but average 20–30 minutes. Serve your veggies hot or at room temperature, straight up or with a vinaigrette, a squeeze of lemon or some grated cheese. Leftovers (if you don't end up eating them all) can be served cold in a salad the next day, or right from the fridge as a snack.

Roast Butternut Squash

SERVES 4

Getting a vitamin A plus was never this easy or yummy. Leftovers warm up easily the next day.

Olive oil cooking spray

1 x 450-g pack cubed peeled butternut squash

2 tablespoons olive oil

1 tablespoon fresh thyme leaves or 1 teaspoon dried thyme

40 g Parmesan cheese, grated

1. Preheat the oven to 200°C/gas mark 6.

2. Coat a 23 x 33-cm baking dish with olive oil cooking spray, then add the squash. Drizzle the olive oil over the squash, scatter the thyme on top and toss gently to coat evenly.

3. Bake the squash for about 25 minutes until tender and golden brown. Scatter the Parmesan over the squash before serving.

NUTRITION INFO: 1 portion provides:

Calcium: ½ serving

Vitamin C: 2 servings

Vitamin A: 4 servings

Fat: ½ serving

Smoky Roasted Carrots with Lime Cream

SERVES 2

If smoky and sweet had a baby (carrot), this would be the delicious result. Warm, roasted spice is cooled by a tangy, creamy topping, with a scattering of almonds adding crunch and a toasty note.

350 g small carrots, peeled and stalks removed
1 teaspoon olive oil
½ teaspoon ground cumin
½ teaspoon smoked paprika
¼ teaspoon chilli powder
¼ teaspoon coarse salt
3 tablespoons light soured cream
1 tablespoon fresh lime juice
4 tablespoons chopped roasted unsalted almonds or shelled pistachios
1 tablespoon chopped fresh coriander leaves

1. Preheat the oven to 220°C/gas mark 7. Line a baking tray with baking paper.

2. Toss together the carrots, oil, cumin, paprika, chilli powder and salt in a medium bowl, rubbing the spices into the carrots. Spread out the carrots on the prepared baking tray in a single layer. Roast for about 15 minutes until tender.

3. Meanwhile, stir together the soured cream and lime juice in a small bowl.

4. Transfer the carrots to a serving platter and top with the soured cream mixture, almonds and coriander leaves. Serve immediately.

NUTRITION INFO: 1 portion provides:

Vitamin A: 3 servings

Fat: ½ serving

Omegas: some

Lemon Carrots with Rosemary

SERVES 2

Baby carrots with a twist of lemon and a sprinkling of aromatic rosemary make a classic companion to roast chicken, whether homemade or ready-prepared. They're also delish with fish.

2 teaspoons olive oil or butter
150 g baby carrots
4 tablespoons low-salt chicken stock or
    vegetable stock
1 clove garlic, very finely chopped
2 teaspoons fresh chopped rosemary or
    ½ teaspoon dried rosemary
1 teaspoon grated lemon zest
Salt and black pepper
Fresh lemon juice

1. Heat 1 teaspoon of the olive oil or melt the butter in a large non-stick frying pan over a medium heat. Add the carrots and cook for about 2 minutes until they begin to soften. Stir in the stock and bring to the boil. Reduce the heat, cover the frying pan and allow the carrots to simmer for about 10 minutes until they are tender. Transfer the carrots to a bowl and set aside, covered, to keep warm.

2. Heat the remaining 1 teaspoon olive oil in the same pan over a medium heat. Add the garlic and cook for about 1 minute until it begins to soften. Add the rosemary and lemon zest. Return the cooked carrots to the pan and stir to coat them.

From the Test Kitchen

Using thyme leaves in the Lemon Carrots in place of the rosemary makes them a perfect partner for poultry. Feeling fishy? Substitute 2 teaspoons chopped fresh dill or ½ teaspoon dried dill.

3. Remove the carrots from the heat. Season with salt, pepper and lemon juice to taste and serve.

NUTRITION INFO: 1 portion provides:

Vitamin A: 3 servings

Fat: ½ serving

Balsamic Braised Red Cabbage

SERVES 4

Braising red cabbage with balsamic vinegar helps preserve its colour and infuses it with a delectably sweet and complex flavour. Fresh and dried cranberries contribute to the colour scheme as well as to the nutritional content and tangy taste. Team this traditional holiday favourite with the Christmas goose or turkey – or Tuesday night's pork chop.

375 g thinly sliced red cabbage
(about 1 small head)
500 ml low-salt vegetable stock or
chicken stock
4 tablespoons balsamic vinegar
1 tablespoon honey
100 g fresh or frozen cranberries
50 g dried cranberries

1. Preheat the oven to 200°C/gas mark 6.

2. Place the cabbage, vegetable stock, balsamic vinegar, honey, and fresh and dried cranberries in a large mixing bowl and stir to mix. Transfer the cabbage mixture to a flameproof baking dish. Bring the mixture to the boil over a medium heat.

From the Test Kitchen

Don't have an hour to spare? Simply place all of the ingredients for Balsamic Braised Red Cabbage in a large saucepan over a medium heat and bring to a simmer. Cover the pan and allow the cabbage to cook for about 10 minutes until tender. Another tip: make this dish up to 2 days in advance – the flavours will deepen. Warm the braised cabbage before serving or allow it to return to room temperature.

3. Carefully cover the baking dish with aluminium foil and transfer it to the oven. Bake for about 45 minutes until the cabbage is tender. Serve warm or at room temperature. The cabbage can be stored in the refrigerator, covered, for up to 2 days.

NUTRITION INFO: 1 portion provides:

Vitamin C: 1 serving

Other fruits and vegetables: 1 serving

Cheesy Roasted Cauliflower

SERVES 4

Even the most resolute vegetable resister will relent to this homey dish of cauliflower topped with a creamy cheese sauce that's packed with calcium and flavour.

1 small head cauliflower, rinsed, patted dry and cut into florets

2 tablespoons olive oil

250 ml milk

2 tablespoons plain flour

115 g Cheddar or Gruyère cheese, grated

Salt and white pepper

1. Preheat the oven to 200°C/gas mark 6.

2. Toss the cauliflower with the oil in a medium-sized bowl until coated. Spread in a single layer on a baking tray and roast for 25–30 minutes until tender and the edges are golden brown.

3. Meanwhile, place the milk and flour in a small saucepan and stir until the flour dissolves. Bring to the boil over a medium-high heat, then reduce the heat and let simmer, stirring occasionally, for about 4 minutes until the sauce thickens.

From the Test Kitchen

Say 'cheese' two ways: you can also use a combination of Parmesan and Cheddar in the sauce for the cauliflower. And because broccoli loves cheese, too, try this cheese sauce on roasted broccoli. Or make a combo of broccoli and cauliflower. Time extra short? Use the cheese sauce over steamed-in-the-bag cauliflower or broccoli.

4. Remove the saucepan from the heat. Add the cheese and stir until it melts. Season with salt and pepper to taste, then pour the sauce over the roasted cauliflower.

NUTRITION INFO: 1 portion provides:

Calcium: 1 serving

Vitamin C: 1 serving

Fat: ½ serving

That's Italian Green Beans

SERVES 2

Any green vegetables take a turn for the Tuscan when prepared with tomatoes, Italian herbs and Parmesan cheese. Steamed broccoli is also tasty prepared this way. Add extra cheese on top for a calcium fix.

225 g green beans, topped and tailed
125 g tinned Italian-seasoned chopped
    tomatoes, drained
1½ teaspoons very finely chopped fresh
    oregano or ½ teaspoon dried
1½ teaspoons very finely chopped fresh
    basil or ½ teaspoon dried
2 tablespoons grated Parmesan cheese
Pinch of dried chilli flakes (optional)

1. Steam the green beans, following the instructions on page 315, for 4–5 minutes until just tender but still crisp.

2. Transfer the green beans to a saucepan, add the tomatoes, oregano, basil, Parmesan and chilli flakes, if using, and stir to mix. Cook over a medium heat for about 1 minute until heated through.

NUTRITION INFO: 1 portion provides:

Vitamin C: ½ serving

Other fruits and vegetables: 1 serving

Vegetables in a Flash

You can't beat steaming when it comes to retaining the nutrients found in vegetables, but you can beat the clock by using a microwave to bring freshly cooked vegetables to the table in 4 minutes or less. When you need to save even more time and effort, choose ready-to-cook vegetables in a bag (you can shave off even more time by buying steam-in-the-bag veggies and zapping them according to the package directions).

Ready to make microwave magic? Arrange the vegetables (the pieces should be uniform in size) in a single layer in a microwave-safe dish. Add 2 tablespoons vegetable or chicken stock (you can also use water). Season the vegetables, if you wish, with herbs, garlic granules, a sprinkle of lemon juice, a dash of salt and pepper, even a spoonful or two of chopped fresh or tinned tomatoes – or nothing at all, if you like your veggies naked, or you'll be adding the steamed veggies to another recipe or topping them with a sauce later. Tent the dish with microwave-safe cling film, punctured to allow steam to escape (don't let the plastic touch the veggies). Or skip the cling film and cover with a microwave-safe plate. Or, best option: invest in a microwave steamer dish that comes with a cover.

Microwave veggies on high for 1½–4 minutes, depending on their thickness, until just tender or how crisp you like them; larger amounts of vegetables may need longer cooking times. Allow the vegetables to stand for 3–5 minutes before serving.

Minty Peas, Carrots and Mushrooms

SERVES 2

The unexpected addition of mint and shiitake mushrooms to peas and carrots gives you a deliciously sophisticated take on the standard school canteen version. You'll eat every carrot and pea on your plate when they're cooked this way. (And make it faster still by using frozen or steam-in-the-bag peas and carrots.)

115 g shelled fresh or frozen peas
60 g carrots, thinly sliced
1 tablespoon olive oil or butter
65 g shiitake mushroom caps, sliced
1 teaspoon very finely chopped shallot
    (optional)
1 tablespoon chopped fresh mint
Salt and black pepper

1. Cook the peas and carrots separately until crisp-tender, following the steaming instructions on page 315 or the microwave oven instructions on the opposite page, for about 2 minutes for steamed peas or 1½ minutes in the microwave, and 3 minutes for steamed carrots or 2½ minutes in the microwave.

2. Heat the olive oil in a saucepan over a medium heat. Add the mushrooms and shallot and cook for about 2 minutes until they begin to soften. Add the peas, carrots and mint and stir gently until heated through. Season with salt and pepper to taste and serve.

NUTRITION INFO: 1 portion provides:

Vitamin C: ½ serving

Vitamin A: 1 serving

Other fruits and vegetables: 1 serving

Fat: ½ serving

Kale and Shiitake Mushroom Salad

SERVES 2

Is it a salad, or is it a stir-fry? Don't try to label it – just enjoy it, along with a day's worth of green and yellow vegetables and a bonus of soy protein.

225 g kale, thick stalks and tough centre
   veins removed, rinsed well
2 tablespoons low-salt vegetable stock
1 tablespoon low-salt soy sauce
1 tablespoon sesame oil
150 g frozen shelled edamame (soybeans)
110 g shiitake mushroom caps, sliced
35 g carrot matchsticks
2 tablespoons seasoned rice vinegar
2 teaspoons olive oil or rapeseed oil
1 tablespoon toasted sesame seeds
   (see page 217)

1. Cut the kale into 1-cm strips.

2. Place the vegetable stock, soy sauce and sesame oil in a large frying pan over a medium-low heat and bring to a simmer. Add the kale and edamame and toss to coat. Cover the pan and cook for just 2–3 minutes until the kale begins to wilt. Transfer the vegetables to a salad bowl.

3. Add the shiitake mushrooms and carrots to the pan and cook for 2–3 minutes until just tender. Add the mushroom mixture to the kale mixture and allow to cool to room temperature.

4. Just before serving, place the rice vinegar and oil in a small bowl and whisk to mix. Drizzle it over the vegetable mixture and toss to coat. Sprinkle the sesame seeds on top and serve.

NUTRITION INFO: 1 portion provides:

Protein: ½ serving

Calcium: 1 serving

Vitamin C: 1½ servings

Vitamin A: 4 servings

Other fruits and vegetables: 1½ servings

Wholegrains and legumes: 1 serving

Iron: some

Fat: 1 serving

Italian Chard

SERVES 2

This tasty side dish brings out the best in sturdy green leafy vegetables; try it with kale, too.

450 g chard, rinsed and patted dry
175 ml low-salt chicken stock or
   vegetable stock
2 teaspoons olive oil
1 clove garlic, very finely chopped
2 teaspoons very finely chopped shallot
25 g Parmesan cheese, grated
2 tablespoons toasted pine nuts
   (see page 217)
Salt and black pepper

1. Slice the leaves off the stalks of the chard. Roughly chop the leaves and cut the stalks widthways into pieces about 1 cm wide and 5 cm long.

2. Place the chicken broth in a small saucepan and bring to a simmer over medium heat. Add the chard stalks, reduce the heat to low and cook for 8–10 minutes until just tender. Drain and set aside.

3. Heat the olive oil in a large non-stick frying pan over a medium-low heat. Add the garlic and shallot and cook, stirring occasionally, for about 2 minutes until softened. Add the chard leaves and cooked stalks and cook, stirring, for 1–2 minutes until the leaves are just wilted.

4. Add the Parmesan and pine nuts to the chard and stir to mix. Season with salt and pepper to taste and serve.

NUTRITION INFO: 1 portion provides:

Calcium: ½ serving

Vitamin C: ½ serving

Vitamin A: 2 servings

Iron: some

Great Greens

Many salad greens that you're used to eating raw in salads wilt well – and tastily. And since the leaves cook down, you can pack far more vitamin power into an average portion. Try rocket or baby spinach, following the recipe for Italian Chard, starting with Step 3, since these do not have tough stems. Tender salad leaves like these wilt in no time. Serve wilted leaves as a side dish or as a delicious bed for fish or chicken.

Oven-Roasted Potatoes

SERVES 2

You don't need a trip through the golden arches when these golden but nearly greaseless potatoes are just 25 minutes from your plate.

Olive oil cooking spray
350 g Maris Piper or red potatoes
   (about 2 medium-sized)
1 tablespoon olive oil
Salt and coarsely ground black pepper

1. Preheat the oven to 220°C/gas mark 7. Coat a large baking tray with olive oil cooking spray.

2. Cut the potatoes into 4-mm-thick slices, then pat them dry with kitchen paper. Place the potatoes in a bowl, drizzle the olive oil over them, then toss to coat evenly.

3. Arrange the potato slices on the baking tray in a single layer and lightly season them with salt and coarsely ground pepper.

4. Bake the potato slices for about 15 minutes until golden on top. Turn the potatoes over and continue baking for a further 10–15 minutes until the second side is golden and the potato slices are tender. If you like crisper potatoes, allow them to bake a little longer, but watch them carefully so they don't burn.

From the Test Kitchen

Chips with that? Cut the potatoes into thick stick shapes. Toss them with olive oil, then place them in a single layer on a baking tray that has been coated with cooking oil spray. Bake the potatoes in an oven preheated to 200°C/gas mark 6 for 15 minutes. Stir the potatoes to turn and continue baking for a further 10 minutes. For extra-crisp potatoes, stir them every 5 minutes. You can shake things up a bit by sprinkling some grated Parmesan cheese, garlic granules or chilli powder over them – or whatever flavour you fancy.

NUTRITION INFO: 1 portion provides:

Vitamin C: 1 serving

Fat: ½ serving

Green Mashers

SERVES 2

Festive on St Patrick's Day, but so delicious you'll want to serve them all year round. The green – and a healthy dose of protein – comes from the edamame the potatoes are mashed with.

150 g frozen shelled edamame
(soya beans)
2 small Maris Piper potatoes,
cut into 2.5-cm chunks
400 ml low-salt chicken stock or
vegetable stock
75 ml milk or buttermilk, plus more as
needed
2 teaspoons olive oil (optional)
25 g Parmesan cheese, grated, or
more to taste (optional)
Salt and black pepper

1. Bring a saucepan of water to the boil over a high heat, add the edamame and return to the boil. Reduce the heat to medium and cook the edamame for about 12 minutes until very soft. Drain and set aside.

2. Place the potatoes and enough stock to cover them in a small saucepan. Bring to the boil over a high heat, then reduce the heat and allow to simmer for 10–15 minutes until the potatoes are tender. Drain, reserving the cooking liquid.

3. Place the milk in a small microwave-safe bowl and microwave at medium-high power for about 45 seconds until heated through (or warm the milk in a small saucepan).

4. Place the cooked edamame and a few tablespoons of the reserved potato cooking liquid in a food processor and process until smooth, then transfer to a bowl. Add the cooked potatoes, warm milk, olive oil and Parmesan, if using. Using a potato masher, mash to the desired consistency, adding more cooking liquid or warm milk as needed. Season with salt and pepper to taste and serve immediately.

NUTRITION INFO: 1 portion provides:

Protein: ½ serving

Calcium: ½ serving if made with Parmesan cheese

Vitamin C: 1½ servings

Wholegrains and legumes: 1 serving

Iron: some

Roasted Herby Sweet Potatoes

SERVES 2

Pop sweet potatoes in the oven when you're roasting poultry or meat, then pop the fragrant, golden brown wedges in your mouth anytime. If you can find them, try using purple sweet potatoes.

Olive oil cooking spray

225 g sweet potato (about 1 medium-
    sized), unpeeled

1 tablespoon olive oil

1 teaspoon chopped fresh rosemary

1 tablespoon chopped fresh oregano or
    1 teaspoon dried oregano

Dash of ground nutmeg

Dash of ground cumin

Salt and black pepper

1. Preheat the oven to 220°C/gas mark 7. Coat a small baking dish with olive oil cooking spray.

2. Cut the sweet potato in half lengthways. Cut each half into 6 wedges.

3. Place the sweet potato wedges, olive oil, rosemary, oregano, nutmeg, cumin and a sprinkle each of salt and pepper in a large bowl and toss gently to coat evenly.

4. Place the sweet potato wedges in the baking dish in a single layer and bake, uncovered, for about 45 minutes until tender and golden in colour, gently stirring them halfway through.

Micro-baked Jacket Potatoes

Craving the creaming comfort of a baked potato without the wait? Skip the baking and head for the microwave instead. To micro-bake a large potato, scrub well, pat dry and poke 4 or 5 times with a paring knife (to allow steam to escape and avoid a potato explosion). Place on a microwave-safe dish. Microwave on high power for about 7 minutes (12 minutes for 2 potatoes), flipping halfway through cooking (use a glove – the potato will be hot). Feeling sweet? You can micro-bake a scrubbed, poked sweet potato on high in 5–6 minutes, flipping carefully halfway through. Check any potato for doneness by sticking a fork in – it should be soft through. If it's too firm, continue microwaving a minute at a time.

NUTRITION INFO: 1 portion provides:

Vitamin C: ½ serving

Vitamin A: 1 serving

Fat: ½ serving

Sweet Potato Crisps

SERVES 2

Bet you can't stop at just one Sweet Potato Crisp – and there's no good reason why you should. You can get a crisps fix and a hefty dose of vitamin A in the bargain.

Olive oil cooking spray
225 g sweet potato (about 1 medium-sized)
1 tablespoon olive oil
2 tablespoons grated Parmesan cheese
1 teaspoon chopped fresh thyme
Salt and black pepper (optional)

1. Preheat the oven to 220°C/gas mark 7. Coat a large baking tray with olive oil cooking spray.

2. Peel the sweet potato, then cut into 4-mm-thick slices. Pat the slices dry with kitchen paper. Arrange the sweet potato slices on the baking tray in a single layer and brush the tops with the olive oil.

3. Bake the sweet potato slices for about 15 minutes until the tops colour slightly. Turn the slices over and continue baking for a further 10–15 minutes until the second side is lightly coloured and the sweet potatoes are tender. If you like crisper sweet potatoes, allow them to bake a little longer, but watch them carefully so they don't burn.

4. Scatter the Parmesan, thyme and salt and pepper, if wished, over the sweet potatoes before serving.

NUTRITION INFO: 1 portion provides:

Vitamin C: ½ serving

Vitamin A: 1 serving

Fat: ½ serving

Roasted Roots

SERVES 4

You'll want to return to these roots over and over again, and to make extra so that you'll have leftovers (served cold, they'd make a delicious addition to a salad or sandwich, too). For easy clean-up, line your pan with baking paper before coating with oil.

Olive oil cooking spray
1 medium-sized sweet potato, halved,
    each half quartered
4 medium-sized parsnips, peeled
4 medium-sized carrots, peeled
225 g beetroot, trimmed, peeled and
    cut into 2.5-cm chunks
1 large fennel bulb, trimmed and
    quartered
2 tablespoons olive oil
1 tablespoon fresh thyme leaves
Salt and freshly ground black pepper
Grated zest of 1 lemon (optional)

1. Preheat the oven to 220°C/gas mark 7. Coat a roasting pan with olive oil cooking spray (or line the pan with baking paper for easier clean-up).

2. Arrange the sweet potatoes, parsnips, carrots, beetroot and fennel in a single layer in the roasting pan. Brush the vegetables with the olive oil and scatter the thyme over them. Season with salt and pepper. Cover the roasting pan with aluminium foil.

3. Roast the vegetables for about 25 minutes until they begin to soften. Uncover the pan and stir the vegetables. Roast them uncovered for a further 20 minutes until tender and golden.

From the Test Kitchen

Roasting brings out the best flavour in just about every vegetable. You can use any of the following in place of, or in addition to, those in Pan-Roasted Vegetables: chunks of red onion, turnips, celeriac, swede, acorn squash and/or butternut squash, and whole peeled baby onions. Just be sure that they are roughly the same size, or cut into comparable-sized pieces.

And don't stop there. Roast cauliflower with cumin seeds, green beans with oregano, tomatoes with basil, and just about any vegetable with rosemary or sage. See page 317 for more.

4. Place the vegetables on a platter and scatter the lemon zest, if using, over them. The vegetables can be refrigerated, covered, for up to 2 days. Reheat in the oven at 180°C/gas mark 4 for about 10 minutes until hot. They can also be enjoyed at room temperature or straight out of the fridge for a snack.

NUTRITION INFO: 1 portion provides:

Vitamin C: ½ serving

Vitamin A: 3 servings

Other fruits and vegetables: 2 servings

Fat: ½ serving

Edamame Succotash

SERVES 4

A twist on an American favourite side dish, this colourful succotash – made with crisp asparagus, bright red pepper, sweetcorn and chewy edamame – is fresh tasting and packed with protein. Terrific, too, as a bed for fish fillets or chicken breasts.

1 tablespoon olive oil
75 g red pepper, chopped
250 ml low-salt vegetable stock
12 asparagus stalks, woody ends
    removed and cut into 1-cm chunks
150 g shelled frozen edamame
    (soya beans)
150 g fresh or frozen sweetcorn kernels,
    thawed if frozen
2 tablespoons chopped fresh flat-leaf
    parsley
Salt and coarsely ground black pepper

Heat the olive oil in a medium-sized non-stick frying pan over a low heat. Add the red pepper and cook for about 3 minutes until it begins to soften. Add the vegetable stock, raise the heat to medium and bring to a simmer. Add the asparagus, edamame, sweetcorn and parsley. Cover the pan, reduce the heat to low and allow to simmer for about 4 minutes until just tender. Season the succotash with salt and coarsely ground pepper to taste before serving.

NUTRITION INFO: 1 portion provides:

Protein: ½ serving

Vitamin C: 1 serving

Vitamin A: 1 serving

Wholegrains and legumes: ½ serving

Other vegetables and fruits: ½ serving

Iron: some

Fat: ½ serving

Grilled Tofu

SERVES 2

Extra-firm tofu takes on an almost meaty texture when it's grilled, making this dish a great vegetarian alternative when you feel like passing on the steak. It's more like a meal than a side dish, especially when served over Spicy Greens with Ginger Dressing (page 256). Don't have a barbecue? Cook this dish on a griddle pan over a medium-high heat on the hob.

400 g extra-firm tofu, drained well on
   kitchen paper
4 tablespoons low-salt soy sauce or
   tamari
2 teaspoons sesame oil
1 teaspoon rapeseed oil
1 tablespoon honey
2 teaspoons very finely chopped garlic
   (optional)
1 teaspoon chilli-garlic sauce, or sriracha
   plus more to taste (optional)

1. Cut the tofu widthways into 8 even slices. Place the tofu slices in a baking dish large enough to hold all of them in a single layer.

2. Place the soy sauce, sesame oil, rapeseed oil, honey, garlic and chilli-garlic sauce or sriracha, if using, in a small bowl and stir to mix. Taste and add more chilli-garlic sauce if wished. Pour the marinade over the tofu slices. Cover and allow to marinate in the refrigerator for 10 minutes, turning the tofu several times.

From the Test Kitchen

For a delicious nutty taste and crunch, try sprinkling the marinated tofu with untoasted sesame seeds before grilling it.

3. Meanwhile, set up the barbecue and preheat it to medium-high.

4. When you're ready to cook, oil the grill rack. Remove the tofu from the marinade and set the marinade aside. Grill the tofu, brushing it with reserved marinade as it cooks, for 3–4 minutes per side until it's heated through and starts to colour.

NUTRITION INFO: 1 portion provides:

Protein: 1 serving

Calcium: ½ serving

Vitamin C: 1 serving

Iron: some

Fat: ½ serving

Broccoli and Tofu Stir-Fry

SERVES 2

You don't have to be a vegan to veg out on this nutritious Chinese favourite. It makes a meaty meatless meal, particularly when it's teamed with brown rice or soba noodles.

200 ml low-salt vegetable stock
2 tablespoons low-salt soy sauce
2½ teaspoons plain flour
2 teaspoons unseasoned rice vinegar
2 teaspoons sesame oil
1 tablespoon rapeseed oil
225 g extra-firm tofu, drained well on kitchen paper and cut into 1-cm cubes
Pinch of salt
150 g broccoli florets
2 teaspoons very finely chopped garlic
1 tablespoon grated peeled fresh ginger (optional)
65 g shiitake mushrooms, sliced
Dried chilli flakes (optional)

1. Place 2 tablespoons of the vegetable stock and the soy sauce, flour, rice vinegar and sesame oil in a small bowl and whisk to mix. Set the sauce mixture aside.

2. Heat the rapeseed oil in a large non-stick frying pan over a medium heat. Add the tofu and salt. Cook, stirring frequently, for about 8 minutes until the tofu is golden all over. Remove the tofu from the pan.

3. Add the broccoli, the remaining stock, the garlic and ginger, if using, to the pan. Cover and cook, stirring occasionally, for about 4 minutes until the broccoli is crisp-tender. Uncover the pan, add the mushrooms and cook for about 2 minutes until softened. Add the sauce mixture and browned tofu to the broccoli and stir gently to coat. Season with chilli flakes to taste, if wished. Cook, stirring occasionally, for about 2 minutes until the sauce thickens.

NUTRITION INFO: 1 portion provides:

Protein: ½ serving

Vitamin C: 2 servings

Vitamin A: 2 servings

Other fruits and vegetables: 1 serving

Iron: some

Fat: 1 serving

Baked Tofu Three Ways

SERVES 2

This simple technique will take your extra-firm tofu to places you never thought possible: crispy, meaty, flavourful. Baked tofu is incredibly versatile – use it with your favourite sauce or in your favourite recipe – from curry to teriyaki. Toss it into your favourite pasta dish, or in place of your usual protein in your sandwich or wrap. Or try it one of three delicious ways suggested here.

1 x 400-g block extra-firm tofu
1 tablespoon oil of your choice
1 tablespoon low-salt soy sauce
1 tablespoon cornflour or arrowroot
    starch

1. Preheat the oven to 200°C/gas mark 6. Line a large baking tray with baking paper.

2. Place the tofu on a clean tea towel or kitchen paper. Cover with another towel and place a frying pan on top to weigh it down. Allow the tofu to drain for at least 10 minutes or up to 30 minutes. Transfer to a chopping board. Cut the block widthways into 2.5-cm-thick slices and transfer to a medium bowl.

3. Drizzle the tofu with oil of your choice and 1 tablespoon low-salt soy

sauce. Scatter with 1 tablespoon cornflour or arrowroot starch and toss gently until the tofu is covered evenly. You can also scatter with seasoning, if you wish – curry powder if you'll be making a curry, a little dried oregano and garlic granules if you're going Italian, chilli powder if you'll be making Mexican.

4. Place the tofu on the prepared baking tray in a single layer. Bake for 25–30 minutes, carefully turning the tofu over halfway, until it is golden in colour and crispy around the edges.

Sprouting Broccoli and Sweet Potatoes

SERVES 2

1 medium-sized sweet potato (peeled or
    unpeeled), sliced lengthways into
    2-cm-thick wedges
2 tablespoons oil
1 teaspoon salt
½ teaspoon pepper
1 large bunch sprouting broccoli

1. Toss the sweet potato wedges in a bowl with 1 tablespoon oil, ½ teaspoon salt and ¼ teaspoon pepper, and place in a baking tray. Transfer to the preheated oven with the tofu and bake for 30–35 minutes, flipping the wedges halfway through.

2. While potato wedges cook, toss the sprouting broccoli with 1 tablespoon oil, ½ teaspoon salt and ¼ teaspoon pepper, and add to the baking tray with the sweet potato wedges about halfway through and cook for the remaining

---

From the Test Kitchen

Leftover baked tofu keeps in the fridge for up to 3 days and reheats well in the microwave. Even better, toss it in the oven or toaster oven to resurrect its crispy edges.

15–20 minutes until the sweet potatoes are coloured and the sprouting broccoli is crisp-tender. If you are using regular broccoli, you'll need to add it a few minutes earlier.

3. Serve with the Baked Tofu along with chopped, salted roasted peanuts (if wished).

NUTRITION INFO: 1 portion provides:

Vitamin C: 1 serving

Vitamin A: 3 servings

Fat: 1½ servings

Iron: some

Peanut Sauce with Red Peppers and Green Beans

SERVES 2

1 large red pepper, sliced
175 g green beans
1 tablespoon oil
½ teaspoon salt
¼ teaspoon pepper
65 g smoooth peanut butter
4 tablespoons well-shaken unsweetened
   canned coconut milk
1½ tablespoons lime juice
1 tablespoon low-salt soy sauce
½ tablespoon sriracha

1. Toss the red pepper with the green beans, oil, salt and pepper. Transfer to a baking tray and put into the preheated oven with the tofu. Cook for 15 minutes, or until the vegetables are crisp-tender.

2. Meanwhile, in a small bowl whisk together the peanut butter, coconut milk, lime juice, soy sauce and sriracha.

3. Serve the roasted vegetables with the Baked Tofu and drizzle with desired amount of peanut sauce.

NUTRITION INFO: 1 portion provides:

Vitamin A: 3 servings

Other: 2 servings

Fat: 2½ servings

Protein: 1 serving

Curried Cauliflower

SERVES 2

1 tablespoon yellow curry paste
1 tablespoon water
1 tablespoon low-salt soy sauce
2 teaspoons soft brown sugar
1 teaspoon chilli-garlic sauce
200 g fresh cauliflower florets
3 tablespoons fresh coriander
2 tablespoons toasted cashews
   (see page 217)

1. In a large bowl, whisk together the yellow curry paste, water, soy sauce, brown sugar and chilli-garlic sauce.

2. Add the cauliflower florets to the bowl and toss until coated with curry mixture. Transfer to a baking tray and add to preheated oven with the tofu. Cook for about 20 minutes until well coloured and crisp-tender.

3. Serve with the Baked Tofu, garnished with the coriander and cashews (see page 217).

NUTRITION INFO: 1 portion provides:

Protein: 1 serving

Vitamin C: 2 servings

Cauliflower Fried 'Rice' with Pickled Peppers

SERVES 2

Never thought of fried rice as health food? Think outside the greasy takeaway box, and take in this tasty dish, packed with flavour and nutrients, but not with fat. The peppers spice things up (and they're pickled, always a pregnancy plus), while the peanuts add crunch. It partners well with chicken, pork, fish or prawns.

3 tablespoons vegetable oil
150 g small broccoli florets
35 g shallots, thinly sliced
2 medium eggs, lightly beaten
1 x 285-g packet riced cauliflower, thawed
    if frozen
2 tablespoons low-salt soy sauce
1 tablespoon sesame oil
¼ teaspoon sugar
¼ teaspoon black pepper
75 g Peppadew piquanté pickled peppers
    or pickled banana peppers
2 tablespoons chopped fresh coriander
2 tablespoons chopped roasted salted
    peanuts

1. Heat 1 tablespoon of the oil in a large non-stick frying pan over a medium-high heat. Add the broccoli and cook, stirring occasionally, for 4–5 minutes until it is bright green and slightly tender. Add the shallots and cook for a further 30 seconds. Remove the pan from the heat and transfer the vegetables to a plate.

From the Test Kitchen

Want some real rice with your veggie rice? Add 100 g of cooked brown or other wholegrain rice, or legume 'rice', after the cauliflower rice is cooked.

2. Wipe the pan clean (take care, it will be hot). Return it to a medium heat and add 1 tablespoon of the remaining oil. Add the eggs and cook, stirring once or twice, for 2–3 minutes until set. Transfer the eggs to a chopping board and cut into 1-cm pieces.

3. Raise the heat under the pan to medium-high. Add the remaining 1 tablespoon oil. Add cauliflower and cook, undisturbed, for about 4 minutes until softened and lightly toasted. Remove from the heat. Stir in the soy sauce, sesame oil, sugar, pepper, broccoli mixture and eggs. Divide between 2 serving plates and top with the pickled peppers, coriander and peanuts.

NUTRITION INFO: 1 portion provides:

Vitamin C: 4 servings

Vitamin A: 2 servings

Fat: 2 servings

Farro Risotto with Mushrooms

SERVES 2

Creamy and cheesy, this dish has all the best elements of a traditional risotto, making it a hearty sidekick for chicken or fish. Or serve the full recipe as a vegetarian main dish for one. The nutritious twist? Farro stands in for Arborio rice, lending more fibre and protein.

1 tablespoon olive oil or butter

1 tablespoon very finely chopped shallot

150 g mushrooms, such as portobello, chestnut, oyster, shiitake or button, roughly chopped

1½ tablespoons chopped fresh flat-leaf parsley

2 teaspoons fresh thyme leaves, or ½ teaspoon dried thyme

2 cloves garlic, very finely chopped

85 g farro

600 ml low-salt vegetable stock or chicken stock, plus more as needed

1 tablespoon tomato purée

60 g Parmesan cheese, grated

Salt and black pepper

1. Heat the olive oil in a medium-sized non-stick saucepan over a medium heat. Add the shallot and cook for about 4 minutes until softened.

2. Add the mushrooms and cook, stirring occasionally, for about 10 minutes until browned.

3. Add the parsley, thyme, garlic and farro, and cook, stirring, for about 1 minute until heated slightly.

4. Add 475 ml of the stock and bring to the boil. Reduce the heat, cover the pan and allow to simmer for 20–25 minutes until the liquid is almost absorbed and the farro is almost tender.

5. Add the remaining 125 ml of stock and the tomato purée. Cook uncovered, stirring occasionally, for about 5 minutes until the farro is tender and creamy. If the farro becomes too dry, add a little more vegetable stock.

6. Stir in the Parmesan and season with salt and pepper to taste. Serve.

NUTRITION INFO: 1 portion provides:

Protein: ½ serving

Calcium: 1½ servings

Other fruits and vegetables: 2 servings

Wholegrains and legumes: 1 serving

Iron: some

Fat: ½ serving

Quinoa with Wild Mushrooms

SERVES 2

This protein-rich grain is easier to cook than to figure out how to pronounce (it's KEEN-wah). And you'll pronounce it delicious alongside poultry or beef.

250 ml low-salt vegetable stock or
    chicken stock
85 g quinoa, rinsed and drained
1 teaspoon fresh thyme leaves
⅛ teaspoon salt
1 tablespoon olive oil
130 g sliced shiitake mushroom caps
1 shallot, very finely chopped
1 tablespoon chopped fresh flat-leaf
    parsley
2 teaspoons sherry vinegar

1. Place the vegetable stock in a medium-sized saucepan and bring to the boil over a high heat. Add the quinoa, thyme and salt, then return the stock to the boil. Reduce the heat to low, cover the pan and cook for about 15 minutes until the quinoa is tender.

2. Meanwhile, heat the olive oil in a non-stick frying pan over a medium heat. Add the mushrooms, shallot and parsley and cook for about 5 minutes until the mushrooms are softened. Add the sherry vinegar and cook for about 30 seconds just until heated through. Toss the cooked quinoa with the mushrooms and serve.

NUTRITION INFO: 1 portion provides:

Protein: ½ serving

Other fruits and vegetables: 2 servings

Wholegrains and legumes: 1 serving

Iron: some

Fat: ½ serving

The Grain Game

There's a whole world of wholegrains. Sure, right now you may not know how to pronounce some of them, never mind cook them, but there's no need to be intimidated. Actually, preparing wholegrains isn't any trickier than preparing pasta, though in some cases the cooking time is a lot longer – from 30 minutes to as much as an hour. To save yourself time, consider cooking large batches, then refrigerating leftovers to be reheated in the microwave for hot cereal, pilau or stuffing, or served cold in salads. They'll keep for up to 1 week. So experiment! Have fun! And remember, no matter how you serve wholegrains, you'll be serving yourself a healthy dose of fibre, protein, B vitamins and trace minerals. Prefer to stay grain-free? Substitute legume 'rice' for any grain – just cook according to packet instructions before saucing.

Leek and Tomato Quinoa

SERVES 2

An easy and cheesy way to explore this intriguing high-protein grain.

85 g quinoa, rinsed and drained
275 ml low-salt vegetable stock
1 tablespoon olive oil
1 large leek (white and pale green parts), trimmed, rinsed well and finely chopped
1 medium-sized ripe tomato, seeded and chopped
2 tablespoons chopped fresh basil or flat-leaf parsley
½ tablespoon fresh lemon juice, plus more to taste
Salt and black pepper
25 g Parmesan cheese, grated

1. Place the quinoa and 250 ml of the vegetable stock in a medium-sized saucepan and bring to the boil over a high heat. Reduce the heat to low, cover the pan and allow to simmer for about 15 minutes until the quinoa is tender (or follow instructions on the packet). Drain if necessary and set aside.

2. Meanwhile, heat the olive oil in a large non-stick frying pan over a medium heat. Add the leek and cook for about 5 minutes until it begins to soften.

3. Add the remaining 25 ml of vegetable stock, cover the pan and allow to simmer for about 5 minutes until the leek is tender.

4. Add the cooked quinoa to the leek and cook, stirring, for about 3 minutes until heated through.

5. Add the tomato, basil or parsley, and lemon juice and gently stir to mix. Taste for seasoning, adding more lemon juice as necessary and salt and pepper to taste. Scatter the Parmesan on top and serve.

NUTRITION INFO: 1 portion provides:

Protein: ½ serving

Calcium: ½ serving

Vitamin C: ½ serving

Wholegrains and legumes: 1 serving

Iron: some

Fat: ½ serving

Red Peppers Stuffed with Quinoa

SERVES 4

These tasty and colourful bundles, packed with the goodness of grains and veggies, make a super side or a super supper (especially if you top with grated cheese before baking, for a calcium and protein boost).

40 g quinoa
250 ml low-salt vegetable stock
Pinch of salt
150 g fresh or frozen sweetcorn kernels, thawed if frozen
2 tablespoons chopped fresh coriander
1 tablespoon fresh lime juice, plus more to taste
1 teaspoon chopped peeled fresh ginger
2 spring onions (white and light green parts), chopped
90 g ripe fresh tomato, chopped
75 g yellow pepper, chopped
1 tablespoon olive oil
Salt and black pepper
2 large red peppers, cut in half lengthways, stalks, seeds and white membrane removed

1. Preheat the oven to 190°C/gas mark 5.

2. Place the quinoa in a large saucepan over a medium heat and cook, stirring frequently, for 5–7 minutes until the seeds are golden in colour and fragrant.

3. Add the vegetable stock and salt and bring to the boil. Cover the pan, reduce the heat to medium-low and allow to simmer for about 20 minutes until the liquid is almost absorbed.

4. Add the sweetcorn to the quinoa and cook for about 5 minutes until heated through. Remove the saucepan from the heat. Add the coriander, lime juice, ginger, spring onions, tomato, yellow pepper and olive oil to the quinoa and sweetcorn mixture and stir gently to mix. Season to taste with salt, pepper and more lime juice if wished. Mound the pilau in the red pepper halves, dividing it evenly between them.

5. Place the stuffed pepper halves on a baking tray and bake for 20–25 minutes until golden in colour.

NUTRITION INFO: 1 portion provides:

Vitamin C: 3 servings

Vitamin A: 1 serving

Other vegetables and fruits: ½ serving

Wholegrains and legumes: ½ serving

Iron: some

Three-in-One Pilau

SERVES 4

Bulgar wheat, quinoa and roasted buckwheat groats team up here for a deliciously different – and nutritious – pilau. Peas or edamame add even more nutrients and a touch of colour.

1 tablespoon rapeseed oil
1 small shallot, chopped
75 g coarse bulgar wheat
40 g quinoa, rinsed and drained
40 g roasted whole buckwheat groats
650 ml low-salt vegetable stock
Salt and black pepper
75 g frozen green peas or shelled
    edamame (soya beans), thawed

1. Heat the oil in a medium-sized non-stick frying pan over a medium heat. Add the shallot and cook for about 2 minutes until it begins to soften.

2. Add the bulgar, quinoa and buckwheat groats to the pan and cook, stirring, for about 2 minutes until coated.

3. Add the vegetable stock and a pinch each of salt and pepper and bring to the boil. Cover the pan, reduce the heat and allow to simmer for about 20 minutes until almost all of the liquid is absorbed and the grains are tender.

4. Add the peas and allow to simmer for about 2 minutes until the peas are heated through. Season with more salt and pepper to taste before serving. Leftovers can be stored, covered, in the refrigerator for up to 3 days.

NUTRITION INFO: 1 portion provides:

Wholegrains and legumes: 1 serving

Iron: some

'Mocktails' and Smoothies

T hink the party's over just because you're pregnant? Not so. Whether you're stocking your bar for a weekend brunch, a bank holiday barbecue or a New Year's open house, don't forget to fill a jug or blender with your favourite 'mocktail' or smoothie so you can toast the occasion, too. But don't wait for a toast to enjoy these drinks. Sip them anytime you're thirsty (or in the case of smoothies, hungry) for a tasty treat. Some make satisfying before-dinner drinks, while others can stand in for – or supplement – breakfast when you're in a hurry or too queasy to face solids.

Iced Watermelon Water

MAKES ABOUT 2.75 LITRES

R efreshingly different – and just plain refreshing. It will be especially soothing to sip when you're queasy.

40 g loosely packed fresh mint leaves
3 tablespoons orange juice (optional)
600 g seedless watermelon flesh, diced
500 g ice cubes

Place the mint and a couple of tablespoons water in a 4-litre jug and muddle them with a wooden spoon. Add the orange juice, if using, the watermelon, ice cubes and 1.4 litres of water. Stir to mix. To serve, pour into glasses. Nibble on the fruit while you sip for a dose of vitamin C.

First Blush

SERVES 2

So sweet and satisfying, your First Blush may lead to a second. Substitute thawed frozen or fresh strawberries and add a little sparkling water if you'd like a more sippable drink.

150 g seedless watermelon flesh, diced
100 g frozen strawberries
250 ml orange juice
8 fresh mint leaves (optional)
125 ml sparkling water (optional)

Place the watermelon, strawberries, orange juice and mint leaves, if using, in a blender or food processor and process until the fruit is puréed and the mixture is well blended. Divide the drinks evenly between 2 tall glasses, stir 4 tablespoons cold sparkling water into each, if desired, and serve.

From the Test Kitchen

Turn your First Blush into a first-class smoothie by adding 240 g vanilla yogurt. You'll also turn a half serving of calcium into a whole one, and add protein if your yogurt is Greek.

NUTRITION INFO: 1 portion provides:

Vitamin C: 2 servings plus

Get Juiced Without the Acid

The high acid levels in orange juice can trigger tummy troubles in some expectant mums, particularly during the queasy early months. If that's true for you, shake up your shake without shaking up your stomach by substituting orange juice with another kinder, gentler juice such as apple juice. Or turn to Iced Watermelon Water (opposite page) minus the orange juice.

Citrus Blueberry Blast

SERVES 2

Very berry, very nutritious, very delicious – blissful blueberries, packed with antioxidants, combine with grape and orange juice to make this 'mocktail' a blast to drink.

155 g frozen blueberries
125 ml unsweetened apple juice
250 ml orange juice
250 ml sparkling water

Place the blueberries, grape juice and orange juice in a blender or food processor and process until the fruit is puréed and the mixture is well blended. Divide the drinks evenly between 2 tall glasses, stir 125 ml sparkling water into each and serve.

NUTRITION INFO: 1 portion provides:

Vitamin C: 1 serving

Other vegetables and fruits: 1 serving

Tropical Temptation

SERVES 1

Drink your vitamins. With a unique combo of flavours – orange, carrot and peach (or mango) – this 'mocktail' provides a taste of the tropics and a whole lot of nutrition.

125 ml orange juice
125 ml carrot juice
150 g stoned fresh ripe or frozen yellow peaches or mango, sliced
1 tablespoon pineapple juice (optional)

Place the orange juice, carrot juice, peaches and pineapple juice, if using, in a blender or food processor and process until the fruit is puréed and the mixture is well blended. Pour into a tall glass and serve.

NUTRITION INFO: 1 portion provides:

Calcium: ½ serving

Vitamin C: 1 serving if made with peaches; 3 servings if made with mango

Vitamin A: 3 servings if made with peaches; 4 servings if made with mango

Other fruits and vegetables: 1 serving if made with peaches

Ocean Breeze Smoothie

SERVES 2

Here's another taste of the tropics, with more vitamins than you can shake one of those little paper umbrellas at. Almond milk can help relieve heartburn, but feel free to use cow's milk instead. For a thicker smoothie, use vanilla Greek yogurt.

150 g frozen mango chunks
240 g frozen pineapple chunks or drained
   canned pineapple
125 ml almond milk or cow's milk
240 g vanilla yogurt
2 fresh mint sprigs

Place the mango, pineapple, milk and yogurt in a blender or food processor and process until the fruit is puréed and the mixture is well blended. Divide the drinks evenly between 2 tall glasses, garnish each glass with a mint sprig and serve.

NUTRITION INFO: 1 portion provides:

Calcium: 1 serving

Vitamin C: 2 servings

Vitamin A: 1 serving

Apple and Spice Smoothie

SERVES 1 VERY GENEROUSLY

Spice up your morning while calming your morning sickness with this big mama smoothie. Add yogurt – and maybe some linseeds (flaxseeds) or wheatgerm – if you'd like to make it a meal. Using frozen banana slices will make the smoothie even thicker.

250 ml pineapple juice
240 g frozen pineapple chunks
1 small apple, peeled, cored and chopped
1 ripe banana, sliced
1 x 2-5-cm piece fresh ginger, peeled and
   thinly sliced

Place the pineapple juice, pineapple, apple, banana and ginger in a blender or food processor and process until the fruit is puréed and the mixture is well blended. Pour into a tall glass and serve.

NUTRITION INFO: 1 portion provides:

Vitamin C: 3 servings

Other fruits and vegetables: 2 servings

Soothing Smoothies

The name says it all – smoothies go down easily even when you're feeling a little rough. They can stand in for a meal when you don't feel like cooking or eating. Here are some general tips for making successful smoothies:

- Start with a liquid: fruit juice, cow's milk, almond milk or plant-based milk. For a smoothie that's more sippable, use at least 250 ml liquid. For a thick smoothie worthy of a spoon – and an extra jolt of calcium – substitute regular or Greek yogurt for part of the liquid or use some in addition.

- To make the smoothie creamy and custardy, use frozen fruits instead of fresh, or freeze cut-up fresh fruit first.

- Boost the smoothie's nutritional profile by adding a tablespoon or two of wheatgerm, oat bran, ground linseeds (flaxseeds) or soft tofu.

- Turn any yogurt smoothie vegan by substituting soft tofu for the yogurt. Just sweeten to taste with your natural sweetener of choice. Or use your favourite vanilla plant-based milk.

- Ginger reduces the queasies for many women; try tossing a tablespoon of sliced peeled fresh ginger into any smoothie before blending.

- Like your smoothies really sweet? Add some honey, maple syrup or other sweetener of choice, from Splenda to Swerve (see page 74). Extra ripe frozen banana also adds sweetness, plus a thick creaminess.

Razzleberry

SERVES 2

Serve this drink thick and creamy – or thin it and make it fizz by adding sparkling water. Either way, it's yummy.

325 g frozen raspberries
250 ml orange juice
12 fresh mint leaves (optional)
2 tablespoons soft tofu
1 tablespoon honey or maple syrup, or to taste
250 ml sparkling water (optional)

Place the raspberries, orange juice, mint leaves, if using, tofu and honey in a blender or food processor and process until the fruit is puréed and the drink is thick and creamy. Divide the drinks evenly between 2 tall glasses. If you want a thinner consistency, add 125 ml sparkling water to each before serving.

NUTRITION INFO: 1 portion provides:

Protein: ½ serving

Vitamin C: 2 servings

It's Easy Being Green Smoothie

SERVES 1

Feeling too green to eat your greens in a salad? Here's your sweet revenge: a green smoothie that doesn't taste like a green smoothie. Switch up the fruit to fit today's preferred flavour profile (that's why you've stashed away so many different varieties in your freezer, right?).

240 g frozen pineapple chunks
30 g spinach (stalks removed), torn into 2.5-cm pieces
250 ml unsweetened almond milk or cow's milk, plus more as needed
1 small ripe banana
1 x 1-cm slice fresh ginger, peeled and grated (optional)

Combine the pineapple, spinach, milk, banana and ginger, if using, in a blender. Blend until combined and smooth, adding additional milk as needed. Serve immediately.

NUTRITION INFO: 1 portion provides:

Calcium: 1 serving

Vitamin C: 2½ servings

Vitamin A: 1 serving

Other fruits and vegetables: 1 serving

Iron: some

Breakfast Booster Shake

SERVES 1 GENEROUSLY

No time to eat breakfast? Drink it instead. This breakfast in a blender may be just the ticket, too, when solids don't appeal – or just aren't staying down.

240 g vanilla yogurt
125 ml almond milk or cow's milk
75 g fresh or frozen mango, cubed
    (about ½ medium-sized mango)
75 g frozen or fresh blueberries
½ ripe banana, sliced (see Note)
3 ice cubes (optional; see Note)

Place the yogurt, milk, mango, blueberries, banana and ice, if using, in a blender or food processor and process until the fruit is puréed and the drink is thick and creamy. Pour the drink into a tall glass and serve.

NOTE: If you like a really thick shake, freeze the banana slices first (you can keep a stash in the freezer). If you are using fresh mango and blueberries and an unfrozen banana, add the ice cubes to chill the shake.

NUTRITION INFO: 1 portion provides:

Calcium: 1½ servings

Vitamin C: 2 servings

Vitamin A: 1 serving

Other fruits and vegetables: 1½ servings

From the Test Kitchen

BOOST YOUR BREAKFAST

Give your shake a bigger boost by trying these tips:

- Add 1–2 tablespoons wheatgerm or ground linseeds (flaxseeds).

- Add 1 tablespoon almond butter or peanut butter.

- Add 60 g soft tofu – you'll get an extra protein boost without any change in flavour.

- Substitute 40 g peach or apricot slices for the mango.

- Sweeten your smoothie, if you wish, with honey, maple syrup or the sweetener of your choice to taste.

Mango Tango

MAKES 1 TALL DRINK

This super-nutritious drink will have your taste buds dancing all the way to the tropics. It's like paradise in a glass.

150 g frozen mango chunks
250 ml chilled pineapple juice
120 g vanilla yogurt
½ teaspoon vanilla extract
2 or 3 ice cubes (optional)

Place the mango, pineapple juice, yogurt, vanilla extract and ice cubes, if using, in a blender or food processor and process until the fruit is puréed and the ice is crushed. Pour into a tall glass and serve.

From the Test Kitchen

For a dairy-free smoothie, substitute 120 g soft tofu for the yogurt. Sweeten to taste with honey or another sweetener, or use vanilla almond milk.

NUTRITION INFO: 1 portion provides:

Calcium: ½ serving

Vitamin C: 4 servings

Vitamin A: 2 servings

Mango and Strawberry Smoothie Bowl

SERVES 1

Cold cereal leaving you cold? Swap out that bowl of ho-hum with this bowl of yum – you'll also be knocking off a couple fruit servings (plus you'll score an A from the mango).

150 g frozen mango chunks
100 g frozen strawberries, plus
    2 to 3 tablespoons for serving
125 ml unsweetened almond milk or
    cow's milk
1 tablespoon maple syrup or honey
1 frozen banana
2 tablespoons chopped walnuts,
    for serving
1 tablespoon desiccated coconut,
    for serving

Combine the mango, 100 g strawberries, milk, banana and maple syrup in a blender. Process on high speed for about 1 minute until smooth. Pour into a serving bowl. Garnish with the remaining strawberries, the walnuts and the coconut.

NUTRITION INFO: 1 portion provides:

Calcium: ½ serving

Vitamin C: 3 servings

Vitamin A: 2 servings

Other fruits and vegetables: 1 serving

Omegas: some

Peanut Butter, Banana and Chocolate Smoothie

SERVES 1

What's peanut butter without banana? And what's either without chocolate? Stop questioning and start blending this match made in smoothie heaven. Add ice to make it thick enough to eat with a spoon – the perfect excuse for scattering salted peanuts and dark chocolate chips on top.

75 g frozen ripe banana slices (about 1 large banana)
120 g Greek vanilla yogurt
2 tablespoons soft peanut butter
1 tablespoon cocoa powder

Combine the banana slices, peanut butter and cocoa in a blender. Blend until combined and smooth. Serve immediately.

NUTRITION INFO: 1 portion provides:

Protein: ½ serving

Calcium: ½ serving

Other fruits and vegetables: 1 serving

Fat: 2 servings

Go Bananas

If there's one smoothie ingredient you should always have to hand, it's frozen ripe bananas. They'll make your smoothie sweet, thick and extra satisfying. Peel ripe bananas (the peels should be well-speckled, without a hint of green) and cut into thirds before storing them in a container or freezer bag. Another use for your frozen banana stash: coat them in melted dark chocolate for a decadent treat.

Carrot Cake Smoothie Bowl

SERVES 1

Craving carrot cake – and a healthy, speedy way to start your day (or to get you through a long afternoon)? Have your cake and drink it, too, in this yummy smoothie.

250 ml unsweetened vanilla almond milk
   or cow's milk
2 tablespoons almond butter
55 g carrot, grated
60 g frozen pineapple
¼ teaspoon ground nutmeg
50 g ice
1 tablespoon raisins
1 tablespoon desiccated coconut
1 tablespoon toasted chopped walnuts
   (see page 217)

Place the almond milk, almond butter, carrot, pineapple, nutmeg and ice in a food processor or blender and process until smooth. Pour into a serving bowl. Garnish with raisins, coconut and walnuts.

Nutrition Info 1 portion provides:

Protein: 1 serving

Calcium: 1 serving

Vitamin C: ½ serving

Vitamin A: 2 servings

Fat: 2 servings

Omegas: some

Desserts

....

Healthy isn't the first thing that usually comes to mind when you think dessert. Sweet, yes. Tempting, yes. But healthy? Not often . . . unless your idea of dessert is a ripe peach. Fortunately, with the recipes in this chapter, healthy desserts aren't just a pipe dream. On the pages that follow you'll find delicious ice lollies, biscuits, cakes, tarts and cobblers designed to fill your nutritional requirements with wholegrains and fruit while filling your sweet tooth with joy. Does having such nutritious treats just a short recipe away (or stashed in the freezer) mean that you'll never want to reach for a truly decadent dessert like that molten chocolate cake or glazed tart? Maybe not. But it's nice to know you can have the option of reaching for a second slice of cake or a third biscuit without a second thought. So dig in!

Fruity Oat Biscuits

MAKES ABOUT 30 BISCUITS

These are way chewier than your average oat biscuit and a lot more nutritious, too. Handle them with care, or you'll find out just how this 'cookie' crumbles (of course, the crumbs taste just as good as the biscuit).

185 g porridge oats
40 g ground linseeds (flaxseeds)
30 g wheatgerm
2 teaspoons ground cinnamon
85 g butter, melted
1 medium egg
250 g honey
75 g raisins, chopped
40 g toasted pecans or walnuts
   (see page 217), chopped

1. Preheat the oven to 160°C/gas mark 3.

2. Place the oats, linseeds, wheatgerm and cinnamon in a large bowl and stir to mix well. Add the butter and stir to combine.

3. Whisk together the egg and honey in another bowl until blended. Pour the egg mixture over the oat mixture and stir well. Add the raisins and nuts and stir to mix.

4. Drop the mixture by tablespoonfuls about 2.5 cm apart onto two non-stick baking trays, then flatten slightly with the back of a fork (wet the fork slightly if the dough sticks to it) to make irregular circles.

5. Bake the biscuits for about 15 minutes until they are lightly coloured and the edges are firm. Allow the biscuits to cool completely on the baking trays before serving. The biscuits can be stored in an airtight container for up to 5 days or frozen for up to 1 month.

NURITION INFO: 1 portion (2 biscuits) provides:

Wholegrains and legumes: ½ serving

Iron: some

Fat: ½ serving

Omegas: some

Cooking with Alternative Sweeteners

Looking to sweeten the pot (or the cake or muffin or pancake mixture) without sugar? Whether you're looking to alternative sweeteners to cut calories or to control blood sugar, it's not just a matter of taste. Some sweeteners are better suited to cooking and baking than others, but happily most (including sucralose, stevia, monk fruit and xylitol) are heat stable. Saccharin (Sweet'n Low) and aspartame (NutraSweet, Equal) aren't, but they're not well suited for pregnancy use, anyway.

Something else to seek in a sweetener: a 1 to 1 ratio when swapping for sugar. If the taste is sweeter, spoon for spoon, than sugar, you'll need to use less. Less sweet than sugar? You'll need to use more. Also look for a taste that approximates sugar well, bearing in mind that taste (and sweetness) can vary from brand to brand.

Finally, if curbing carbs is your goal – especially if it's on doctor's orders – be mindful of the carb count. Scan the Nutrition Facts to get the scoop on the sweetener you're scrutinising. Some sweeteners, particularly baking blends, may contain some sugar.

For more about alternative sweeteners, see page 74.

Gingerbread Mum

MAKES 1 x 23-CM CAKE (8–12 SERVINGS)

Ginger makes this cake especially soothing for a queasy tummy – and especially hard to resist.

Cooking oil spray
240 g wholemeal flour
40 g ground linseeds (flaxseeds)
25 g porridge oats or wheatgerm
2 teaspoons ground ginger
1 teaspoon ground cinnamon
2 teaspoons bicarbonate of soda
160 g molasses or treacle
110 g soft brown sugar
2 medium eggs
4 tablespoons rapeseed oil
2 teaspoons minced peeled fresh ginger

1. Preheat the oven to 180°C/gas mark 4. Lightly coat a non-stick 23-cm-square cake tin with cooking oil spray.

2. Combine the flour, linseeds, oats, ground ginger, cinnamon and bicarbonate of soda in a medium-sized bowl.

3. Place the molasses, brown sugar, eggs, oil and ginger in another bowl and beat with an electric whisk on a low speed or with a hand whisk until well mixed.

4. Add the flour mixture to the molasses mixture, beating at a low speed just until thoroughly blended. Pour the mixture into the prepared cake tin.

5. Bake for about 30 minutes until the top of the cake springs back when lightly pressed.

6. Allow the cake to cool slightly in the tin before turning it out on to a wire rack to cool completely, or allow it to cool and serve straight from the pan. For instructions on storing the cake, see the box below.

NUTRITION INFO: provides:

Wholegrains and legumes: 1 serving

Iron: some

Fat: ½ serving

Pop Them into Your Freezer

No one expects you to eat an entire cake at one sitting (though you might be tempted to do so every now and then). Instead, bake the cake, cut it into individual servings, wrap the pieces in aluminium foil and store them in the freezer for an easy dessert or anytime snack. (Don't forget to eat one slice first!) The cake slices will keep for up to a month in the freezer. To serve, simply let cake slices thaw at room temperature or in the fridge.

Almond Flour Brownies

MAKES 9–12 BROWNIES

These chewy, gooey brownies are gluten-free, but no one will notice. Plus, almond flour adds protein power, scoring you extra brownie points, even if you're not adding gluten.

Cooking oil spray
225 g semisweet chocolate chips
150 g soft brown sugar
2 medium eggs
5 tablespoons avocado oil (or rapeseed oil)
1 teaspoon vanilla extract
80 g blanched almond flour
2 tablespoons cocoa powder
½ teaspoon baking powder
¼ teaspoon salt

1. Preheat the oven to180°C/gas mark 4. Lightly coat a non-stick 20-cm-square cake tin with cooking oil spray.

2. In a small saucepan, melt 115 g of the chocolate chips over a low heat until smooth and glossy. Remove from the heat and set aside to cool slightly.

3. Whisk together the brown sugar, eggs, oil and vanilla in a medium-sized bowl. Stir the almond flour, cocoa, baking powder and salt together in a small bowl. Slowly whisk the flour mixture into the egg and sugar mixture. Whisk in the melted chocolate.

4. Fold in the remaining 110 g chocolate chips. Pour the mixture into the prepared tin and smooth the surface with a rubber palette knife. Bake for 20–24 minutes until the edges are set and the centre is still ever so slightly underdone and a skewer inserted in the centre comes out with a few moist crumbs stuck to it. Allow the brownies to cool in the tin before cutting into squares. Store in an airtight container for up to 3 days.

NUTRITION INFO: 1 portion (1 x 5-cm brownie) provides:

Fat: ½ serving

Omegas: some

Not Nuts for Nuts?

Nuts provide a healthy host of vitamins, minerals and vital fatty acids. But if you'd like to leave them out of these recipes because you're not nuts for the taste, you have a nut allergy or your doctor has advised you to avoid nuts during pregnancy, go right ahead.

Omitting chopped nuts from a recipe won't affect the outcome significantly (toss in desiccated coconut if you wish). If a recipe calls for ground nuts, substitute an equal amount of ground linseeds (flaxseed), wheatgerm, oats or flour.

Poached Pears with Ginger

SERVES 4

Yes, these elegant pears are perfect for company. But why should company have all the fun? They're easy enough to make midweek, too. Have the leftovers for breakfast or as a snack.

4 Bosc pears

700 ml unsweetened apple juice

50 g soft brown sugar

1 teaspoon vanilla extract

1 x 2.5-cm piece fresh ginger, peeled and thinly sliced

4 small wedges mature Cheddar cheese (30–40 g each)

1. Peel the pears, then arrange them, stalk end up, in a deep saucepan just big enough to hold them tightly in place. Add the apple juice, sugar, vanilla, ginger and just enough water to cover the pears.

2. Place the saucepan over a medium-high heat and bring the poaching liquid to the boil. Reduce the heat, partially cover the pan and allow the pears to simmer for about 20 minutes until soft but not mushy.

3. Allow the pears to cool to room temperature in the poaching liquid. Remove them and set aside.

4. Place the saucepan over a high heat, bring the poaching liquid to the boil and continue boiling for about 10 minutes until reduced by half.

5. To serve, place the pears on serving plates and drizzle some of the poaching liquid over them. Serve a wedge of Cheddar alongside each pear.

NUTRITION INFO: 1 portion provides:

Calcium: 1 serving

Vitamin C: 1 serving

Other fruits and vegetables: 2 servings

Strawberry Mint Slushie

SERVES 1

Not your average syrupy slushie, this one delivers icy refreshment that's just sweet enough, especially if the strawberries you use are extra ripe. Frozen strawberries will work, too, as will frozen or fresh blueberries. But why stop with berries? Just about any fruit is nice with ice.

225 g ripe fresh or frozen strawberries
2 teaspoons fresh mint
225 g ice
4 tablespoons sparkling water (or more, as needed)

Combine strawberries, mint and ice in a food processor or blender and process until the ice is completely crushed (some larger, crushed pieces may remain), stopping as needed to scrape down the sides. Pour sparkling water in and process for a few more seconds until the consistency resembles a slushie. Add more sparkling water as needed to reach desired consistency.

From the Test Kitchen

Not sweet enough after all? Add a sprinkle of your favourite sweetener.

NUTRITION INFO: 1 portion provides:

Vitamin C: 4 servings

Yogurt Banana Ice Lollies

MAKES 8 ICE LOLLIES

Searching for a sweet frozen treat that's actually healthy to eat? You'll go bananas for these easy-to-prep ice lollies – keep a stash for dessert, snacks . . . hey, even breakfast.

600 g ripe bananas, sliced
    (about 2 large bananas)
50 g sugar (or Splenda or Swerve)
120 g natural full-fat Greek yogurt
3 tablespoons double cream

1. Place the bananas and 25 g of the sugar in a blender and blend, stopping to scrape down the sides as needed, for about 1 minute until smooth.

2. Place the yogurt, double cream and the remaining 25 g of sugar in a bowl and stir to mix well. Add the banana purée and whisk to mix well. Spoon the mixture into 8 x 115-g ice lolly moulds. Insert ice lolly sticks into the moulds and freeze for at least 4 hours to over-night until solid.

From the Test Kitchen

Swap out 150 g of bananas for 150 g of your favourite fruit. Strawberries or blueberries for a berry blast or mangoes or pineapple if you're feeling tropical.

3. Just before serving, run the moulds briefly under hot water to release the ice lollies.

NUTRITION INFO: 1 portion (1 ice lolly) provides:

Other fruits and vegetables: ½ serving

Spicy and Sweet Ice Lollies

MAKES 8 ICE LOLLIES

Cool, creamy and sassy with a balance of sweet and heat, in case you're craving both. Substitute chopped raspberries or blueberries.

225 g fresh or frozen strawberries
1 tablespoon soft light brown sugar
5 tablespoons honey
½ teaspoon cayenne pepper
2 x 5-cm-long strips lemon peel
540 g natural full-fat Greek yogurt

1. Place the berries and brown sugar in a small saucepan over a medium heat. Cook, stirring occasionally to mix well and pressing to break up the berries, for 10–12 minutes until they fully release their juices. Cool completely.

2. Meanwhile, place 80 ml water, the honey, cayenne and lemon peel in a small saucepan. Cover and bring to the boil over a medium-high heat. Remove from the heat and allow to stand for 15 minutes. Pour the syrup through a fine-mesh seive into a bowl; discard the solids. Allow to cool completely for about 10 minutes.

3. Stir the yogurt into the syrup. Alternately spoon the yogurt and the berry mixtures into 8 x 115-g ice lolly moulds, beginning and ending with the yogurt mixture. Insert ice lolly sticks into the moulds and freeze for at least 4 hours to overnight until solid.

4. Just before serving, run the moulds briefly under hot water to release the ice lollies.

NUTRITION INFO: 1 portion (1 ice lolly) provides:

Calcium: ½ serving

Vitamin C: ½ serving

Conversion Table

Approximate Equivalents

1 medium eating apple (without core) = 100 g

1 large banana (without skin) = 120 g

1 kiwi fruit (without skin) = 60 g

1 mango (without stone or peel) = 150 g

5 asparagus spears = 125 g

1 small beetroot = 35 g

1 broccoli spear = 45 g

1 medium button mushroom = 10 g

1 medium onion = 150 g

1 medium pepper = 160 g

1 medium tomato = 85 g

Weight Conversions

METRIC	IMPERIAL	METRIC	IMPERIAL
15 g	½ oz	200 g	7 oz
30 g	1 oz	225 g	8 oz
45 g	1½ oz	250 g	9 oz
55 g	2 oz	280 g	10 oz
70 g	2½ oz	310 g	11 oz
85 g	3 oz	350 g	12 oz
100 g	3½ oz	375 g	13 oz
115 g	4 oz	400 g	14 oz
140 g	5 oz	450 g	16 oz
175 g	6 oz	500 g	1 lb 2 oz

NOTE: All conversions are approximate but close enough to be useful when converting from one system to another.

Liquid Conversions

METRIC	IMPERIAL	US
30 ml	1 fl oz/2 tbsp	2 tbsp
45 ml	1½ fl oz/3 tbsp	3 tbsp
60 ml	2 fl oz/4 tbsp	¼ cup
75 ml	2½ fl oz/5 tbsp	⅓ cup
90 ml	3 fl oz	⅓ cup + 1 tbsp
100 ml	3½ fl oz	⅓ cup + 2 tbsp
125 ml	4 fl oz	½ cup
150 ml	5 fl oz	⅔ cup
175 ml	6 fl oz	¾ cup
200 ml	7 fl oz	¾ cup + 2 tbsp
250 ml	8 fl oz	1 cup
275 ml	9 fl oz	1 cup + 2 tbsp
300 ml	10 fl oz	1¼ cups
325 ml	11 fl oz	1⅓ cups
350 ml	12 fl oz	1½ cups
375 ml	13 fl oz	1⅔ cups
400 ml	14 fl oz	1¾ cups
450 ml	15 fl oz	1¾ cups + 2 tbsp
500 ml	16 fl oz	2 cups (1 pint)
600 ml	20 fl oz (1 pint)	2½ cups
900 ml	1½ pints	3¾ cups
1 liter	1¾ pints	4 cups

Oven Temperatures

°C	GAS	°F	°F	GAS	°C
120	½	250	200	6	400
140	1	275	220	7	425
150	2	300	230	8	450
160	3	325	240	9	475
180	4	350	260	10	500
190	5	375			

NOTE: Reduce the temperature by 14°C (25°F) for fan-assisted ovens.

Index

A

A2 milk, 37, 63, 150
Acai berries, 66
Acesulfame-K, 74; *see also* Sugar
    substitutes
Acidic foods, 118
Acidophilus, 149; *see also* Probiotics
Acne, 129
Activity restrictions, 160–161
Additives, 59, 78; *see also* Chemicals
Adequate Intake (AI), 11
Agave, 28, 155; *see also* Sugar substitutes
Air fryers, 137
Alcohol, 2, 79–80
    aversion to, 117
    breastfeeding and, 172,173, 175
    calcium absorption and, 39
    cooking with, 79
    elimination of, 2, 79–80, 146
    substitutes for, 79, 80, 146
Allergens, 151
Allergies
    advice for food, 153–154
    in breastfed babies, 171
    gluten, 151–152
    milk, 36, 39
    peanut, 36
    plant milks and, 38–39
    preventing in baby, 19, 25, 36
    probiotics to reduce, 25
    sugar and, 28
Almond milk, 38, 40
Almonds, for heartburn relief, 124–125
Amaranth, 48; *see also* Wholegrains
Amino acids, 15, 33–34; *see also* Protein
Anaemia
    extreme fatigue and, 127
    iron intake and, 7, 30, 48, 167
    nutrients that prevent, 7, 16, 17, 20, 30, 8
    pica and, 116

postnatal, 165, 167
Animal products
    nutrients found only in, 12, 16, 42
    organic, 60–64
    selecting, 60–64
    see also Dairy products; Eggs; Poultry;
        Fish; Meats
Ankles, swollen, 129
Anorexia nervosa, 102–103; *see also*
        Eating disorders
Antacids, 49, 122, 125, 150
Antenatal care, 2
Antenatal vitamin supplements
    in Daily Dozen, 33
    DHA in, 52
    folic acid in, 5
    gluten-free diet and, 152
    morning sickness and, 112–113
    multiples and, 157
    overview of, 53–55
    weight-loss surgery and, 95
Anthocyanin, 66
Antibiotics in animal products,
        60, 63
Antioxidants, 25, 64, 66
Appetite, 105, 107, 142, 158
    B vitamins and, 12–13
    fluctuations in, 90, 99
    loss of, 22
    snacks and, 100
Appetite suppressants, 102
Artificial preservatives, 58
Artificial sweeteners
    breastfeeding, 175–176
    safety of, 28, 74–75, 175
    in fizzy drinks, 22
    types of, 74–75
    see also Sugar substitutes
Aspartame (Equal, Nutrasweet), 74;
    see also Sugar substitutes
Attention deficit hyperactivity disorder
    (ADHD), 17

Aversions. *See* Food aversions

B

Bacne, 7, 129
Bacteria
  beneficial, 25, 121, 149, 160
  in cacao powder, 77
  in cheese and dairy products, 81–82
  in deli meats, 83
  E. coli, 63, 84, 182
  eggs and, 186–187
  in fish and seafood, 81, 183, 184, 186
  fluids to prevent, 160
  food safety and, 178–179, 181–182, 184,
    186
  in kombucha, 84
  Listeria, 81–82, 83, 84, 183
  in meat and poultry, 183, 184, 186
  pasteurisation to eliminate, 63, 81–82
  on produce, 67, 181–182, 214
  in protein bars, 55
  in raw foods, 31, 81–82
  in raw juices, 84
  in spirulina, 76
  in sprouts, 84
  toxoplasmosis, 183
  in wheatgrass, 66
Bariatric surgery, 95
Barley, 48
  breast milk supply and, 172–173
  see also Wholegrains
Bars
  lactation, 172
  nutrition, 55
  protein, 36
Beans
  gas and bloating, 123, 196
  protein source, 34–35
Bed rest, 160–161
Bedtime snacks, 108, 109, 124, 126, 156
Beef. *See* Meats
Beer, 79, 80, 118, 173
  breast milk supply and, 172–173
  see also Alcohol
Beta-carotene, 64–65; *see also* Vitamin A
Betacyanin, 66

Binge eating. *See* Eating disorders
Binge drinking, 79; *see also* Alcohol
Biotin, 15
Birth defects, 5, 12, 16, 17, 24
  eating disorders and, 102
Birth injuries, 93
Birthweight, 5, 18, 24, 25, 52, 77, 90, 93, 150
  of multiples, 156
Black cohosh, 72, 141
Blenders, 137
Bloating, 122–123
  dairy and, 149, 150
  see also Constipation; Swelling Blood
    glucose
  carbohydrates and, 154–155
  chromium deficiencies and, 20
  gestational diabetes and, 154–156
  low levels of, 128–129
  mini-meals and, 165
  sugar substitutes and, 28
Blood pressure, 23, 49; *see also*
    Hypertension
Blue cohosh, 72
BMI. *See* Body mass index
Body image issues, 91, 102–103
Body mass index (BMI)
  calculating, 86–87
  weight gain recommendations and, 87
Bone growth (baby's), 7, 8, 12, 13, 14, 15, 18,
    22, 24, 37
Bone health (mum's), 3, 4, 8, 19, 37, 166
Bowel movements. *See* Constipation
BPA, 77
Brain development
  alcohol and, 79
  exercise and, 98
  iodine deficiency and, 50
  lead exposure and, 77
  nutrients for, 13–17, 20, 25, 51
Brain, pregnancy, 16
Bread, 67, 142, 185
Breakfast, 126, 135, 191
Breastfeeding
  alcohol and, 173, 175
  allergies in baby and, 154, 171
  caffeine and, 175
  calcium and, 166
  calories and, 164

Daily Dozen for, 164–168
DHA and, 51, 167
eating while, 168–176
fish safety and, 72, 176
fluids while, 167–168
foods to limit/avoid while, 173, 175–176
herbs and, 71, 169–170, 175–176
lactation boosters and, 169–173
multiples, 164, 166
myths about, 170, 173
probiotics and, 25
sugar substitutes and, 175
supplements and, 168, 169–170, 175
vitamin supplements during, 168
weight loss and, 174
Breast milk supply, 168–173
Breast milk, colour of, 169
Breast milk, flavour of, 6, 169–170
British Nutrition Foundation, 11
Buckwheat, 48; see also Wholegrains
Budget, eating well on a, 132–134
Buffets, 146–147, 180
Bulgar wheat, 48; see also Wholegrains
Bulimia, 102–103; see also Eating disorders
B vitamins. See Vitamin B

C

Cacao powder, 77
Caesarean delivery, 18
Caffeine, 175
    amounts in foods, 70, 72, 77
    blood sugar and, 129
    calcium absorption and, 39
    as diuretic, 52–53
    energy from, 127
    headaches and, 128
    moderate intake of, 69–71, 175
    mood swings and, 129
    postnatal and, 175
    reducing, 2, 26, 131
    sleep and, 126
Cage-free eggs, 62, 187
Calcium
    absorption of, 18, 22, 39
    bone health (baby's), 7
    bone health (mum's), 8, 19–20

in Daily Dozen, 33, 37–41
dairy-free sources of, 43; see also
    Plant milks
developing baby's need for, 3, 97
fizzy drinks and, 22
multiples and, 103
need for, 19, 37
postnatal, 166
RNI for, 20
reserves of, 4
sources of, 37–41, 43, 150
supplements, 54, 150
teeth and gum health, 128
vegetarians/vegans and, 43
Calories
    baby's brain development and, 5
    counting, during pregnancy, 33
    in Daily Dozen, 34
    empty, 28–29
    fatigue and, 125–126
    multiples pregnancy and, 156–157
    need for extra, 33
    postnatal, 163, 164, 166
    weight gain, 96–97, 100–101
Carbohydrates
    gestational diabetes and, 154–155
    morning sickness and, 109–110
    simple, 28
    see also Complex carbohydrates
Carbonated drinks, 123
Carotenoids, 65
Carpaccio. See Raw foods
Car travel, 144
Cashew milk, 39
Castor oil, 141
Caviar. See Raw foods
Cereals, 67, 165; see also
    Carbohydrates
Cheese
    calcium in, 37
    lactose-free, 37, 149
    lactose intolerance and, 149
    raw/unpasteurised, 81–82
    see also Calcium; Dairy products
Chemicals
    in animal protein, 60–61
    natural and synthetic, 78
    see also Additives; Pesticides; Organic

Chewing, to prevent wind 122
Chewing gum, to prevent heartburn
    124
Chia, as fibre source, 76
Chicken. *See* Poultry
Chlorine in tap water, 77
Chocolate, dark, 6, 32, 77
Cholesterol, 192
Choline, 16
Chopping boards, 179; *see also*
    Kitchen safety
Chromium, 20
Cleft palate, 54
Coconut milk, 38
Coconut water, unpasteurised 63
Coeliac disease, 99, 150–153
Coffee, 160
    aversion to, 117
    avoiding, with UTIs, 160
    caffeine in, 70
    limiting intake of, 69–71
Cold meats, 82, 83–84, 186
Colds, 158
Colic, 171
Complex carbohydrates
    benefits of, 28
    morning sickness and, 109–110
    postnatal, 163
    sources of, 47–49
Complications, from excessive
    weight gain, 93
Constipation, 52, 119–122, 160–161
Convenience foods, 133, 137–138
Copper, 20
Corn, wholegrain 48; *see also*
    Wholegrains
Corn syrup, 155
Cramps, leg, 128
Cravings. *See* Food cravings
Cross contamination
    coeliac disease or gluten sensitivity
        and, 151
    kitchen safety and, 179
Cruise travel, 144
Cured fish, 81
Cured meats, 83

D

Daily Dozen, 13, 32–56
    antenatal vitamin supplement, 33, 53–55
    breastfeeding and, 169
    calcium, 33, 37–41
    calories, 33, 34
    fat and high-fat foods, 33, 50–51
    fluids, 33, 52–53
    fruits and vegetables, 33, 42–47
    iron-rich foods, 33, 48–50
    omega-3 fatty acids, 33, 51–52
    overview of, 33
    postnatal, 164, 166–168
    protein, 33–35
    for vegetarians and vegans, 42–43
    vitamin A, 33, 41–42
    vitamin C, 33, 40–41
    wholegrains and legumes, 33, 34–36,
        47–49
Dairy-free milk alternatives, 38–39
Dairy products, 37–39
    as calcium sources, 37–40
    food safety and, 186
    lactose intolerance and, 148–149
    mouldy, 185
    pasteurised, 63
    problems handling, 148–150
    raw/unpasteurised, 81–82
    selecting, 63–64
    sell-by date for, 180
    see also Cheese; Milk
Dark chocolate, 6, 32, 77
Dates, to induce labour, 140
Dates on food labels, 180, 181, 183
Defrosting foods, 183–184
Delivery. *See* Labour and delivery
Desserts, 143, 147
DHA, 25
    in antenatal supplements, 51–52
    in eggs, 62
    in dairy, 63
    postnatal, 167
    see also Omega-3 fatty acids
Diabetes
    extra weight and, 93
    linseeds (flaxseed) and, 75

gestational, 28, 154–156
predisposition to, 6
type 1, 29
type 2, 5, 8, 154
Diarrhoea,
castor oil and, 141
excess fibre and, 120
food poisoning and, 146
stomach bug and, 159
Diet
influence on health, 3
see also Postnatal diet; Pregnancy diet
Dietary Reference Values (DRVs), 11
Digestive system, 122–123
Dining out, 140–143; *see also* Parties
Distracted eating, 97–98
Diuretics
calcium absorption and, 39
caffeine as, 52–53
eating disorders and, 102–103
Dizziness, 128
Down syndrome, folate intake and, 17
Dried fruits, 64
Drinking. *See* Alcohol

E

Eating disorders, 91, 102–103
Eating efficiently, 27, 100
postnatal, 163
Eating habits, baby's future, 6
Eating out, 140–143; *see also* Parties
Eating well
at parties, 146–147
at work, 131–132
basic principles for, 26–32
on bed rest, 160–161
benefits for baby, 3–7
benefits for mum, 7–8
while breastfeeding, 168–176
on a budget, 132–134
choosing food for, 57–68
with coeliac disease or gluten sensitivity,
150–153
while eating out, 140–143
for energy, 165
feeling unwell and, 105–129

with food allergies, 153–154
food aversions and, 117–119
food cravings and, 113–116
with gestational diabetes, 154–156
with IBS, 152–153
lactose intolerance and, 148–150
morning sickness and, 106–113
multiples and, 156–157
for next baby, 175
planning for, 134–135
postnatal, 162–176
time constraints and, 135–139
when sick, 158–160
while travelling, 143–146
E. coli, 63, 84,182; *see also* Food safety
Efficient eating, 27, 100, 163
Eggs
food safety and, 184, 186–187
free-range 62, 187
omega-3, 52
pasteurised, 63, 82
raw, 82–83
selecting, 62, 180
Electrolyte drinks, 172
Energy drinks, 71
Enriched wheat, 67–68
Enrichment of food, 23, 43; *see also*
Food fortification
Environmental Health Department
on water safety, 76–77
EpiPen, 154
Equal (aspartame), 74; *see also*
Sugar substitutes
Erythritol, 75; *see also* Sugar substitutes
Essential fatty acids, 50–51; *see also* DHA;
Omega-3 fatty acids
Evening primrose, to induce labour, 141
Exercise
on bed rest, 161
gestational diabetes and, 154
postnatal, 174
weight gain and, 98, 100

F

Family-style eating, 32, 164
Farmers markets, 29–30

washing fruit and vegetables from, 67, 182
Farro, 48; *see also* Wholegrains
Fast foods, cooking, 137
Fat-free foods, myths and facts about, 98
Fatigue
    postnatal, 165
    pregnancy 7, 125–127
Fats
    adding, 100
    benefits of, 50–51
    cutting, 97
    in Daily Dozen, 33, 50–51
    foetal development and, 97
    morning sickness and, 110
    myths and facts about, 98–99
    postnatal, 167
    sources of, 51
Fat-soluble vitamins, 12
Fenugreek, breast milk supply and, 169–170
Fibre
    adding to diet, 123, 153
    calcium absorption and, 39
    in complex carbs, 28
    functions of, 25
    in grains, 46, 120, 206
    lack of, and constipation, 30, 47, 120
First trimester
    foetal development during, 14–15
    lack of appetite in, 99–100
    morning sickness in, 106
    weight gain during, 89, 99–100
    weight loss during, 89
Fish
    to avoid, 74, 81
    doneness of, 184
    food safety and, 183–186
    limiting intake of, 72–74
    mercury in, 72, 167, 176
    myths about eating, 4
    raw/rare, 81, 167, 185–186
    selecting, 61–62
    smoked and cured, 81
    wild, 62
Fizzy drinks, 22, 39, 71
Flavonoids, 25, 66
Flavour learning, 6
Flax milk, 39

Flaxseeds. *See* Linseeds
Flour
    enriched, 68
    stone-ground wheat, 68
    wheat, 67
    white, 46
    wholemeal, 46, 68
Flu, 158
Fluids
    bed rest and, 160–161
    constipation and, 121
    in Daily Dozen, 33, 52–53
    fatigue and, 127
    on flights, 144
    heartburn and, 124
    morning sickness and, 111
    multiples and, 157
    need for, 131
    night-time, 126
    postnatal, 167–168
    when sick, 158, 159, 160
    while travelling, 145
Fluoride, 20–21
Foetal alcohol syndrome, 79
Foetal development, 14–15
    brain development, 5, 51
    eating well and, 3–7
    first trimester, 14–15
    highlights of, 14–15
    nutrition for, 97
    organs, 4–5
    second trimester, 15
    third trimester, 15
Folate (folic acid), 16–18, 72
    deficiency, 5, 6, 129
    green tea and, 72
    overview of, 16–18
Food allergies, 25, 36, 151, 153–154;
    see also Allergies
Food aversions, 117–119
Food-borne illnesses, 183
    myths about, 178
    see also Food poisoning; Food safety;
    Kitchen safety
Food cravings, 32, 113–116, 164
Food enrichment, 23, 46
Food fortification, 23, 40
    food labels and, 59

Food labels, reading, 58–59
  coeliac disease or gluten sensitivity, 151
  see also Dates on food labels
Food myths, 4
Food poisoning, 159; *see also* Food-borne
  illnesses; Food safety; Kitchen safety
Food preparation, 177–187
Food processors, 137
Food recalls, 182
Foods
  to avoid, 78–84
  convenience, 133, 137–138
  enriched, 23, 43, 67–68
  fat-free, 98
  fortified, 23, 40
  freeze-dried, 64
  gluten-free, 99
  GMO, 65
  to limit during pregnancy, 69–78
  low-carb, 98
  refreezing, 181
  reheating, 180, 270
  snacks, 138–139
  spicy, 4, 124, 141
  store-brand, 133
  see also Frozen foods; Processed
    foods
Food safety, 177–187, 212
Food selection, for eating well, 57–68
Food Standards Agency,
  and dairy, 63
  and labelling, 151
Food temperatures
  safety and, 179
  for fish, meat, and poultry, 184–185
Foremilk, 169
Fortified foods. *See* Food fortification
Free-range
  eggs, 62
  on food labels, 61
Freeze-dried foods, 64
Freezing foods
  bulk cooking and, 138–139
  freezer temperature, 179
  meat, poultry and fish, 183
  for safety, 180, 181
Freshness, of produce, 29–31
Frozen foods

  on a budget, 133
  convenience and, 138
  defrosting, 136, 183–184
  fish, 62
  freshness of, 30–31
  fruit, 110, 111, 199
  lifespan of, 180
  morning sickness and, 110, 111, 112
  smoothies, 110
  see also, Freezing foods
Fruit juices, 155
Fruit preserves, 201, 205
Fruits 163–164, 165
  blue, 66
  choosing, 29–31
  constipation and, 120
  in Daily Dozen, 33, 42–47
  dried, 64
  fluids in, 52
  food safety and, 181–183
  freeze-dried, 64
  frozen, 30–31, 110, 111, 199
  gestational diabetes and, 155
  increasing intake of, 29, 44–45, 163–164,
    165
  mouldy, 185
  morning sickness and, 109–110
  organic, 29, 66–67, 133
  postnatal, 166–167
  purple, 66
  red, 64
  seasonal, 133
  selecting, 64–67
  tips for increasing intake of, 44–45
  vitamin A–rich, 43–45, 64–65
  vitamin C–rich, 18, 40–41
  white, 66
  see also specific types

G

Garlic
  benefits of 66
  breastfeeding and, 170
  myth about, 46
  smell, 108
Gas and bloating, 122–123

in baby, 171
constipation and, 120
dairy and, 148
IBS and, 152–153
Six-Meal Solution and, 107
Gastroesophageal reflux disease
(GERD), 123
GD. *See* Gestational diabetes
Genetically modified organisms
(GMOs), 65
Gestational diabetes, 154–156
sugar substitutes and, 28, 75
Ginger,
morning sickness and, 108, 109,
111–112
stomach bug and, 159
Gluten, 151–152
Gluten-free diet, 150–153
Gluten-free foods, 99
Gluten sensitivity, 150–153
Glycaemic load, 154–155
GMOs, 65
Goitre, 21
Grains, 36–37
refined, 46, 47
see also specific types; Wholegrains
Gram (g), 13
Grass-fed meats, 61, 63
Greek yogurt, 27, 36, 41
postnatal, 163
Green tea, 72
Grocery shopping, 57–68
buying in bulk, 133–134
dairy, 63–64
eggs, 62
fish, 61–62
fruits and vegetables, 64–67
loyalty programmes, 135
meal planning and, 135–136
meat and poultry, 60–61
online, 135, 136
planning for, 134
tips for, 57–60
wholegrains, 67–68
Growth hormones, 63
Gum problems, 128

H

Haemorrhoids, 7
Hair problems, 129
Handwashing, 178
Headaches, 128
Health, baby's long-term, 6–7
Health foods, to limit during pregnancy,
75–78
Healthy eating. *See* Eating well
Heartburn, 7, 123–125
cold foods and, 111
Six-Meal Solution and, 107
postnatal, 161
Heart disease, 166
Hemp, 76
Hemp milk, 39
Herbal tea, 71–72, 141, 170
Herbs
breastfeeding and, 169–170, 175
during pregnancy, 71
to induce labour, 141
High blood pressure. *See* Hypertension;
Pre-eclampsia
High-fat foods, 33, 50–51
postnatal, 167
High-protein diets, 34
Hindmilk, 169
Holidays, eating well, 147
Hormones
consumed in diet, 60
cravings and, 113
in dairy products, 63
digestion and, 120
food aversions and, 117
headaches and, 128
leg cramps and, 128
metallic taste and, 118
morning sickness and, 101–102, 106
puffiness and, 50
skin problems and, 129
Hyperemesis gravidarum, 89
Hypertension, 6, 93

I

Ice chewing, 116
Immune system, 158
Immunity boosters, 159
Infants
  full-term, 6, 90
  low birthweight, 90
  overweight, 93
  preterm, 5–6, 90
Ingredients list, 58; *see also* Labels on food
Insomnia, 126
Instant pot, 137
Intrauterine Growth Restriction (IUGR), 5
Iodine, 21, 50, 54, 166
Iron
  caffeine and, 70
  deficiency, 5, 8, 21, 127, 129
  need for, with multiples, 157
  in oats, 170–171
  overview of, 21–22
  sources of, 43, 49–50, 170
  supplements, 21, 48–49, 54, 121, 127, 157
  vegetarians and, 43
Iron-rich foods
  in Daily Dozen, 33, 48–50
  postnatal, 167
Irritable bowel syndrome (IBS), 152–153
Italian food, to induce labour, 141

J

Jasmine, 175
Juices
  fruit, 155
  pasteurised, 63
  raw/unpasteurised, 84

K

Kamut, 48; *see also* Wholegrains
Keto diet, 30
Ketones, 30
Kidney infection, 160
Kitchen equipment, 136–137

Kitchen safety, 178–179
Kiwi fruit, constipation and, 121
Knives, 137
Kombucha, 84

L

Labour and delivery, 8
  complications, from excessive weight
    gain, 91
  foods to induce, 140–141
Lactation boosters, 169–173
Lactose intolerance, 36, 37, 148–149
Large for gestational age (LGA), 93
Laxatives, eating disorders and,
    102–103
Lead, in drinking water, 76–77
Leeks, 66
Leftovers, 135, 137, 139, 180; *see also*:
    Freezing foods; Reheating foods
Leg cramps, 128
Legumes
  in Daily Dozen, 33, 34–35, 47
  pasta, 68
  postnatal, 167
  wind and, 123
Lemons, morning sickness and, 108, 111,
    112
Limes,
  morning sickness and, 111, 112
  myths about, 20
Linseeds, 75–76, 206
Liquorice, to induce labour, 140
Listeria, 81, 82, 83, 84, 183
Listeriosis, 82
Low birthweight, 5, 51, 90
Low-carb diets, 30
Low-carb foods, 98
Low-fat diet, 155
Low-FODMAP diet, 153
Low glycaemic index foods, 154–155
Lunch
  bringing from home, 131, 132–133
  ideas for, 132
  planning for, 135

M

Maca, 77
Magnesium
  constipation and, 126
  deficiency, 8
  leg cramps and, 121, 128
  overview of, 22
Male foetuses, weight gain and, 101
Manganese, 22
Mannitol, 75; *see also* Sugar substitutes
Marinating, safety of, 184
Matcha, 72
Meals,
  small and frequent, 107, 155–156
  at work, 131–132
Meal planning, 134–136, 139
Meal prepping, 138–139
Meal skipping, 27–28, 155
  postnatal, 163
Meats
  cold, 83–84
  doneness of, 184, 185
  food safety and, 183–186
  freshness of, 180
  grass-fed, 61
  raw or rare, 83, 185
  red, 269
  selecting, 60–61
  smoked and cured, 83
Mercury, in fish, 72, 167, 176
Metallic taste, 118
Microgram (mcg), 13
Microwave cooking
  potatoes, 328
  fish, 299
  to minimise odours, 108,
  tips for, 136
  vegetables, 322
Milk
  A2, 37, 63, 150
  colds and, 158
  dairy-free alternatives, 38–39
  lactose intolerance, 37, 63, 148–150
  to soothe heartburn, 125
  in soups, 223
  as source of calcium, 37–38, 166

  use-by date for, 180
Milk supply, foods that boost,
    170–173
Milled grains, 49, 68
Millet, 48–49; *see also* Wholegrains
Milligram (mg), 13
Mindful eating, 97–98, 161
Minerals, 19–24, 157
Mini-meals
  blood-sugar regulation and, 155–156
  for extra calories, 157
  to fight fatigue, 126–127, 165
  to reduce mood swings, 128–129
  to reduce nausea, 108
  suggestions for, 107
  see also Snacks; Six-Meal Solution
Mocktails, 146
Molybdenum, 22
Mood swings, 128–129
Moringa, 77–78
Morning sickness, 7
  alleviating, 108, 111–112
  antenatal vitamins and, 112
  eating well and, 106–113
  fluids and, 111
  medications for, 113
  odour sensitivity and, 106–107
  pregnancy hormones and, 101–102
Mould, on food, 182, 185; *see also* Food
    safety
MTHFR gene, 17
Multiple gestation
  breastfeeding and, 172
  eating well and, 156–157
  weight gain recommendations and, 87, 89,
    101–104
Myths, pregnancy. *See* Old wives' tales

N

Natural sweeteners, 28, 75; *see also*
    Sugar substitutes
Nausea, 106, 108–109, 116; *see also*
    Morning sickness
Neonatal intensive care unit (NICU), 5
Neural tube defects, 5, 16
Newborns

sleep habits of, 6
    see also Infants
Niacin, 14
Night-time snacks, 108, 109, 124, 126, 156
Nitrates, 83–84
Norovirus, 144
NutraSweet, 74; *see also* Sugar substitutes
Nutrients, 10–25
    distribution of, 3
    fibre, 25
    for foetal development, 4–7
    minerals, 19–24
    omega-3 fatty acids, 25
    phytonutrients, 25
    postnatal, 166-168
    probiotics, 25
    for vegetarians and vegans, 42–43
    vitamins, 11–19
    see also specific types
Nutrition information, on food labels,
    58–59
Nuts and seeds, protein in, 37

O

Oats, 49
    breast milk supply and, 170–172
    coeliac disease and gluten sensitivity, 151
    see also Wholegrains
Obesity, 5
    BMI and, 86–87
    risk for, 7
    weight gain recommendations and, 87
Odours, sensitivity to, 106, 108
Oedema, 128; *see also* Swelling
Office meals, 131–132
Old wives' tales
    about food cravings, 115
    about salt, 24
    about sour milk, 173
    about spices, 170
    about spoiled food, 179
    about water, 54
    Chinese, 41
    on gender, 46
Omega-3 fatty acids
    benefits of, 25

brain development and, 5
    in Daily Dozen, 33, 51–52
    in dairy products, 63
    in eggs, 62
    foetal development and, 97
    in grass-fed meats, 61
    in linseeds (flaxseeds), 75
    in meats, 61
    postnatal, 167
    to regulate moods, 129
    sleep habits and, 6
Online supermarkets,
    saving money and, 134
    saving time and, 136
Organ development, 4–5
Organic
    dairy products, 63
    eggs, 62
    fish, 62
    meats, 60–61
    produce, 29, 66–67, 133, 182
Osteoporosis, 7, 8
Overeating, 108
Overweight
    babies, 93
    BMI and, 86–87
    weight gain recommendations and, 87

P

Paleo diet, 30–31
Pantothenic acid, 19
Parties, eating well at, 146–147
Pasta
    chickpea, 27
    legume, 68
    lentil, 27
    wholegrain, 27
Pasteurisation, 63, 81–82
Pasture-raised animals, 61
Pea milk, 39
Peanut butter, allergies and, 36
Peanut allergy, 36
Perishable foods, 179, 180; *see also*
    Food safety
Pesticides, 29, 66, 67; *see also* Chemicals;
    Organic

Phosphorus, 22–23
Phytoestrogens, 75
Phytonutrients, 25, 41–42, 66
Pica, 116
Pineapple, to induce labour, 141
Placenta, 16
Plane travel, 143–144
Plant milks. *See* Dairy-free milk alternatives
Portion sizes
　assessing, 35
　cravings and, 116
　morning sickness and, 107
　restaurants and, 142
　see also Serving sizes
Postnatal Diet, 163–168
Postnatal period, 8
　Daily Dozen in, 164, 166–168
　eating well during, 162–176
　fatigue in, 165
　weight loss during, 91, 93, 103, 166, 174
　see also Breastfeeding
Potassium, 23, 128
Poultry
　doneness of, 184
　food safety and, 183–186
　selecting, 60–61
Pre-eclampsia, 18, 20, 37, 89
Pregnancy
　advice given during, 4
　benefits of eating well during, 3–8
　comfort during, 7
　complications during, 7–8
　complications in future, 93
　eating disorders and, 102–103
　exercise during, 98
　extra calories in, 33, 34
　foods to limit during, 69–78
　uncomfortable, and excessive weight gain, 91
　weight gain during, 85–104
Pregnancy Daily Dozen. *See* Daily Dozen
Pregnancy Diet, 19, 26–56
　basic principles for, 26–32
　Daily Dozen, 32–56
　eating good enough and, 56
Premature delivery, 5–6
　eating well to avoid, 8, 18
　lack of weight gain and, 90

Pressure cookers, 137
Preterm infants, 5–6, 51, 90
Preterm labour. *See* Premature delivery
Probiotics, 25, 121, 149, 153, 160
Processed foods
　cheese, 82
　chemicals in, 78
　cold meats, 83–84
　enriched, 23, 43, 67–68
　fat-free or low-carb, 98–99
　food labels and, 59
　fortified, 23, 40
　gluten-free, 99, 152
　iodine in, 21
　postnatal, 164
　sodium in, 24, 50
　sugar substitutes, 74–75
Produce
　food safety and, 181–183
　organic, 29, 133, 182
　washing, 181–182, 212
　see also Fruits; Vegetables
Protein
　bars, 55
　brain development and, 5
　diet high in, 30–31
　in Daily Dozen, 33–35
　low-cost sources of, 133
　morning sickness and, 110
　postnatal, 166
　supplements, 36
　for vegetarians and vegans, 42
　whey, 36
Prunes, 121
Pyridoxine, 14–15

Q

Quinoa, 49; *see also* Wholegrains

R

Rare food
　fish, 81, 167, 185–186
　meats, 83
　postnatal, 167, 173

see also Food safety; Raw foods
Raspberry leaf tea, 72, 141
Raw foods
  cacao powder, 77
  dairy products, 81–82
  diet, 31
  eggs, 82–83
  fish and seafood, 81, 167, 185–186
  juice, 84
  meats, 83, 185
  postnatal, 167, 173
  sprouts, 84
  see also Food safety; Rare food
Recalls, food, 182
Reference Nutrient Intakes
  (RNI), 11
Red Tractor stamp, 61
Refined grains, 46, 47
Refreezing foods, 181; *see also* Freezing foods
Refrigeration
  eggs and, 186–187
  food safety and, 179, 180
  travel and, 145
Reheating foods, 180, 270
Rehydration solution, 146, 159
Rennie
  calcium and, 150
  heartburn and, 125
Restaurants, eating well at, 140–143
Riboflavin, 13–14
Rice, 49
  reheating, 270
Rice milk, 38–39
Rolaids
  heartburn and, 125
  calcium and, 150
'RSCPA Assured' stamp, 61

S

Saccharin, 74, 176; *see also*
  Sugar substitutes
SI (Safe Intake), 11
Salads, 142
  adding fat to, 51
Salmon, 27, 84
  calcium absorption and, 39

cravings for, 24, 50, 115
myths about eating, 4
postnatal, 166
swelling and, 128
Salt, 39, 50, 128, 166
Sashimi. *See* Fish, raw
Sausages, 83
  postnatal, 186
Seafood. *See* Fish
Seasonal produce, 133
Second trimester
  foetal development during, 15
  weight gain during, 89
Selenium, 23–24
Serving sizes, 35, 58, 142; *see also*
  Portion sizes
Sex, predictions about baby's, 104
Shopping for food. *See* Grocery
  shopping
Sickness, eating well and, 158–160
Simple carbohydrates, 28
Six-Meal Solution, 107, 127, 129
Skin problems, 129
Skipping meals. *See* Meal skipping
Sleep deprivation
  postnatal 165
  see also Fatigue
Sleep habits, of newborns, 6
Slow cooker, 135, 136–137
Small for gestational age (SGA),
  5, 90
Smell 106, 108, 114; *see also* Odours
Smoked fish, 81
Smoked meats, 83
Smoking, 2
Smoothies, 110, 159
Snacks
  to fight fatigue, 126–127
  ideas for, 138–139
  multiples and, 157
  night-time, 108, 109, 124, 126, 156
  planning for, 134
  to reduce nausea, 108, 109
  to regulate blood sugar, 128, 156
  for weight gain, 100
  while travelling, 143, 144, 145
  at work, 131
  see also Mini-meals

Sodium, 24, 50, 166; *see also* Salt
Sorbitol, 74–75; *see also*
    Sugar substitutes
Soup, 142, 158
Sour foods
    metal taste and, 118
    morning sickness and, 108, 111, 112
Soya beans, GMOs and, 65
Soy milk, 38
Soy products, nutrients, 42–43
Spelt, 49; *see also* Wholegrains
Spicy foods
    heartburn and, 124
    to induce labour, 141
    myths about, 4
Spider veins, 129
Spina bifida, 5, 16, 17, 24, 54
Spirulina, 76
Splenda (sucralose), 74; *see also*
    Sugar substitutes
Spoiled foods, 181
Sprouts, raw 84, 167
Stevia, 75; *see also* Sugar substitutes
Stomach bug, 158–160
Stomach upset. *See* Nausea; Vomiting
Sucralose (Splenda), 74; *see also*
    Sugar substitutes
Sugar, 28–29
    fatigue and, 165
    gestational diabetes and, 155
    ingredient lists and, 58
    mood swings and, 129
    substitutes, 28, 74–75
    postnatal intake and, 163, 165
    reducing, 28–29, 155, 163
Sugar alcohols, 74–75; *see also*
    Sugar substitutes
Sugar substitutes
    natural, 28
    safety of, 74–75
    safety while breastfeeding, 175–176
Sunett, 74; *see also* Sugar substitutes
Superstitions. *See* Old wives' tales
Supplements, 2
    calcium, 150
    DHA, 52
    iron, 21, 48–49, 54, 121, 127, 157
    postnatal, 168

    protein, 36
    see also Antenatal vitamin supplements
Sushi. *See* Fish, raw
SweetLeaf, 75; *see also* Sugar substitutes
Sweet'N Low, 74, 176; *see also*
    Sugar substitutes
Sweeteners. *See* Sugar substitutes
Sweets, 28–29, 127, 147; *see also* Gestational
    diabetes; Sugar
Swelling, 7, 50, 52, 99, 128
    activity restriction and, 160–161
Swerve, 75; *see also* Sugar substitutes

T

Taste buds, 6, 114
Tea, 160
    green, 72
    herbal, 71–72
Thiamin/thiamine, 12–13
Third trimester
    foetal development during, 15
    weight gain during, 89
Time constraints, eating well and,
    135–139
Time-saving ingredients, 138–139
Tinned foods, 181
Tooth and gum problems, 128
Train travel, 144
Traveller's tummy, 145–146
Travelling, eating well while,
    143–146
Triplets, 101; *see also* Multiple
    gestation
Truvia, 75; *see also* Sugar substitutes
Twins, 87, 101–104; *see also* Multiples
Type 1 diabetes, 29
Type 2 diabetes, 5, 8, 154

U

Unpasteurised dairy products, 81–82
Use-by dates. *See* Dates on food labels
Urinary tract infections (UTIs),
    52, 160

V

Varicose veins, 129
Vegans, 42–43
    breastfeeding and, 168
    dairy-free alternatives, 38–39
    omega-3 supplements, 53
    vitamin B_{12}, 16, 42
Vegetables, 29–31, 120, 163–164
    in Daily Dozen, 33, 42–47
    fats with, 51
    fluids in, 52
    food safety and, 181–183
    freeze-dried, 64
    green, 65–66
    growing own, 135
    increasing intake of, 29, 163–164
    mouldy, 185
    organic, 66–67, 133
    'other', in Daily Dozen, 45–47
    postnatal, 166–167
    purple, 66
    red, 64
    seasonal, 133
    selecting, 64–67
    tips for increasing intake of, 44–45
    vitamin A-rich, 64–65
    white, 66
    see also specific types
Vegetarians, 42–43
    omega-3 supplements, 53
Vitamin A, 12, 55
    in Daily Dozen, 33, 41–45
    in fruits and vegetables, 64–65
    postnatal, 166
    supplements, 54
Vitamin B
    breast milk supply and, 48–49
    complex carbohydrates and, 28
    dry scalp and, 129
    gluten-free foods and, 99, 152
    low-carb diets and, 30
    morning sickness and, 112
    overview of, 12–18, 19
    antenatal vitamins and, 112
    sources of, 47, 48, 76, 171, 172, 269
    vegan and vegetarian diets and, 42

Vitamin B_1 (thiamin, thiamine), 12–13
Vitamin B_2 (riboflavin), 13–14
Vitamin B_3 (niacin), 14
Vitamin B_4 (choline), 16
Vitamin B_6 (pyridoxine), 14–15, 129
    morning sickness and, 112
Vitamin B_7 (biotin), 15
Vitamin B_{12}, 15–16
    in antenatal supplements, 54
    breastfeeding and, 168
    postnatal weight loss, 95
    sources of, 42
    vegans/vegetarians and, 42
Vitamin C, 12, 18, 78, 129
    in Daily Dozen, 33, 40–41
    deficiency, 8
    iron and, 54
    postnatal, 166
    sources of, 41
Vitamin D, 12, 18, 55
    deficiency, 8
    sources of, 42, 150
    vegans/vegetarians and, 42
Vitamin E, 12, 19
Vitamin K, 12, 19
Vitamins, 11–19
    antenatal, 5
    antenatal supplements, 52, 53–55, 152,
        157
    deficiencies, 3, 8
    fat-soluble, 12
    postnatal supplements, 168
    storage of, 12
    supplements, 12, 95
    water-soluble, 12
    when sick, 158, 159–160
    see also Antenatal vitamin supplements
Vomiting, 106, 146, 159; see also Morning
        sickness; Nausea

W

Water
    bottled, 77, 145
    breastfeeding and, 167–168
    distilled, 78
    intake, 52–53

morning sickness and, 111
sparkling, 145
tap, 76–77, 145
tips for increasing intake of, 53
Water retention, 128
Weight control, gestational diabetes and, 156
Weight gain, 34, 85–104
    after weight-loss surgery, 95
    appropriate amount of, 85–88
    bed rest and, 161
    BMI calculation, 86–87
    distribution of, 92
    dos and don'ts for checking, 89
    eating disorders, 91, 102–103
    excessive, downside of, 91–93
    in first trimester, 89, 99–100
    gender of baby and, 101
    inadequate, downside of, 90
    multiples and, 87, 89, 101–104, 156
    plotting your, 94
    postnatal loss of, 91, 93, 103
    predictions about baby's sex and, 104
    pre-pregnancy weight loss and, 100
    psychological factors in, 91, 102–103
    recommended rate of, 88–90
    too fast, tips for, 96–99
    too slow, tips for, 99–101
    weighing in and, 93, 95–96
    when to check with practitioner about,
        99, 101
Weight loss
    breastfeeding and, 174
    during first trimester, 89
    eating disorders, 91, 102–103
    postnatal, 91, 93, 103, 166, 174
    pre-pregnancy, 100

Weight-loss surgery, 95
Wheatberries, 49; see also Wholegrains
Wheatgrass, 77
Whey protein, 36
White flour, 46
White wholemeal, 68
Wholegrain pasta, 27
Wholegrains
    benefits of, 46
    in Daily Dozen, 33, 47–49
    for energy, 165
    fibre in, 120
    nutrients in, 163
    postnatal, 167
    selecting, 67–68
    servings of, 36–37
Wholemeal flour, 46, 68
Wine, 79; see also Alcohol
Woks, 137
Workplace eating, 131–132

X

Xylitol, 75; see also Sugar substitutes

Z

Zinc, 24
    deficiency, 5, 8

Recipe Index

A

Alfredo light, 241
Almonds
  almond flour brownies, 355
  gluten-free carrot and almond muffins, 206
  power breakfast bars, 202
Apples
  apple and spice smoothie, 345
  pork fillet with sweet potato and, 279
Apricot ginger glazed chicken, 282–283
Asparagus
  and Parmesan curls, 316
  salmon salad Niçoise, 264
Avocado
  better BLT, 210
  Mediterranean salad, 254
  tomato soup with, 227

B

Bacon, better BLT, 210
Banana
  apple and spice smoothie, 345
  breakfast booster shake, 347
  green smoothie, 348
  peanut butter, banana and chocolate smoothie, 350
  yogurt banana ice lollies, 358
Bars and bites
  almond flour brownies, 355
  no-bake energy bites, 203
  power breakfast bars, 202
Basil
  pesto with sunflower seeds, 245
  salmon with, and tomatoes, 304
Basque chicken, 286
Beans
  better BLT, 210

black bean quesadilla, 218
black beans in lime and cumin vinaigrette, 219
breakfast burritos, 196
chicken enchiladas, 285
Italian green beans, 322
roasted Mediterranean sea bass with red pepper and white beans, 298
seared scallops on white beans and kale, 308
taco salad, 260
turkey chilli, 232
vegetable and edamame soup, 230
white bean spread, 211
Beef
  kebabs with cumin marinade, 274
  many peppers steak bake, 273
  Mexican lasagne, 276
  slow-cooker beef stew, 272
  steak salad, 261
  stir-fry, ginger, 269–271
  taco salad, 260
  tomato-layered mini meat loaves, 275
Beetroot, roasted, 330
Beverages
  citrus blueberry blast, 344
  first blush, 343
  iced watermelon water, 342
  mango tango, 349
  razzleberry, 347
  tropical temptation, 344
  see also Smoothies
Black beans
  breakfast burritos, 196
  chicken enchiladas, 285
  in lime and cumin vinaigrette, 219
  quesadilla, 218
BLT, Better, 210
Blueberries
  any day breakfast parfait, 199
  breakfast booster shake, 348
  citrus blueberry blast, 344

ginger-blueberry wholemeal pancakes, 201
spicy and sweet ice lollies, 359
triple blueberry muffins, 205
Bread
    prawn remoulade toast, 311
    stuffed eggy toast, 198
Breakfast
    any day breakfast parfait, 199
    baby's big bite, 197
    booster shake, 348
    burritos, 196
    cafe eggs, 191–192
    egg bites, 194
    mango and strawberry smoothie bowl, 349
    mushroom and spinach omelette, 193
    no-bake energy bites, 203
    power breakfast bars, 202
    stuffed eggy toast, 198
    wholemeal buttermilk pancakes, 200
Broccoli
    cauliflower fried 'rice' with pickled peppers, 336
    and cheese soup, 231
    with chicken and penne, 238–239
    ginger beef stir-fry, 269–271
    roasted vegetable soup, 229
    and tofu stir-fry, 333
    tomato and mozzarella salad, 255
    vinaigrette, 315
Brownies, almond flour, 355
Buckwheat, three-in-one pilau, 341
Bulgar wheat, three-in-one pilau, 341
Burgers, chicken, with mango relish, 212
Burritos, breakfast, 196
Butternut squash
    and pear soup, 222–223
    roast, 317

C

Cabbage
    balsamic braised red, 320
    oriental slaw, 256
Caesar
    chicken Caesar wrap, 214

prawn Caesar salad, 262
simple dressing, 263
tangy dressing, 263
Cake, gingerbread, 354
Cantaloupe, ginger melon salad, 248–249
Carrots
    coconut chicken, 293
    curtido, 258
    and ginger soup, 224
    gluten-free carrot and almond muffins, 206
    lemon, with rosemary, 319
    minty peas, carrots and mushrooms, 323
    oriental slaw, 257
    roasted, 330
    roasted vegetable soup, 229
    salmon poached in Thai carrot broth, 305
    smoky roasted, with lime cream, 318
    tropical temptation, 344
    warm lentil ragout, 301
Cauliflower
    cheesy roasted, 321
    fried 'rice' with pickled peppers, 336
Chard, Italian, 329
Cheddar cheese
    macaroni and cheese, 243
    poached pears with ginger, 356
    savoury spinach Cheddar muffins, 207
    taco salad, 260
    tomato-layered mini meat loaves, 275
    turkey chilli, 232
Cheese
    Alfredo light, 241
    black bean quesadilla, 218
    broccoli and cheese soup, 231
    cheesy roasted cauliflower, 321
    macaroni and, 243
    Mediterranean salad, 254
    savoury spinach Cheddar muffins, 207
    taco salad, 260
    see also specific types
Chicken
    apricot ginger glazed, 282–283
    Basque, 286
    broccoli with chicken and penne, 238–239
    burgers with mango relish, 212
    chicken Caesar wrap, 212

chickpea pasta with chicken, tiny tomatoes, and spinach, 237
coconut, 293
curried chicken salad, 259
enchiladas, 285
lettuce wraps, buffalo, 290–291
Mexican tortilla soup, 233
mole, slow-cooker, 289
oven-fried, 281
Parmesan, chunky tomato, 282
penne with chicken and tomato sauce, 240
rosemary lemon, 280–281
satay lettuce wraps, 290
tandoori, 292
teriyaki, 283
Chickpeas
  Alfredo light, 241
  crunchy, 252
  Mediterranean salad, 254
  pasta with chicken, tiny tomatoes and spinach, 237
Chilli, turkey, 232
Chocolate
  almond flour brownies, 355
  no-bake energy bites, 203
  peanut butter, banana and chocolate smoothie, 350
Chowder, fish and potato, 234
Cobb salad, 266
Coconut chicken, 293
Coleslaw
  carrot, 256
  curtido, 258
  oriental slaw, 256
Conversion table, 361
Cookies, fruity oat, 352–353
Courgette, creamy linguine with prawns and red pepper, 244
Crisps, sweet potato, 329
Cucumbers
  coconut chicken, 293
  curried chicken pitta, 215
  gazpacho, 226
  ginger cucumber salad, 256–257
  Greek salad sandwich, 220–221
  Mediterranean salad, 254
  sauce, 295

watermelon, cucumber and feta salad, 248
Curtido, 258

D

Desserts
  almond flour brownies, 355
  fruity oat cookies, 352–353
  gingerbread, 354
  poached pears with ginger, 356
  spicy and sweet ice lollies, 359
  yogurt banana ice lollies, 358
Dinner salads, 259–268
Dips and spreads
  creamy kale pesto, 216–217
  mango relish, 212
  not honey mustard, 211
  white bean spread, 211
Dried fruit
  no-bake energy bites, 203
  power breakfast bars, 202

E

Edamame
  and corn salsa, 288
  green mashers, 326
  kale and shiitake mushroom salad, 324
  red pepper and edamame peanut noodles, 242
  succotash, 331
  three-in-one pilau, 341
  and vegetable soup, 230
Eggs
  baby's big bite, 197
  breakfast burritos, 196
  cafe, 191–192
  egg bites, 194
  mushroom and spinach omelette, 193
  salmon salad Niçoise, 264
  spicy egg salad, 221
  tomato and roasted red pepper frittata, 195
Eggy toast, stuffed, 198
Enchiladas, chicken, 285

F

Farro risotto with mushrooms, 337
Fennel
    roasted, 330
    rocket, with shaved fennel and roasted
        pepper salad, 253
Feta cheese
    Greek salad sandwich, 220–221
    Greek salad snapper, 297
    prawns with, 310
    watermelon, cucumber and feta salad,
        248
Fettucine, with turkey and wild
    mushrooms, 236
Fig and rocket salad with Parmesan
    shavings, 252
Fish
    ginger-steamed halibut, 294–295
    Greek salad snapper, 297
    Instant Pot salmon with sweet potatoes
        and kale, 300
    marinated salmon fillets with ginger and
        lime, 299
    microwaved, 299
    mustard glazed salmon, 303
    pan-fried trout with tomatoes and
        spinach, 312–313
    and potato chowder, 234
    red snapper with mango salsa, 296
    roast, 302
        roasting techniques, 303
    roasted Mediterranean sea bass with red
        pepper and white beans, 298
    roast salmon on bed of lentils, 301
    roasted salmon with mild mustard crust,
        302–303
    salmon cakes with tropical salsa, 306
    salmon poached in Thai carrot broth, 305
    salmon parcel, 216
    salmon salad Niçoise, 264
    salmon with basil and tomatoes, 304
Flageolet beans. See White beans
Flaxseeds. See Linseeds
Frittata, tomato and roasted red pepper,
    195
Fruit preserve, 201, 205

Fruits
    any day breakfast parfait, 199
    fruity oat cookies, 352–353
    fruity turkey salad, 220
    ginger melon salad, 248–249
    see also specific fruits

G

Gazpacho, spiced-up, 234
Ginger
    apple and spice smoothie, 345
    apricot ginger glazed chicken, 282–283
    beef stir-fry, 269–271
    and carrot soup, 224
    cucumber salad, 259
    ginger-blueberry wholemeal pancakes,
        201
    gingerbread, 354
    ginger-steamed halibut, 294–295
    marinated salmon fillets with ginger and
        lime, 299
    melon salad, 248–249
    poached pears with, 356
    sauce, 271
    sesame ginger vinaigrette, 265
    spicy salad leaves with ginger dressing,
        256
Grains, 338
    Farro risotto with mushrooms, 337
    leek and tomato quinoa, 339
    quinoa with wild mushrooms, 338
    red peppers stuffed with quinoa, 340
    three-in-one pilau, 341
Green beans, Italian, 322

H

Halibut, ginger-steamed, 294–295

I

Ice lollies
    spicy and sweet, 359
    yogurt banana, 358

Instant Pot
  buffalo chicken lettuce wraps, 289
  lemony salmon with sweet potatoes and
    kale, 300

K

Kale
  creamy kale pesto, 216–217
  lemony salmon with sweet potatoes and,
    300
  seared scallops on white beans and, 308
  and shiitake mushroom salad, 324
Kebabs
  beef, 274
  pork, 278
  prawn and watermelon, 309
Kidney beans
  taco salad, 260
  turkey chilli, 232

L

Leek and tomato quinoa, 339
Lemons
  lemon carrots with rosemary, 319
  rosemary lemon chicken, 280–281
  vinaigrette, 253
Lentils
  ragout, 301
  red lentil and tomato soup, 228
  roast salmon on bed of, 301
Lettuce wraps
  buffalo chicken, 290–291
  chicken satay, 290
Linseeds
  no-bake energy bites, 202
  triple blueberry muffins, 205

M

Macadamia nuts, mango salad, 249
Macaroni and cheese, 243
Mango
  any day breakfast parfait, 199

breakfast booster shake, 348
  chicken burgers with mango relish, 212
  mango tango, 349
  ocean breeze smoothie, 345
  and orange salad, 250
  prawn and mango salad, 264–265
  red snapper with mango salsa, 296
  relish, 211
  salad, 251
  salmon cakes with tropical salsa, 306
  and strawberry smoothie bowl, 349
  tropical temptation, 344
Melons
  ginger melon salad, 248–249
  iced watermelon water, 342
  prawn and watermelon kebabs, 309
Mexican lasagne, 276
Mint
  iced watermelon water, 342
  minty peas, carrots and mushrooms, 323
Mocktails
  citrus blueberry blast, 344
  first blush, 343
  iced watermelon water, 342
  tropical temptation, 344
Mozzarella cheese, broccoli, tomato and
    mozzarella salad, 255
Muffins
  gluten-free carrot and almond, 206
  pumpkin, 209
  raisin bran, 208
  savoury spinach Cheddar, 207
  storing and reheating, 207
  triple blueberry, 205
Mushrooms
  beef kebabs with cumin marinade, 274
  broccoli and tofu stir-fry, 333
  Farro risotto with, 337
  fettucine with turkey and wild
    mushrooms, 236
  ginger-steamed halibut, 294
  kale and shiitake mushroom salad, 324
  minty peas, carrots, and, 323
  mushroom and spinach omelette, 193
  quinoa with wild, 338
  steak salad, 261
  turkey steaks in mushroom sauce, 287
Mustard

glazed salmon, 302
roasted salmon with mild mustard crust,
302–303

N

Nectarines, any day breakfast parfait, 199
Noodles
chicken satay lettuce wraps, 290
red pepper and edamame peanut, 242
Nuts and seeds
fruity oat cookies, 352–353
pesto with sunflower seeds, 245
raisin bran muffins, 208
toasted, 217
see also specific types

O

Oat bran
pumpkin muffins, 209
raisin bran muffins, 208
Oats
fruity oat cookies, 352–353
no-bake energy bites, 203
power breakfast bars, 202
raisin bran muffins, 208
triple blueberry muffins, 205
Olives
Basque chicken, 286
Greek salad sandwich, 220–221
Greek salad snapper, 297
Mediterranean salad, 254
salmon salad Niçoise, 264
Omelette
egg white, 192
mushroom and spinach, 193
Orange juice
citrus blueberry blast, 344
first blush, 343
iced watermelon water, 342
low-acid, 343
razzleberry, 347
tropical temptation, 344
Oranges, and mango salad, 250
Oriental slaw, 256

P

Pancakes
add-ins, 200
ginger-blueberry wholemeal, 201
wholemeal buttermilk, 200
Parcel meals, 284
Parmesan cheese
asparagus and, 316
chunky tomato chicken Parmesan curls,
282
crisps, 252
fig and rocket salad with, 252
steak salad, 261
Parsnips
roasted, 330
roasted vegetable soup, 229
Pasta
Alfredo light, 241
broccoli with chicken and penne,
238–239
chickpea, with chicken, tiny tomatoes and
spinach, 237
creamy linguine with prawns and red
pepper, 244
easy prep, 235
fettuccine with turkey and wild
mushrooms, 236
macaroni and cheese, 243
penne with chicken and tomato sauce,
240
red pepper and edamame peanut
noodles, 242
sauces, 245–246
types of, 239
Peaches
any day breakfast parfait, 199
tropical temptation, 344
Peanut butter
banana, and chocolate smoothie,
350
chicken satay lettuce wraps, 290
no-bake energy bites, 203
red pepper and edamame peanut
noodles, 242
Pears
and butternut squash soup, 222–223

poached, with ginger, 356
salad, crunchy, 250
Peas
   carrots, and mushrooms, minty, 323
   three-in-one pilau, 341
Pecans, fruity oat cookies, 352–353
Peppers
   rocket, with shaved fennel and roasted
      pepper salad, 252
   Basque chicken, 286
   beef kebabs with cumin marinade, 274
   cafe eggs, 191–192
   chicken Caesar wrap, 212
   creamy linguine with shrimp and red
      pepper, 244
   edamame succotash, 331
   gazpacho, 234
   ginger beef stir-fry, 269–271
   ginger-steamed halibut, 294
   Mediterranean salad, 255
   Mexican lasagne, 276
   oriental slaw, 256
   penne with chicken and tomato sauce,
      240
   pork kebabs, 278
   prawn Caesar salad, 262
   red pepper and edamame peanut, 242
   red peppers stuffed with quinoa, 340
   red snapper with mango salsa, 296
   roasted Mediterranean sea bass with red
      pepper and white beans, 298
   salmon cakes with tropical salsa, 306
   many peppers steak bake, 273
   steak salad, 262
   taco salad, 261
   tomato and roasted red pepper frittata,
      195
   turkey chilli, 232
Pesto
   creamy kale, 216–217
   with sunflower seeds, 245
Pickled vegetables, 268
Pineapple
   apple and spice smoothie, 345
   green smoothie, 347
   mango tango, 349
   ocean breeze smoothie, 345
   pork kebabs, 278

salmon cakes with tropical salsa, 306
Pinto beans, taco salad, 260
Pomegranate salad, 251
Pork
   kebabs, 278
   medallions with rocket and tomatoes, 277
   fillet with sweet potato and apple bake,
      279
Potato crisps, 325
Potatoes
   cafe eggs, 191–192
   and fish chowder, 234
   green mashers, 327
   microwaved, 328
   oven-roasted, 326
   salmon salad Niçoise, 264
   see also Sweet potatoes
Poultry. *See* Chicken; Turkey
Prawns
   Caesar salad, 262
   creamy linguine with shrimp and red
      pepper, 244
   with feta, 310
   and mango salad, with sesame ginger
      vinaigrette, 264–265
   remoulade toast, 311
   and watermelon kebabs, 309
Pumpkin muffins, 209

Q

Quesadilla, black bean, 218
Quinoa
   leek and tomato, 339
   red peppers stuffed with, 340
   three-in-one pilau, 341
   with wild mushrooms, 338

R

Raisins
   no-bake energy bites, 202
   power breakfast bars, 202
   raisin bran muffins, 208
Ranch dressing, 291
Raspberries, razzleberry, 347

Red peppers. *See* Peppers
Red snapper
    Greek salad, 297
    red snapper with mango salsa, 296
Relish, mango, 212
Risotto, Farro, with mushrooms, 337
Roast beef in tomato sauce, 272
Roasted vegetables, 317
Rocket
    crunchy pear salad, 248
    and fig salad, 253
    pork medallions with rocket and
        tomatoes, 277
    with shaved fennel and roasted pepper
        salad, 252
    steak salad, 262
Romaine lettuce
    chicken Caesar wrap, 214
    coconut chicken, 293
    Greek salad sandwich, 220–221
    Mediterranean salad, 254
    salmon salad Niçoise, 264
    taco salad, 260
Russian dressing, 266–267

S

Salad dressings
    American Southwest Russian, 266–267
    lemon vinaigrette, 253
    ranch, 291
    sesame ginger vinaigrette, 266–267
    simple Caesar, 263
    tangy Caesar, 263
Salad leaves
    mango salad, 251
    pomegranate salad, 250
    spicy, with ginger dressing, 256
    wilted, 329
    see also specific types
Salads
    broccoli, tomato and mozzarella salad,
        255
    Cobb, 266
    crunchy pear, 250
    curried chicken, 259
    curtido, 258

dinner, 259–268
fig and rocket, 252
fruity turkey salad, 220
ginger cucumber, 256–257
ginger melon salad, 248–249
Greek salad sandwich, 220–221
kale and shiitake mushroom, 324
mango and orange, 250
mason jar salads, 267
Mediterranean, 254
oriental slaw, 257
pomegranate, 251
prawn and mango, 264–265
prawn Caesar, 262
ranch, 289
rocket, with shaved fennel and roasted
    pepper, 252
salmon salad Niçoise, 264
serving sizes, 247
side, 247–258
spicy egg salad, 221
spicy salad leaves with ginger dressing, 256
steak, 261
taco, 260
watermelon, cucumber and feta, 248
Salmon
    with basil and tomatoes, 304
    cakes, with tropical salsa, 306
    fillets, with ginger and lime, 299
    Instant Pot, with sweet potatoes and kale,
        300
    mustard glazed, 302
    parcel, 216
    poached in Thai carrot broth, 305
    roast, on bed of lentils, 301
    roasted, with mild mustard crust, 302–303
    salad Niçoise, 264
Salsa
    mango, 296
    speedy, 307
    sweetcorn and edamame, 288
    tropical, 306
Sandwiches
    better BLT, 210
    chicken burgers with mango relish, 212
    chicken Caesar wrap, 214
    curried chicken pitta, 215
    Greek salad, 220–221

ideas for, 213
salmon parcel, 216
spicy egg salad, 221
turkey salad, 220
Sauces
cucumber, 295
ginger, 271
hiding vegetables in, 246
pesto with sunflower seeds, 245
turkey Bolognese sauce, 246
Scallops
seared, on succotash, 307
seared, on white beans and kale, 308
Sea bass, roasted Mediterranean, 298
Seafood
creamy linguine with prawn and red
pepper, 244
prawn and watermelon kebabs, 309
prawn remoulade toast, 311
prawns with feta, 310
seared scallops on white beans and kale,
308
seared sea scallops on succotash, 307
see also Fish
Seeds. See Nuts and seeds
Sesame ginger vinaigrette, 265
Shakes. See Smoothies
Shiitake mushrooms. See Mushrooms
Side salads, 247–258
Slow cooker
chicken mole, 289
slow cooker beef stew, 272
Smoothies
apple and spice, 345
breakfast booster shake, 348
green, 347
mango and strawberry smoothie bowl,
349
mango tango, 349
ocean breeze, 345
peanut butter, banana and chocolate, 350
soothing, 346
Soups
broccoli and cheese, 231
butternut squash and pear, 222–223
creamy, 223
fish and potato chowder, 234
gazpacho, 226

ginger and carrot, 224
Mexican tortilla, 231
red lentil and tomato, 228
roasted vegetable, 229
sweet potato vichyssoise, 225
tomato, with avocado, 227
vegetable and edamame, 230
Spinach
chickpea pasta with chicken, tiny
tomatoes and spinach, 237
creamy kale pesto, 216–217
crunchy pear salad, 250
green smoothie, 347
mushroom and spinach omelette, 193
pan-fried trout with tomatoes and,
312–313
savoury spinach Cheddar muffins, 207
Sprouting broccoli and sweet potatoes,
baked tofu with, 334–335
Squash
butternut squash and pear soup, 222–223
roast butternut, 317
Steak
many peppers steak bake, 273
salad, 261
Steamed vegetables, 315
Stir-fry
broccoli and tofu, 333
ginger beef, 269–271
vegetables for, 271
Strawberries
any day breakfast parfait, 199
first blush, 343
mango and strawberry smoothie bowl,
349
and mint slushy, 357
Succotash
edamame, 331
seared scallops on, 307
Sugar snap peas, ginger-steamed halibut,
294–295
Sunflower seeds, pesto with, 245
Sweetcorn
and edamame salsa, 288
Mexican lasagne, 276
red peppers stuffed with quinoa, 340
Sweet potatoes
baked tofu with sprouting broccoli and,

334–335
crisps, 329
lemony salmon with kale and, 300
pork fillet with apple and, 279
roasted herby, 328
vichyssoise, 225

T

Taco salad, 260
Tandoori chicken, 292
Teriyaki chicken, 283
Tofu
    and broccoli stir-fry, 333
    baked, with sprouting broccoli and sweet
        potatoes, 334
    curried broccoli and, 335
    grilled, 332
    razzleberry, 347
Tomatoes
    Basque chicken, 286
    beef kebabs with cumin marinade, 274
    broccoli, tomato and mozzarella salad,
        255
    chickpea pasta with chicken, tiny
        tomatoes, and spinach, 237
    chunky tomato chicken Parmesan, 282
    gazpacho, 226
    Greek salad sandwich, 220–221
    leek and tomato quinoa, 339
    Mediterranean salad, 254
    pan-fried trout with tomatoes and
        spinach, 312–313
    penne with chicken and tomato sauce,
        240
    pork medallions with rocket and, 277
    prawn Caesar salad, 262
    and red lentil soup, 228
    salmon salad Niçoise, 264
    salmon with basil and, 304
    slow cooker beef stew, 272
    soup with avocado, 227
    taco salad, 260
    tomato and roasted red pepper frittata,
        195
    tomato-layered mini meat loaves, 275
    turkey Bolognese sauce, 246

Tortillas
    black bean quesadilla, 218
    breakfast burritos, 196
    chicken Caesar wrap, 214
    chicken enchiladas, 285
    Mexican lasagne, 276
    Mexican tortilla soup, 233
Trout, pan-fried, with tomatoes and
    spinach, 312–313
Turkey
    Bolognese sauce, 246
    chilli, 232
    with sweetcorn and edamame salsa, 288
    fettucine with turkey and wild
        mushrooms, 236
    fruity turkey salad, 220
    steaks in mushroom sauce, 287

V

Vegetables
    microwaved, 322
    pickled, 268
    roasted, 317
    roasted root, 330
    roasted vegetable soup, 229
    steamed, 315
    vegetable and edamame soup, 230
    see also specific vegetables
Vinaigrette
    broccoli, 315
    lemon, 253
    lime and cumin, 219
    sesame ginger, 265

W

Walnuts
    creamy kale pesto, 216–217
    crunchy pear salad, 250
    fruity oat cookies, 352–353
    mango and strawberry smoothie bowl,
        349
    power breakfast bars, 202
Watermelon
    first blush, 343

ginger melon salad, 248–249
iced watermelon water, 342
kebabs, prawn and, 309
watermelon, cucumber and feta salad,
    248
White beans
  better BLT, 210
  roasted Mediterranean sea bass with red
    pepper and white beans, 298
  seared scallops on white beans and kale,
    308
  spread, 211
  vegetable and edamame soup, 230

Y

Yogurt
  any day breakfast parfait, 199
  banana ice lollies, 358
  breakfast booster shake, 348
  cucumber sauce, 295
  ocean breeze smoothie, 345
  peanut butter, banana, and chocolate
    smoothie, 350
  ranch dressing, 291
  spicy and sweet ice lollies, 359